Family Constellations

Family Constellations

A Breakthrough in Psychotherapy and Human Sciences

Damian Janus
Translated by Barbara Gąstoł

LEXINGTON BOOKS
Lanham • Boulder • New York • London

Published by Lexington Books
An imprint of The Rowman & Littlefield Publishing Group, Inc.
4501 Forbes Boulevard, Suite 200, Lanham, Maryland 20706
www.rowman.com

6 Tinworth Street, London SE11 5AL, United Kingdom

British Library Cataloguing in Publication Information Available

Library of Congress Cataloging-in-Publication Data

Names: Janus, Damian, 1969- author. | Gąstoł, Barbara, translator.
Title: Family constellations : a breakthrough in psychotherapy and human sciences / Damian Janus ; translated by Barbara Gąstoł.
Other titles: Ustawienia systemowe Berta Hellingera
Description: Lanham : Lexington Books, [2022] | Includes bibliographical references and index. | Summary: "In Family Constellations: A Breakthrough in Psychotherapy and Human Sciences, Damian Janus examines family constellation theory in comparison with other therapeutic approaches. Janus argues that the findings derived from family constellations offer new understandings for the fields of psychotherapy, psychology, anthropology, and religious studies"— Provided by publisher.
Identifiers: LCCN 2021039592 (print) | LCCN 2021039593 (ebook) | ISBN 9781793627421 (cloth) | ISBN 9781793627438 (ebook)
Subjects: LCSH: Family psychotherapy. | Family constellations (Families)
Classification: LCC RC488.5 .J3517 2022 (print) | LCC RC488.5 (ebook) | DDC 616.89/156—dc23
LC record available at https://lccn.loc.gov/2021039592
LC ebook record available at https://lccn.loc.gov/2021039593

Contents

Introduction

The axis of this book is the therapeutic method referred to as family constellations or systemic constellations, founded in the late 1970s and early 1980s by Bert Hellinger (1925–2019)[1] and further developed by him in the 1990s. I discuss this method extensively in my book *Systemic Constellations: Theory, Practice, and Applications* (Janus 2021). I invite both the reader who has not encountered systemic constellations and the reader who is familiar with the method but would like to deepen their understanding of the processes behind it.

Family constellations are more than just another psychotherapeutic method. The extraordinary nature of the processes they involve, the technical simplicity and full repeatability of the phenomena occurring, together with the great therapeutic effectiveness of this method, demand that they be considered a major step toward discovering human psychology and even nature.

In the first part of the book, I discuss the relationships between the theory and practice of family constellations and psychodrama, psychoanalysis, family therapy, and other therapeutic approaches, including those referred to as unconventional (such as neoshamanism or Christian intergenerational healing). I identify similarities and common paths, but I also show where and how family constellations surpass the achievements of other therapies.

In the second part of the book, I address the application of the processes discovered through systemic constellations in the fields of psychology, cultural anthropology, religious studies, and philosophy. From a new perspective and with previously unavailable tools, I explore such diverse issues as beliefs of traditional cultures, theories of psychological development and the process of nurturing, the question of motivation and ethics, and the very structure of the human psyche.

What are family constellations? Hellinger built on and modified some of the earlier observations and conclusions of family therapists who had worked using techniques that were prototypes of constellations (Virginia Satir, Thea Schönfelder, Ruth McClendon, Leslie B. Kadis, and others). He founded his discoveries on the use of an unusual effect: strangers—referred to as representatives—"set up" as the father, mother, brother, or wife of a given client reveal their true emotions and the existing family relations. Thanks to this phenomenon it has become possible to make detailed observations of the processes occurring in families over several generations.

Both the factors that caused suffering and destroyed relationships and those that led to order and well-being became identifiable. These factors were brought to light by the representatives and not by the actual family members, but hundreds of constellations proved that they were a perfect reflection of what was happening in the psyche of the actual family members. This was also supported by the fact that the client felt clearly relieved when the problematic issues were being solved. What is more, the client's relatives not present in the constellation session also experienced its effect.

How is it possible that people who do not know the client or his family accurately show the truth? We do not know the details of this phenomenon, which is called the knowing field (German: *das wissende Feld*). Despite its seemingly esoteric nature, this term is extremely apt. A constellation works just as if the representatives are surrounded by an invisible field from which they draw information. The condition is to refrain from speculation and to have a neutral intention ("Now I am your father"). The representative does not think about his role, and standing as somebody's alcoholic father, he does not imagine a staggering person with a bottle in his hand, nor does he judge him negatively. It turns out to be easier than it seems, because if we just internally express this type of intention, the knowing field captivates us and we are able to show the inner state and relationships of another person. In such a situation, there may be "substitutes" of illnesses and bodily symptoms in the person represented. The representative may feel some kind of suffocation when the person represented suffers from lung disease or feel that his leg is stiff if it has been amputated or if the person represented limps. There are many more such convergences, and, what is important, they are not exceptions but occur in many constellations. The information is so precise that it reveals, for example, concealed adoptions, existence of siblings, or abortions.

Showing important facts from the lives of clients and their ancestors is only a part of constellations; one could say it is their diagnostic side. The other side of constellations, closely connected with the first one, is their therapeutic effect. It is achieved through the mere observation of the constellation by the client and as a result of the fact that the emotions (as well as thoughts and tendencies), which vibrated in a latent way in his family system, are allowed to manifest themselves. And the most important healing factor is bringing about the so-called orders of love (German: *Ordnungen der Liebe*). The orders of love are based on respecting the basic system dynamics: belonging, bond, hierarchy, and balance. They also include the reconciliation between perpetrators and victims and the acceptance of one's parents and own life with gratitude. These orders are not arbitrary; they emerge in a completely spontaneous way among the representatives in a constellation. The representatives notice that something is pushing them to bow to the parents, to move away from the deceased, to approach the representative of the aborted child, to embrace someone, or to stand behind him as his support. The spontaneous emergence of the orders of love, that is, the image of resolution in the constellation, may be particularly evident in the so-called New Family Constellations (silent family constellations), in the course of which the therapist hardly intervenes. Most of the therapeutic work is carried out by the representatives who, guided by the knowing field, move from the image of the problem to the final solution.

How do we know that this is the solution and that something has changed? The representatives rid themselves of previous negative or chaotic feelings and instead feel peace, joy, and love. The client, who just watched the constellation or entered it at the end, feels the same—lightness, completeness, love, strength, and hope. And this state persists—according to the accounts of countless clients, a constellation has changed their lives.

The basic principle the family system is driven by is the right to belong. It does not matter to the system—or, more precisely, to our hidden conscience—whether the family member is a person that is "widely respected and admired" or an aborted fetus that has never existed as a social person. All those who have appeared in the system—due to blood ties or certain specific events—have the same right to belonging, respect, and memory. The system "remembers" all its members equally, regardless of the value we attribute to them. Yet someone is excluded all the time. Ex-wives and ex-husbands are excluded as if the new relationship was the first. After divorce, fathers are excluded as if their children no longer needed them or could replace them with new ones. Aborted children may be excluded as if they never existed. Dead children may also be excluded, because their death became such a great trauma that no one is able to think about them any longer. Sometimes siblings are excluded as if they were not "real." The sick, handicapped, alcoholics, those who lived a short life or suffered a hard lot are excluded. Victims of homicides and accidents are excluded, as they are not remembered due to the horror they cause. Also, killers are excluded due to moral outrage and contempt for their actions.

When someone is excluded, this has consequences. In family constellations, we refer to them as entanglement. What is entanglement? It is the unconscious identification with someone older in the family, often a person who died before we were born. Those whose lot was difficult, who were excluded, and about whom we sometimes know nothing have the strongest effect on us. Being entangled, we are tied to that person from the past without knowing it. We want to "be close" to him, by making our own fate similar to his fate. Because of this unconscious love, we bring trouble upon ourselves. For entanglements lead to many problems, from difficulties at work to serious illnesses.

Why do entanglements occur? Through constellations we have found out that we all tend to unconsciously take the burdens, traumas, or faults of our ancestors. This process is actually the strongest pathogenic effect discovered by constellations. The child subconsciously knows about the burdens, guilt, or depression of his parents and other ancestors. He imagines that he can carry their difficulties for them or together with them. That is why he falls ill or causes trouble, and as an adult, he suffers defeats. There is a tremendous force within us, referred to as the family conscience, commanding us to interfere in the affairs of the older ones, just as if we were more competent to solve them.

One of the most important processes of constellation therapy, almost the essence of it, is "giving back" the concerns that are not one's own to one's ancestors and turning toward one's own life, with the awareness and respect for one's bond with them. In bringing about these orders and changing our inner attitude, so-called sentences of strength (German: *Sätze der Kraft*) help. Among them, there is one we can consider particularly important. It reads: "You have a good place in my heart, and I'm leaving your fate with you, with respect." This sentence helps to solve a great many psychological problems, because very often they boil down to an unconscious bond with an ancestor. The more the bond is negated (when the person from the past is forgotten, rejected, or his meaning is belittled), the more the bond is fateful. The above sentence is so powerful because, leading to one's autonomy, it affirms this bond. There are therapies and therapists who find that someone is "too strongly attached to his mother," "has not cut his umbilical cord," and so on. And although there may be much truth in this statement, these therapies offer an impossible or destructive solution for the client—they say that he should "cut himself off." Thanks to constellations, we know that there is a psychological level within us that does not tolerate such a cut-off. And when the cut-off takes place, it will "punish" us with depression, illness, or life weakness. The sentence "You have a good place in my heart, and I'm leaving what's yours with you" honors the deep love we have for the members of our family system and at the same time frees us to go into our own lives. Even though I have worked with constellations for many years, I am still impressed by the impact of this phrase and the internal act that follows it.

Through systemic constellations, we have also learned about the other principles that operate in the family system, or—if we look at it from a different perspective—in the hidden part of our conscience. It turns out that we all want to submit to the hierarchy of seniority within the system, even though, for various reasons, we often violate it. But when we live without respecting it, when, for example, we become overly concerned with our parents or reject them, then the hidden conscience activates and demands that we pay. When we violate the hierarchy, also the flow of strength from our ancestors to us is blocked.

Another manifestation of the operation of conscience is the mechanism of balancing. When we wrong someone, we want to suffer defeat, hence the various forms of atonement that we are aware of to various degrees. Similarly, when we feel that we cannot reciprocate to someone, particularly a person close to us, we desire to compensate through the evil that befalls us. All these processes, despite their individual shades, are universal and can be easily identified and felt during family constellations.

Family constellations show what is universal and, in a sense, closest to man, and what has been mostly hidden. This method does not need complex conceptual constructs or elaborate techniques to bring out things of fundamental life significance. The insights and effects it brings seem to eclipse anything that other methods of working with a man can offer.

NOTE

1. He was originally a monk and a priest, and a school principal in Africa, who familiarized himself with the concept of group dynamics and used this knowledge in his work in school. His interest in psychotherapy deepened and he eventually left the order. He was trained in several therapeutic approaches, and in 1979 he began to work with his own method, which he constantly developed (Hellinger and Heilmann 2018).

Part I

FAMILY CONSTELLATIONS AND OTHER THERAPEUTIC METHODS

Chapter 1

Family Constellations and Psychodrama

THEATER AND THE PSYCHE

Family constellation therapy is related in many ways to other psychotherapeutic methods. These connections are genetic in nature—because certain concepts were the starting points and inspirations for the developer of constellations, as well as logical—because there are similarities in approaching problems and working on them in constellations and in other therapeutic methods. When considering the context that other therapeutic methods provide for constellations, one should begin by presenting psychodrama.

The author of this method is Jacob Levy Moreno, an Austrian psychiatrist, who already as a teenager, in 1911, observed that encouraging children to spontaneously play their life problems has a therapeutic effect (Czapów and Czapów 1969, 74). Psychodrama involves working on our inner experiences not only through words but also space, body, and movement. Moreno said that it can be called a method that "explores the truth of the soul through action" (Ameln and Becker-Ebel 2020, 3). Tian Dayton, a psychodrama practitioner, writes:

> Many traumas are preverbal—experiences that occurred before we learned to express ourselves through speech. It is difficult to reach these wordless places and reflect upon them exclusively through the use of language. But when our bodies are engaged, we can move through the memory and show what happened rather than try to reconstruct it through words. (Dayton 1994, xix)

As systemic constellations, psychodrama also uses the space of the outside world to see the inner world of our psyche. By engaging the body, we enhance our perception capabilities. During a psychodrama, we reach the memories that would be impossible to extract in a different way and discover deeper levels of our feelings and relationships.

Moreno put emphasis on stage architecture, auditorium, props, and lighting, hence psychodrama resembles theater. All the same, the most important aspect of his method was spontaneity. Moreno noted that man's spontaneity, expressed in spontaneous acting, goes further than we would expect. When true spontaneity was shown to the audience in the Theatre of Spontaneity (*Stegreiftheater*) started by Moreno, they thought that the performances had been rehearsed earlier (Stadler 2018, 24). During constellations, it sometimes happens that the surprised client asks if the representatives were instructed in advance how they should act.

In the theater, we can find elements resembling psychodrama, especially in the activities of Russian theater director and theorist Konstantin Stanislavski (Stanislavski 2010). At the turn of the nineteenth and twentieth centuries, this theater reformer changed the way an actor approached his role, creating an original psychotechnique of acting. In general, his method of mastering the role and acting craft instructed not to think about the new role or try to understand the actions of the character purely intellectually. Stanislavski advised not to create complex ideas about a given scene, behavior, and motivation of the character in advance. He recommended that one start immediately with real, even the simplest, activities, such as entering a room in an inn. By involving the body and movement, the actor "analyzed" the character through "an inner and outer analysis" of himself as a human being "in the life of the role" (Stanislavski 2010, 68).

Interestingly, in this initial period of work on a role, Stanislavski treated the actor's feelings, thoughts, and associations that appeared when he played the part as more important than the author's script. When the elements of the role that he referred to as "the life of the human body," that is, the actor's real psychophysical response in stage conditions, appeared, then the actor's "psyche, to a certain extent, merged with the role" (Stanislavski 2010, 55). This is indeed a revolutionary approach, which would be completely unjustified if Stanislavski had recognized the ordinary perspective on mind and perception. If this had been the case, an actor unfamiliar with the role could not add anything significant. However, Stanislavski's perspective was not ordinary. He wrote:

> What are the ways to set our creative nature to work? You know that you must give it and your creative subconscious free rein.
>
> Here, too, my technique can be of help.
>
> Just as you are drawn towards psychical actions so you are drawn away from your own subconscious forces. In that way you grant them freedom of action and draw them into creative activity. In other words concentrate your attention on creating "the life of the human body." In this way you grant your nature total

> freedom, which will help you, without realizing it, create, stimulate, animate, and justify your physical actions.
>
> The workings of nature and the subconscious are so subtle and profound that you do not even notice them when working.
>
> When I was experimenting with Khlestakov, starting with physical actions to create "the life of the human body," I was unaware of what was going on inside me. I naively imagined that physical actions created themselves, and that I was directing them. But it turned out that they were only the external. Reflex expression of the life, the creative work that, unawares, was being carried out by my subconscious forces.
>
> It is not within the capabilities of consciousness to carry out that hidden work and so what seems beyond us, is done by our nature. What persuades nature to do this work? My technique for creating "the life of the human body." It brings into play by normal, natural means subtle forces of nature not susceptible calculation. (Stanislavski 2010, 69)

Stanislavski "analyzed" the character based on his own feelings and spontaneous behaviors. After a short rehearsal for the role of Khlestakov—the main character of Nikolai Gogol's comedy *The Government Inspector*—in which he unconventionally enacted his behavior, Stanislavski deliberates (in Stanislavski's text, a fictitious theater director, Tortsov, acts and speaks on his behalf):

> What prompted me to make such a entrance? What memories? Perhaps the combination of the puerile braggart and coward, that is Khlestakov's inner nature? Where did my feelings come from? (Stanislavski 2010, 54)

He continues:

> What did I just do? I analyzed what I felt by chance and what happened as a result by chance. I analyzed my physical actions in the given circumstances but not just coldly, intellectually. All the elements helped me. I analyzed my mind and body. (Stanislavski 2010, 54)

Stanislavski treated seriously what appeared "by chance" when he tested a role. His spontaneous behavior could—as one can see—surprise himself, but on this basis he drew conclusions about the psychology of a given character.

The processes Stanislavski addresses are essentially the same processes we encounter during constellations. Even the language used to describe them, when the author talks about the creative and subconscious forces of nature, is similar to Hellinger's language. By putting together the subconscious, body, nature, and creativity, he points to the same factors that we consider to be important in systemic constellations. What is also important for Stanislavski—it could not be otherwise, considering the nature of his technique—is movement:

> "I feel," he said, without interrupting what he was doing, "that long periods have been created out of individually different actions, and an unbroken line of logical and sequential actions out of those periods. They are pushing forward and that produces movement, and movement, a genuine inner life." (Stanislavski 2010, 57)

We see movement in the same way during constellations. Subjecting our body to the field triggers movement, this movement leads us further, it does not stop and does not lose its inner logic. This movement is accompanied by feelings, through which a representative reveals the inner life of a given person. The similarity between Stanislavski's technique and thought and family constellations goes even further. Stanislavski writes:

> Yes! Our deeply hidden secrets only open up when an actor's inner and outer experiencing work in accordance with the laws laid down for them, when there is absolutely no forcing, no deviation from the norm, when there are no clichés and conventions, etc. In a word, when everything is true up to very extreme of ultra-naturalism.
>
> But all you have to do is disturb our nature in the slightest degree and that is enough to kill all the elusive subtleties of subconscious experiencing. (Stanislavski 2010, 66)

Jerzy Grotowski and his Laboratory Theatre followed a similar path. Grotowski consistently tried to make theatrical performance an exposure of a certain truth, to make it "being" and not "playing a part." His activities were described with such terms as collective psychotherapy, psychoanalysis, existential psychology, theater clinic, and psychodramatic social system. Indeed, they departed from ordinary performances and moved toward specific psychological workshops for actors and audiences. The actors of the Laboratory Theatre underwent systematic psychophysical trainings; they discovered "various faces of their personality" and "transformed not only as actors but also as humans" (Osiński 1980, 255).[1] Grotowski stated:

> I do not put on a play in order to teach others what I already know. It is after the production is completed and not before that I am wiser. Any method which does not itself reach out into the unknown is a bad method. (Grotowski 2002, 130)

He too, like Stanislavski, conducted "research on theater," in this case of a psychological, anthropological, and cultural nature. There is nothing here but seeing the fact that a play can bring new information about man and life (psychodramatist Eva Røine thinks that psychodrama could contribute to research studies by identifying common themes of various problems, such as drug addiction, hysteria, fear of authority, and other; Røine 1997, 169). Zbigniew Osiński writes that in the Laboratory Theater the "man-actor does not illustrate or present or tell, but calls into being a [. . .] fact whose basis lies in the hidden but inherent powers of man" (Osiński 1980, 283).

In Grotowski's opinion, the director, working with the actor, plays the auxiliary role, the role of an obstetrician. His job is to remove obstacles so that the actor's spontaneity could emerge. He referred to this attitude—totally corresponding to "helping from the last row" advocated by Hellinger—as "a state of idle readiness." Osiński writes that this type of approach to work requires that the director "bring his mind into a state that is as passive as possible, but at the same time receptive" and prepare himself "to receive 'messages' from the world that is both in him, in his 'unconscious' and 'conscious,' and outside him," that emerges at the intersection of two realities—that of the actor and of the director (Osiński 1980, 276).

Grotowski aimed at a "poor theater," eliminating scenography and purely theatrical elements, such as music. This is a similar way to the one from Moreno's psychodrama to systemic constellations, which could be referred to as "poor psychodrama" (already the French school of psychodrama branched off from using many props; Pawlik 2012, 19).

The same elements—perhaps difficult to define precisely, but constantly recurring—are present in both psychodrama and in Stanislavski's and Grotowski's work with actors: spontaneity that brings out unexpected contents, the hidden cognitive abilities of man, the subconscious that seems to transcend the boundaries of the individual and link him to some broader reality. Hellinger, through family constellations, addressed these phenomena, showing that they can be trusted as therapeutic tools.

MAN IN RELATIONSHIPS

An important term coined by Moreno is "social atom," that is, the configuration of individuals directly or indirectly relating to each other and emotionally connected at a given time (Czapów and Czapów 1969, 68–69). Moreno says that man, from the moment of his birth, is part of a social atom and is subject to a network of interpersonal relations "between him and his mother, father, grandmother, or grandfather, and then: neighbors, acquaintances, and friends" (Czapów and Czapów 1969, 69). According to Moreno, the social atom is as necessary for man as the body, and its decay is almost equivalent to the dying of the organism. Moreno was the founder of sociometry, a method of studying relations in groups. He also used the term to define the arrangement of interpersonal relations that we carry in our minds. This inner arrangement affects our behavior. As Dayton states, we bring this "interior sociometry (our internalized original cast of characters and states of relatedness with them) to any situation," in which we in turn encounter "another's interior sociometry." Psychodrama always sees the individual in the context of his internal relationships, "even in a one-to-one therapeutic situation, and even as an isolate in a context" (Dayton 1994, 42).

The more the so-called telic sensitivity—allowing him to become the subject and object of the process of *tele*—is developed in man, the more he becomes part of the social atom. The term *tele* is an interesting element of Moreno's thought and is associated with phenomena close to telepathy, which, according to Moreno, play a role in interpersonal relations. This is how Moreno describes it:

> Tele is defined as a feeling process projected into space and time in which one, two, or more persons may participate. It is an experience of some real factor in the other person and not a subjective fiction. It is rather an inter-personal experience and not the affect of a single person. It is the feeling basis of intuition and insight. It grows out of person-to-person and person-to-object contacts from the birth level on and gradually develops the sense for inter-personal relationships. (Moreno 2019, 350)

It is interesting that the process of *tele*—that is, the intuitive and telepathic connection between people—is, according to Moreno, the main factor determining our functioning in groups. In family constellations, we can see that such processes—involving the knowing field and the interpersonal transmission of psychic material—are decisive when it comes to the development of an individual in the family. Telic sensitivity emerges primarily during intense contact between the infant and the mother and continues in adult life as a certain tendency. Dayton tries to explain the concept of *tele* by referring to our responses to strangers—even though we have no information about them, we feel comfortable with some and uncomfortable with others, some seem familiar to us even though we have never met them before. She states that these "nonverbal responses are a part of *tele*, or a sort of telepathic sensory awareness" (Dayton 1994, 28). "It is two-way empathy, a sensing the reality of who someone else is; it is the bonding that holds people together" (Dayton 1994, 28).

As we can see, Moreno's perspective on interpersonal relationships is not typical. He considers the processes that are not mentioned in academic lectures on interpersonal communication or psychology of relationships to be among the most important factors. However, Moreno emphasizes the objectivity of the process of *tele*, pointing out that it is not a "subjective fiction," but a shared reality.

BEYOND THE INFORMATION PROVIDED

The basic premise of psychodrama is that the playing process reveals the psychological truth; it brings out unconscious knowledge and suppressed memories. Whereby the truth about oneself and one's relationships is not only learned directly but also through so-called "auxiliary egos," members of the group who play the persons important to the "protagonist" (client), and through "doubles," that is, representatives of the client himself. Psychodramatist, Anna Bielańska, writes that "through the occurrence of 'tele,' stage magic, even those emotions and behaviors of the protagonist that were not previously manifested or mentioned are often acted out" (Bielańska 2009, 65).

To explain the phenomenon occurring during a psychodrama, Moreno coined concepts such as *surplus reality* and *tele* discussed above. He noted that in a psychodrama one can go beyond ordinary reality and experience a new, more complex reality. This complex reality, which can be shown by a psychodrama, is the actual area of its healing influence that can change the "course of an individual" in an instant (Røine 1997, 70). Surplus reality is a specific experiencing of time, space, others, and oneself.

Røine states that one of Moreno's most genius techniques is the empty chair and that "when no one is sitting in the empty chair, the level of surrounding surplus reality becomes particularly high" (Røine 1997, 122). There is no one in the chair, but there is an idea that someone/something could be there. This is enough to trigger the effect of perceiving through the field.

Tele, as a process of telepathic connection between people, enables, as Moreno argued, an insight into the real situation of another person. One of the basic psychodramatic techniques, which is role reversal (e.g., the parent and the child can exchange their roles on stage), seems to use this process. In this technique, protagonists "go beyond projecting onto or empathizing with" and "actually experience being" another person (Dayton 1994, 69). Røine writes that *tele* is "transference of thoughts and emotions" between two persons, which "Moreno calls 'Zweifühlung' as opposed to 'Einfühlung' (empathy in English)" (Røine 1997, 77).

In the technique called doubling, the double "speaks the unconscious of the protagonist, bringing the material that is lodged in the background to the foreground" (Røine 1997, 66). This is what Røine writes about doubling:

> A description of being a double can sound like a mystic experience. In fact, just what happens when a person assumes the role of another person's alter ego is still

> a mystery. [. . .] Of the two kinds of doubling, the simplest is based on asking a group member to stand behind the protagonist and express spontaneous opinions about whatever problems the protagonist is struggling with. (Røine 1997, 130–31)

The second form of doubling is that the double, in repeating movements of the protagonist,

> is able to register the inner anxiety of the protagonist. [. . .] the double acquires information about an inner reality that might not have been gained by standing behind the protagonist. [. . .] The transmission of information from the protagonist to the double is difficult to explain. [. . .] Empathy and tele are qualities that can be improved by training. [. . .] The experience of being a double could be described as a temporary absence from one's self. (Røine 1997, 132–33)

The concepts of *surplus reality* and *tele* are not easy to define. However, it is clear that they are based on the experiences that, in systemic constellations, we would associate with the knowing field. When working with constellations, we also feel that the space "changes," for example, where we feel that someone is missing and that some deceased person should lie down on the floor. In psychodrama, it is believed that surplus reality comes from the protagonist's psyche, while we know that it has its source in the knowing field (that is why it can "change" around the empty chair). Røine states that "empathy and tele are qualities that can be improved by training," with which one must agree. One can only add that this training is amazingly easy and fast, which is demonstrated by even completely inexperienced representatives. Both during psychodramas and constellations, we are in some surplus reality, we bring unnoticed or unknown relationships and events to light. The body and movement—as observed by Moreno—helps us to reach this information in an unexpected way.

The phenomenon of extrasensory access to knowledge during the work of actors using Stanislavski's method was also mentioned by writer Aleksandr Blok in his diaries:

> The actors (mostly young) are given an outline, a theme, a scheme that gets "concentrated." The person who provided the scheme (the writer, for example) knows exactly how it develops, but the *words* are provided by the *actors* [. . .] They also rehearse Molière (!), without knowing the lines: after the characters and situations are precisely described, the *actors* are asked to fill the silence with words; Stanislavski says that they are getting close to Molière's text. (Blok 1974, 125–26)

Back to Moreno, in the context of the psychodrama with Hitler (sessions with a patient who believed himself to be Adolf Hitler that began in 1939; Janus 2021, 155–56), he stated:

> A magnificent panorama of the world of our time emerged in bold relief, as if caught in the miniature mirror of this group. Careful analysis of the responses, as well as of the production, suggested that the real Adolf Hitler might have profited greatly if he had had participated in psychodramatic sessions during his adolescence. [. . .] On the deeper level of the structure we saw the familial figures in Hitler's life reflected in their relationship to the corresponding figures in the life of each member of the group. But we also saw the figures of the larger world—emperors and kings, autocratic rulers of nations like Stalin and Mussolini, rulers of free governments like Roosevelt and Churchill. (Moreno and Moreno 2011, 199)

As we can see, Moreno took seriously what the psychodramas revealed. He claimed that he learned something about Hitler based on the play of his psychotic patient, and that he even learned about the people who had affected the dictator's life. Such an attitude must seem insane to the one who sees psychodrama or systemic constellations as just manifestations of participants' subjectivity. Psychodramatists observed that some psychodramas seem to refer to the times and places completely unknown to their participants, which is why they described them as transpersonal psychodramas (Røine 1997, 193–95).

Another observation made by psychodramatists is the phenomenon of the objective meaning of spatial arrangements such as the side on which the protagonist's father and mother stand in relation to each other. This is the same principle as the one emphasized by Hellinger: the father's place is on the right and the mother's on the left. Røine writes:

> Experience has shown that the father is placed on the right and the mother on the left. If the protagonist is convinced that the father should be on the left, this usually implies that the father has been an absent figure, weak or, perhaps, a distracted artist. If the mother is placed on the right side, she has been the dominant person. Without being able to explain it, this has proven itself true time after time—it might have to do with the concept of energy, but this idea bears no scientific significance. (Røine 1997, 188)

The concept of "energy" understood in this way has indeed found no place in science, but it is one of the most important aspects of constellations. A constellation is of an informative and energetic nature because certain significant spatial arrangements (closer—further, on one side or on the other, higher—lower, etc.), acquired information, and internal attitudes translate into clear feelings, some of which are of precisely an "energetic" nature (feeling the "energy").

HEALING ON STAGE

One of the fundamental functions of psychodrama is to give the participant a cathartic and corrective experience of his basic and original interpersonal relationships that determine his behavior (Czapów and Czapów 1969, 34). Constellations show that these basic interpersonal relationships that determine our behavior concern the family. Psychodrama takes a very similar approach to working with these factors. Dayton states that the way to find a solution to our difficulties caused by growing up in a "destructive family system" is to explore the impact of the system on us. The way is to "understand the full generational system," not to make "an alcoholic father the problem, or an abusive sister the problem," which would be a straight path to a therapeutic impasse. She writes that psychodrama:

> offers a method of dealing with the family system *as it is stored and lives within our psyches*. Though we may not have the original cast of characters to work with, we do have the ability to concertize our inner truth and to bring our family of origin from the darkness of memory to the psychodramatic stage. (Dayton 1994, 119–20)

Dayton identifies the factors that we also consider to be healing in constellations. She says, for example, that thanks to the understanding of the generational system, we take pressure off from the parents or other people, which is a way toward developing and getting better. She continues with these words:

> In psychodrama the person can play out the introjected parents from both his point of view and from theirs. Spending time in the role of the parents helps to bring the personality of the parent that lives within the protagonist to a conscious level. [. . .] Spending time in the role of the protagonist helps that person to give back to the parent such feelings as shame, anger and even love, which he has carried in silence within him because the empathic bond between the parent and child was not sufficiently intact to contain these emotions. (Dayton 1994, 222–23)

The point is to adequately perceive one's own family system and experience the relationship with the parents and the related emotions that could not be expressed, including love. We also have here, known from constellations and extremely important, "giving back" (leaving with them) to the parents their feelings, such as shame. Recognizing the need for love, the bond with the parents and loyalty, as well as the possibility and necessity of "corrective work" in this regard is an important part of psychodrama. Røine states that "it is the mother and father 'in ourselves' that have to be united" (Røine 1997, 197).

The need to rebuild the bond in order to become able to autonomize is even a credo of family constellations. Dayton also writes that "we must first successfully bond before we can successfully individuate" (Dayton 1994, 224).

Dayton states that "psychodrama helps protagonists to 'get what they never got'" and "by using surrogates" it provides "a feeling of love, acceptance and support" (Dayton 1994, 224). We know from family constellations that these experiential kinds of processes are real. The child can establish the parent and ancestor within himself as a source of strength. Dayton writes that "when the parent is intact within the child, the child can then move out into the world with an inner point of reference—a sense of being loved and held; he can learn to love and hold himself and recognize other people and experiences that provide that same feeling" (Dayton 1994, 225).

The technique is very similar to that used by Hellinger to restore the original movement toward the mother or father. The author makes the same point as Hellinger: approaching the areas of "void" causes pain, but only confrontation with that pain can lead to healing. In systemic constellations—which is odd to some people—we recognize those who have died as equally important as the living. And how is it in psychodrama? Bielańska writes that Moreno signalled the importance of the dead:

> For him, the dead play an important role among the living—they are, as it were, constantly present among them. That is why there is always room for them on the psychodramatic stage. They can become present here and enter into dialogue with the living. Rejecting their presence and meaning disrupts the social atom—it disrupts the whole. (Bielańska 2009, 39)

This is the same perspective on the question of the dead that Hellinger presented. Psychodramatists consider the connectedness with the dead to be an important factor in our mental life:

> In many psychodramas deceased persons assume a place on the stage as if it were the most natural thing in the world. [. . .] Very often, if we get the departed person on the stage, and the protagonist is willing to work within the dimension of death, the entire group will experience recovery. [. . .] It might seem strange when a protagonist, in the role of his dead father, says that he wants to hug his son. When this occurs, the auxiliary ego can hold the protagonist in his arms and bring about a scene of reconciliation based on a deep longing rather than sentimentality. (Røine 1997, 178)

Røine emphasizes that what happens on stage is not sentimentalism but comes from deep layers of emotions and from ties. Interestingly, she mentions that accepting the deceased makes the whole group feel better. Looking from the perspective of constellations, we see this act as consistent with the orders of love, so it is understandable that the participants feel a sense of relief. The author also notes that it is often the case that, precisely because the given people are dead, "it is possible to repair some fragments from a ruinous family life" (Røine 1997, 190). Our view is different from the common belief that only relationships with the living people can be repaired, whereas in relation to the dead, one can only change one's attitude, start thinking about them differently, and so on.

Psychodramatists realize that in fact in such situations something more happens than a mere mental change. During a psychodrama, close contact (which has never existed before) with the parent is established:

> The very body seems to undergo some kind of structural change on a molecular level. Something is added that has been missing throughout the person's life. We can observe backs straightening and voices strengthening. (Røine 1997, 197)

Psychodrama uses rituals; frequently there are reconstructions of funeral rituals, which are helpful, for example, for those who could not participate in the funeral and mourning process. Ritual forms are also present in constellations, although they are reduced to elementary actions such as bowing. Dayton writes:

> For most Americans, the idea of ritual is obscured by vague visions of ancient rites and elaborate ceremonies. We have, as a society, divested ourselves of cultural and family rituals, and thus may lack clear connection with our deeper selves, our spiritual paths, and the society in which we live. Our lack of meaningful ritual often causes us to reach for objects outside ourselves to achieve a sense of grounding [. . .]. Eventually, we may experience a spiritual crisis in which we lose our inner sense of being a part of something larger than ourselves. Rituals in longstanding cultures are, in some sense, scripted psychodramatic events. We can use psychodrama in a similar way to ritualize or concretize an important passage, event or stage. (Dayton 1994, xx)

Dayton proposes a psychodramatic exercise for dealing with abortion, which is to help cope with the pain and bid goodbye to the unborn child. The exercise indicates similarities in the process of getting out of this kind of trauma in psychodrama and systemic constellations. The therapist suggests the following steps:

1. Ask the protagonist to choose someone to play the child, or use an object [. . .] or an empty chair.

2. Allow the protagonist to hold, grieve for, talk to, or otherwise interact with the child.
3. Allow the protagonist to reverse roles with the child.
4. Allow full time for the protagonist to share the hopes and dreams she had for the child—all that will not be, from both the viewpoint of the mother, and, if desired, from the viewpoint of the child (in role reversal).
5. Ask the protagonist to end the scene in any way she wants. (Dayton 1994, 156)

The author also writes:

> A mother often has a name for an unborn child. Ask the protagonist to use the name in the drama, if she chooses, and the child can use Mother. Often the mother will ask forgiveness from the child or will grant it to herself from the position of role reversal if there is guilt associated with the abortion. This exercise can be used with fathers in the same way. In either case the spouse can be represented in the drama, or anyone the protagonist needs to be present. (Dayton 1994, 156)

The child gets a name, the mother is called a mother and reactivates the bond with the child, she forgives herself. A person or an object representing the child can be used here. This exercise can heal because the mother comes in contact with the real child. It is not a conversation about the abortion and the child, but an experience of the relationship. Constellations prove that this experience is much deeper than merely symbolic—the mother really contacts the child's soul (the soul as it manifests itself through constellations—it is not a religious or spiritual vision).

GOD ON STAGE

Moreno did not see man only from a psychosocial perspective. He believed that we are connected with the universe and God. He understood human creativity, and thus also the ability to know the sources of problems and to recover, as a manifestation of the divine power acting through man (Stadler 2018, 43). Moreno perceived man in personal, social, and cosmic dimensions, he stated that "the cosmos should be included in the therapeutic process as one of the basic values in human life" (Bielańska 2009, 23). He encouraged one to "stand firmly on the ground and try to solve problems by 'reaching for the stars' because everything is interconnected," and "people are 'cosmic' beings, that is, they see everything that happens also outside the therapeutic office" (Bielańska 2009, 23). Finnish psychodramatist Martti Lindqvist writes that

> the roots of Morenian drama are deeply philosophical—even theological. The basis of Moreno's cosmology is the concept of a continuous cosmic drama, which God himself both directs and acts. (Lindqvist in: Holmes, Karp, and Watson 2005, 144)

The "cosmos," the "interconnectedness" of all things, and the ability of people to "see" what happens "outside the therapeutic office." These elements may seem surprising in the context of a psychotherapeutic method that is supposed to be close to ordinary life. It turns out that when working with groups and with what spontaneously manifests itself in people we are confronted with a reality different from the ordinary one.

Moreno noticed that what was previously associated with the artistic activities of the few, namely spontaneity and creativity, is part of the essence of every man (Czapów and Czapów 1969, 61). We also learn that from constellations in which we see how ordinary people spontaneously express, often in subtle and diverse ways, deep deposits of human experience. Since the essence of God and the universe—according to Moreno—is endless spontaneity and creativity, it is through spontaneity and creativity that the divine and cosmic dimension of man is revealed in psychodrama.

Obviously, God, or more precisely the idea of God, gets embodied in the actions and feelings of a particular person, which makes it possible to reflect on it and capture its individual meaning. We deal here with experimental theology, whose main tool is the exchange of roles with God. Moreno "wanted to find a new understanding of God as an active, all-encompassing, creative principle in the world" (Czapów and Czapów 1969, 21). Referring to man as connected into the "cosmic drama," Moreno talked about the same as Hellinger, who argued that we are grasped by something bigger, by the creative spirit. One of psychodrama participants writes:

> We felt we were part of something bigger. [. . .] I'm not saying that psychodrama is magic. [. . .] If they are able to connect the session's personal drama with the universal drama, then sometimes the universal will get plugged into the personal. (Sprague in: Holmes, Karp and Watson 2005, 22)

Røine writes that psychodrama "is hardly the Orthodox Jewish or Christian view of truth. Tolerance, compassion, love, and forgiveness are all by-products of a good psychodrama" (Røine 1997, 169). The same is true for systemic constellations.

PSYCHODRAMA AGAINST THE BACKGROUND OF FAMILY CONSTELLATIONS

Psychodrama is an important method of therapy and self-development that brings great benefit to people who participate in it. It has numerous similarities to what is known to people familiar with family constellations, uses similar techniques, and can be applied in similar fields (we can work with the client individually, using figurines or objects, work with larger systems such as organizations, etc.). Psychodrama theory involves a broad, "cosmic" view of man and uses unusual processes in therapy, normally referred to as parapsychological (*tele*). However, although Moreno's concepts are close to Hellinger's understanding and psychodrama often delves into the same processes as constellations, the method does not know the orders of love or the concept of the knowing field.

Psychodrama participants have the possibility to put into order what in normal life is considered past or unattainable, like a conversation with the dead father or aborted child, but the therapeutic change is based on known psychological processes. These include abreaction, getting insight, looking from a different perspective, sometimes a reconciliation or a goodbye. To reach a solution in a psychodrama, we start from the current situation about which we learned through the patient's social atom and we look for the desired state, that is, the change the patient expects. To do this, we position both "atoms" on stage: the current state atom and the desired state atom. Next, the psychodramatist together with the patient is working on "how the current state atom could turn into the desired state atom" (Stadler 2018, 80).

In constellations, we can also talk about a transition from the present picture to the picture of resolution (Janus 2021, 7). However, we do not construct these pictures. They emerge spontaneously if we can provide the conditions for that (appropriate attitude, not omitting any important element of the system, patience). Psychodrama involves more rational thinking and conscious planning and does not focus on unconscious processes that much. At a certain point, the client and the therapist, as well as other members of the group, integrate the information obtained during the spontaneous process into the sphere of their deliberations and seek a solution based on this. During constellations, both the diagnostic data and the solution path appear spontaneously, and the therapist's rational thinking helps to remove the obstacles and facilitate the process.

Although Moreno saw the fact that surprising and new information and feelings emerge during role-playing, which he tried to encapsulate in the term *surplus reality*, contemporary psychodramatists do not address this issue thoroughly. They assume that when, for example, role feedback does not confirm the protagonist's opinion of the person being acted out, this does not show the reality of that person, but the client's hidden attitude (Stadler 2018, 102). So they assume a hypothesis of a kind of telepathy between the protagonist (the client) and his auxiliary ego (the one who plays the role). Constellations have shown clearly enough that this is a different process, a specific connection to the information field (the knowing field). For the information about people other than the client, even those completely unknown to him, is regularly confirmed as true.

NOTE

1. All quotations from non-English sources throughout the book have been translated by Barbara Gąstoł.

Chapter 2

Family Constellations and Family Therapy

MAN IN THE CONTEXT OF THE FAMILY

Family therapy, in its various forms, has many common elements with family constellations in terms of both theory and therapeutic treatment. The beginnings of this therapy were observations of people suffering from schizophrenia—it was observed that their condition changes in the presence of family members. Thus, schizophrenia became perceived not as a simple mental illness but as a reaction to such and no other family environment. Unfortunately, this could also be interpreted to mean that families are responsible for sustaining the disease, and this was the view held by some therapists and psychiatrists.

Family therapy went further. Not only was there a focus on the familial determinants of mental disorders, but the entire family was recognized as an entity that could be treated, and then its healing potential was recognized. Family therapists have become aware that they cannot try to replace the client's important family members:

> One of the basic premises of family therapy is that people should be helped to fill their emotional needs, literally, through their intimates, through the people who matter the most, rather than through a therapist, a parental surrogate whose association with the patient is necessarily limited, professional and *as if*. (Framo 1992, 10–11)

Virginia Satir, the "mother of family therapy," originally conducted individual psychotherapy and was inspired to change her approach by calls from her patients' relatives. Satir noticed that among the complaints about her therapy, and even threats, there were masked requests for help:

> It became clear that any individual's behavior is a response to the complex set of regular and predictable "rules" governing his family group, though these rules may not be consciously known to him or the family. From this point of view, we can begin to stop seeing relatives' activities only as dangers, and look at them as forces for growth and indications of the power of interactional transactions in relation to shaping the behavior of the individuals that are a part of the system. (Satir 1983, ix)

The patient's family was no longer isolated and treated as disrupting the therapy process. It was taken seriously in its dilemmas, grievances, expectations, and concerns. This became possible because the behaviors and words of family members were understood as a manifestation of certain paramount patterns functioning in the family. In this way, these were no longer personal grievances, which needed to be ignored for the sake of the patient—instead these reactions began to be seen as important information about the principles governing the family. These principles, observed by the first family therapists, can be regarded as prefigurations of the systemic orders discovered by Hellinger.

Because each person's reactions were considered a manifestation of the influence of the family context, the mind itself began to be seen as "external" in a sense, and this significantly changed the understanding of pathology. The founder of structural therapy, Salvador Minuchin, wrote:

> When the mind is viewed as extracerebral as well as intracerebral, to locate pathology within the mind of the individual does not indicate whether it is inside or outside the person. Pathology may be inside the patient, in his social context, or in the feedback between them. (Minuchin 1975, 9)

Pathology ceased to be an internal matter of the individual and became partly "externalized." The same paradigm is used in family constellations. We know that the mind is in constant interaction with something that is beyond it, with the family field. Therefore, the traditional approach to what is in the environment and what is in the mind is no longer adequate. The mind of the individual has become an element of the system.

Gregory Bateson, an anthropologist, contributed to treating the family as a system. He transplanted the ideas of Norbert Wiener, the founder of cybernetics, into the social sciences. Therapists inspired by the theory of systems saw the family as a complex entity that consists of the sum of activities of interconnected elements, that is, family members. Family members, interacting with one another, create a system that is governed by its own laws. Their behavior (also feelings, mood, thoughts) is determined by the system—something beyond their individual mind. This is a fundamental observation—the same one that is used by systemic constellations. We see that in families there are forces that are superordinate to the will of individuals, and we call the whole of these forces the soul of the family.

The fact that family interactions follow fixed patterns was first identified by Don D. Jackson in the marital dyad (Goldenberg and Goldenberg 2008, 81–82). He found that the interactive behaviors of family members are determined by internal rules and repetitive behavioral sequences and not by their personality traits or needs. This was a step toward discovering the invisible world of systemic orders. Hidden system dynamics have a stronger impact than overt behaviors and messages. If, for example, in the parents' generation these orders are disturbed, it will have a negative impact on the children even when the parents try very hard to be good parents. The founder of family systems therapy, Murray Bowen, writes:

> The striking observation was that when the parents were emotionally close, more invested in each other than either was in the patient, the patient improved. [. . .] When the parents were emotionally close, they could do no wrong in their "management" of the patient. The patient responded well to firmness, permissiveness, punishment, "talking it out," or any other management approach. When the parents were "emotionally divorced," any and all "management approaches" were equally unsuccessful. (Bowen 2004, 68)

Note that Bowen highlights that "management approaches," that is, specific external behaviors of the parents, do not affect the child as strongly as their emotional closeness. In other words, he states that systemic factors—in this case the unity of the parental couple—outweigh the behavioral ones. In a constellation, we see such mechanisms directly, for example, in the immediate tranquility displayed by the child's representative when the mother expresses respect for his father. Jacek Kubitsky points out that systemic therapists treat emotions as secondary and do not analyze them, believing that they are a resultant of the structure of the family system (Kubitsky 2010, 97). Therefore, in the systemic approach, laws, orders, and structures are more important than emotions, judgments, and behaviors.

Thinking in terms of systems makes it possible to look for general laws, system isomorphisms that manifest themselves within very different formations, such as bacterial populations or human communities, economics, or chemistry. Ludwig von Bertalanffy made an attempt to identify such patterns in the so-called general system theory (Bertalanffy 2015). Whereas, in psychology, Bowen saw human functioning as part of a natural system, following the same laws as the rest of nature (Goldenberg and Goldenberg 2008, 177). We know that the orders identified by Hellinger not only govern the functioning of the individual in the family system but also apply to other human systems.

LOVE AND THE ORDERS IN THE FAMILY

Love and the Bond

In Helingerian therapy, we see four fundamental dynamics present in family systems and interpersonal relationships—bonding, belonging, balancing, and hierarchy. What primarily ties the family system together is love. This bond is the fundamental force shaping relations within the family. It may lead to problems and even to death when someone wants to share the fate of someone dead, but it also makes it possible to solve difficulties. Has the basic and multidimensional effect of love been noticed by traditional family therapists? Cloé Madanes discovered what family constellations also show—that the ground of complicated events and relationships in the family is not manipulation, power struggles, or selfish demands for attention, but the love-driven consideration of one for the other. Family members "almost telepathically" sense their relatives' problems and are "willing to sacrifice themselves if it will only make things a bit easier for their families" (Simon 1992, 123). Family constellations corroborate the therapist's observations that the bond with family members can be at the root of even destructive behaviors. Madanes states:

> Love is complex and it sometimes involves hurting oneself or hurting the object of one's love. . . . A daughter may make a suicide attempt so that her depressed mother will pull herself together to take care of her daughter and in so doing will come out of her depression. Violence toward others may also have the function of obtaining or of giving love. (Simon 1992, 123)

Madanes understands love as a binder and a powerful force motivating family members who are constantly engaged in the process of protecting one another. This is done even through quite destructive behaviors and symptoms whose unconscious aim is to try to protect one of the family members, the parental couple, to change someone's behavior, and so on.

John Elderkin Bell, the pioneer of family group therapy, wrote:

> Some of my friends who have worked with the families of schizophrenics, report that withdrawn and seemingly unrelated individuals experience the intensity of love and respect we see in the families of normal or neurotic people. This bond is not only of a biological nature; it is based on the long history of group process, even though the group is disturbed. The group has a meaning, a kind of appropriateness in the individual's mind, that makes him want to continue his membership in it. After the unpleasant truths come out, love and respect show themselves. If the unpleasantness is not expressed, then the love is hidden too. Revealing the intensity of disruptive forces in the family seems a necessary step

> toward discovering the strength of the bonds that tie the family together. (Bell 1975, 199)

As one can see, Bell accentuates love, bond, desire to belong, and respect. The importance of love was also emphasized by the founder of family-of-origin therapy, James L. Framo, who invited his client's parents or grandparents to sessions. He believed that only in such a context can problems be properly shown and solved because on a deep level, everyone wants reconciliation with their loved ones. This is what he wrote:

> Consider this aspect of the innate nature of family life: Families can provide the deepest satisfactions of living: unreserved and unconditional love; gratifying bonding; measureless sacrifice; enduring dependability; compassionate belonging; the joys and warmth of family holidays, dinners and vacations; the fun and play; the give and take; and knowing your family is always there when needed. Still, the hurts and damage that family members can inflict upon one another are infinite: scapegoating; humiliation and shaming; parentification; crazymaking; physical, sexual, and psychological abuse; cruel rejections; lies and deceit; and the manifold outrages against the human spirit.
>
> [. . .] No matter how enraged people are at their parents and siblings, the deepest part of themselves yearns to love and to be loved by these irreplaceable figures. In this context positive feelings can emerge such that mothers, fathers, sons, daughters, brothers, and sisters can understand, reconnect, come to terms with and, finally, forgive each other. (Framo 1992, 6–7)

Kurt Ludewig states that although many therapists, when addressing anorexia, emphasize the patient's refusing to take on the role of a woman and her rivalry with her siblings, he believes that what is important in this disorder is feelings of love and mutual care. He rejects interpretations that say that love in families affected by anorexia is not authentic, asking what feelings would be more authentic than the ones that involve giving up one's own self-fulfillment or may even lead to death, which can happen in the case of an anorexic (Ludewig 1995, 170). What we have here is recognition of the fundamental importance of love, which is not a choice in the family, but a biological imperative. The family as a whole is always characterized by feelings of love.

We know from working with constellations that autonomy can only be achieved by accepting the deep bond that connects us to our family of origin and can never be achieved through rejection and cutting ourselves off, for example, from our parents. This was noted to some extent by Bowen, who argued that as we live in the family, we are simultaneously influenced by the push and pull forces, togetherness and distance, symbiosis and autonomy, and it is the individual's task to balance these processes so as to be able to maintain intimacy with his loved ones and differentiate at the same time (Goldenberg and Goldenberg 2008, 176).

Belonging

Through family constellations, we learned how powerful the dynamics of belonging is—one belongs to the family system regardless of one's personal merit, age, or role in it.

Traditional family therapists noticed that the family is the kind of system where none of its members can be replaced by someone else. For example, if a parent leaves the family and another person comes in his place, he will not replace the absent person, even if he tries hard. The Goldenbergs write that "loyalty, and a continuity or durability of membership characterize all families" (Goldenberg and Goldenberg 2008, 4). As we know, some people from outside the family group also belong to the family system, such as the parents' former partners, and it is part of the orders of love to acknowledge their existence and the fact that in creating a new family, we do not start from scratch. These relationships were observed by Satir:

> One of my suggestions when working with people who are preparing for a blended family life [adoption, patchwork family] is that they constantly keep in mind that each had a life before and much of what goes on in the present life will have a reference point in the past. [. . .] It is important that everybody is clear about what has happened and straight about his or her way of communicating it. [. . .] we can't fall of the face of the earth, or destroy or get away from all that we had yesterday. We need to include and integrate the things that belong to yesterday. (Satir 1988, 165–66)

Satir mentions three basic types of blended family: when a woman with children marries a childless man, when a man with children marries a childless woman and when each partner already has children. She writes:

> In the first case, the blended family consists of the wife, the wife's children, husband, and wife's ex-husband. In the second case, the unit is husband, husband's children, wife, and husband's ex-wife. In the third case, the family consists of wife, wife's children, wife's ex-husband, husband, husband's children, and the husband's ex-wife.
>
> Even though these people may or may not (and probably don't) all live under one roof, they are in each other's lives, for better or worse. Room has to be made for all of them. Each member is significant to the growth and success of

> the blended family. Many people in the blended families try to live as though other members didn't exist. (Satir 1988, 161–62)

The therapist believed that there was a network of invisible connections between family members, which she called the family map:

> I believe that anyone who has ever been part of a family leaves a definite impact. A departed person is often very much alive in the memories of those left behind. Frequently, too, these memories play an important role—often a negative one—in what is going on in the present. [. . .] If the departure has not been accepted, for whatever reason, the ghost is still very much around and often can disrupt the current scene. (Satir 1988, 185)

Satir notes that "anyone who has ever been part of a family leaves a definite impact," which is a kind of prefiguration of the Hellingerian right to belong that says that everyone who has ever belonged to the family system has an equal right to belong. The therapist says that the departed person is "alive in the memories" of those who remain, and at the same time states that it is their "ghost" that stays with them. This ambiguity stems from the fact that, without using the concept of field, she needs to somehow express this "indirect" state of existence of the departed one, whose impact—which she probably observed—goes beyond the effect of memory.

Satir distinguishes between an "accepted" departure and one that has not been accepted, stating that in the latter case, the "spirit" of the absent person has a destructive effect on the family. Here we deal with the partially recognized issue of exclusion. In constellations, we see that such an unacceptable departure can be death, such as that of a mother or child. It causes a lack of mourning, and this entails a lack of acceptance of the departed as departed, and thus de facto excluding him from the family.

Hierarchy

The importance of family hierarchy is highlighted by the structural school of family therapy. Minuchin observes that patterns of behavior in the family are governed by a certain rule that "well-functioning families should be hierarchically organized, with the parents exercising more authority and power than the children and the older children having more responsibilities as well as more privileges than their younger siblings" (Goldenberg and Goldenberg 2008, 241). Moreover, Minuchin points to the father as playing the leading role in a well-functioning family. The latter is in line with the view of Hellinger, who points out that the one who externally provides for the family has priority over the one who organizes its interior. This role is usually fulfilled more successfully by the father. It should be noted, however, that this pattern is not one of the systemic orders (orders of love) in the strict sense, as opposed to the hierarchy resulting from chronology—the older ones have more life significance for us than the younger ones.

According to structural therapists, the boundaries in the family should be clear and the family should not be a totally democratic organization. In families with problems, there is a lack of clarity as to the hierarchy, and thus the struggle for power and excessive taking on or avoiding the responsibility (Górniak and Józefik 2003, 104). Hierarchy, as intergenerational separation, is also addressed by Carl Whitaker's symbolic-experiential therapy (Namysłowska 1997, 77). Most family therapists also point to the harmful influence of parentification, that is, reversing the hierarchy of care in the family.

Although family therapists have recognized the fact that such a thing as family hierarchy exists and serves some dynamic function in the family life, it must be emphasized that they have not grasped its essence and depth. They have understood hierarchy primarily as a distribution of power within the family and not, as in systemic constellations, as an invisible transmission of heritage, a one-way transmission of what strengthens as well as what burdens.

Balance

Hellinger pointed to the principle of involuntary "balancing" of the ratio between gains and losses that occurs in human relationships. He noted that the relationship can last and develop only when there is a mutual exchange—when gifts are received and reciprocated, and faults are compensated. When there is a stagnation in this harmonic flow, or its direction becomes one-sided, the relationship at the emotional level withers. William J. Lederer and Don D. Jackson wrote about something similar in *The Mirages of Marriage*:

> In this book we shall demonstrate the necessity for "equality" in marriage. This kind of equality is not based on the absurd belief that spouses need to have the same IQ or the same interests, or to work equally hard. It is based on the more subtle notion that close, enduring human relationships depend on an interplay of behavior which signals to each spouse that whatever he receives has been forthcoming in response to something given. In other words, a *quid pro quo* (something for something) agreement is in effect: to live in a reasonable harmony the spouses negotiate with respect to their behavior and responsibilities. Perhaps this kind of relationship appears selfish and unromantic, yet in our view it is the single most required and most overlooked aspect of any marriage. It seems all too clear that most Americans believe that "love" and "romance" plus plenty of gadgets will keep a couple happy. Americans tend

to enter marriage with a grinning, false-face concept of what married life will be like. From this delusion has come our mass marital failure. (Lederer and Jackson 1990, 16–17)

As one can see, Jackson and Lederer identified a kind of principle of balance in marriage, and they consider its dynamics to be more important for the functioning of marriage than superficial similarities and equality of spouses. Conventional family therapists observe—at least in part—the dynamics of balance and their impact on changes in our mood and self-judgment. An example is the clinical vignette presented by Kubitsky, where the husband felt like an "innocent" because of his wife's aggressiveness (Kubitsky 2010, 166–67). When his wife stopped harassing him, he realized he was losing this position. Here, we see the dynamics of the victim feeling superior.

CONVERGENCES OF THE THERAPEUTIC TECHNIQUES

Bert Hellinger is not the only discoverer of family constellations. Ruth McClendon and Leslie B. Kadis, from whom he learned, carried out family constellations and found solutions, but worked intuitively and could not identify their patterns (Hellinger 2001, 437–38). An important technique of family therapy is role-playing, which is obviously related to the technique of systemic constellations. Many therapists underline the strong impact of role-playing; for example, Satir says that

> everyone is capable (and I know this without ever asking anyone anything) of experiencing the feelings of somebody else and portraying them. Role-playing has two very important aspects. Through role-playing a person is, in effect, demonstrating than he knows more than he thought he did. That is Number One. It is fascinating, for instance, when you ask the son, in the family where there has been trouble between a father and son, to role-play his idea of how his father feels. I have had some fantastic things happen when I said, "It looks like at this point in time you don't really know what it is like to be in each other's shoes, so let's reverse things for a moment. You, John, be your father, and you, Father, be John. Now how would you two deal with the son asking to use the car?" The results can be incredible. (Satir, Stachowiak, and Taschman 1990, 138)

And further on she writes:

> All the forms of role-playing make it possible for the person to use his own self-knowledge on the feeling level to be able to understand what it is like to walk in somebody else's shoes. For example, if you were to role-play your

> mother right now, you would bring a lot more to the role than you would have before you started thinking of her as a person. (Satir, Stachowiak, and Taschman 1990, 139)

David Kantor developed the technique of sculpting. Kantor and his colleagues noticed that work in space provides the most adequate view of complicated, multi-person dependencies in the family, related to closeness and distance, power and subordination, activity and passivity, as well as other dimensions. They write about it as follows:

> Sculpture is a dynamic, active, nonlinear process that portrays relationships in space and time so that events or attitudes may be perceived and experienced simultaneously. It is meant to provide the meanings, metaphors, and images of relationships in a way that can be shared by all who participate and observe. Information is not talked about but experienced through action and observation. An opportunity is provided for the presentation of a map rather than word description. It restates in action patterns behavior that language has used as metaphor. "I can't get close to him." "He turned his back on me." "I've felt distant since he said that." All these are colorful phrases into which sculpture breathes life again. (Duhl, Kantor, and Duhl 1973, 52)

Satir together with Richard Bandler and John Grinder say that sculpturing is "one of the most powerful techniques to achieve the perspective of process" (Bandler, Grinder, and Satir 1976, 158). The authors understand the process as a set of patterns and ways of interaction within the family (as opposed to the content communicated by its members). Satir often used "sculpturing" the family, also calling it "posturing" (Satir 1983, 250). The therapist "sculptured," for example, communication in a family, asking its members to take certain positions and make symbolic gestures, such as crouching and curling up or pointing a finger in someone's direction in an accusatory gesture. The sculptures were created on the basis of observations and interpretations of Satir herself, but they were accompanied by elements added spontaneously by the family members as well as by their own emotions.

The technique of sculpturing is evidently connected with family constellations—the instruction "Set up your inner picture of the family," which was originally used in constellations, derives directly from this technique. It was only later that it was observed that this kind of symbolic projection is not necessary, as information about the family picture will be provided by the knowing field anyway.

Sharon Wegscheider-Cruse developed her own version of this technique, which she referred to as family portrait. It is not much different from the sculpture, but the therapist, after setting up the picture of the family—which is done by one of its members—asks the others to change their places and poses to those they would like to see in the family picture. When we compare it with constellations, we can see that such a modification is a step toward creating the picture of resolution (the sculpture itself or the first phase of the family portrait can be considered the picture of the problem).

Satir also initiated the technique called family reconstruction, which involves acting out the members of the client's family by the volunteers. She wrote:

> All of us were born little, without any little bag of direction about how to grow and develop as people. For all of us, our major resources were the people who were around and saw to it that we survived. The chances are good that the ways you learned to survive are what you are now using [. . .]. Children grow up with some very peculiar ideas about what motivates their parents and what explains their behavior. How many adults feel comfortable in telling their children what is really going on, that they are hurting or afraid or have made a mistake? The parent's hiding or withholding their own inner experiences is more likely to be the case. [. . .] the child puts together the discrepancy he or she experiences as a way of understanding self and others and this becomes the operating model for assessing oneself. Family reconstruction is a method I developed to help a person go back and pick up the missing pieces. (Satir in: Wegscheider-Cruse et al. 1994, 1–3)

During reconstruction, when the client is emotionally blocked or feels confused, the double is asked how he would feel or react in a given situation. The tasks of the double are very similar to those of the client's representative in systemic constellations.

Mara Selvini Palazzoli brought rituals into therapy. Using them aimed at transferring therapeutic interventions from the verbal level to the level of uniting and changing the family. The therapist and her colleagues explain that "the term *family ritual* refers to an action or series of actions, usually accompanied by verbal formulas or expressions, which are to be carried out by all members of the family" (Selvini Palazzoli et al. 1978, 95).

Alongside recommendations, such as that the family gathers together on a daily basis and that each member of the family speaks for fifteen minutes, expressing emotions—which have little to do with the orders of love—there are also those that aim to reaffirm the bonds, accept a person into the family, forgive, reconcile, or end mourning.

BODY, SPACE, FIELD

Bodily Sensations and the Knowing Field

Satir emphasized the informative role of bodily feelings in working with families:

> The atmosphere in a troubled family is easy to feel. Whenever I am with such a family, I quickly sense that I am uncomfortable. Sometimes it feels cold, as if everyone were frozen [. . .]. Sometimes it feels as if everything were constantly spinning, like a top; you get dizzy and can't find your balance. [. . .] Sometimes the air is full of secrecy, as in a spy headquarters.
>
> When I am in any of these kinds of troubled atmospheres, my body reacts violently. My stomach feels queasy; my back and shoulders soon ache, and so does my head. [. . .]
>
> As a therapist I have learned to be tuned in to these feelings in myself and to recognize the signs of them in my patients. They tell me a good deal about what is actually going on between us. (Satir 1972, 10-11)

Satir relates her own psychophysical feelings to what is really happening in the family. So she assumes the existence of some kind of message from the family system and its reception by her own organism. Satir also states that this reception can also concern family members, which—lasting permanently—causes their ills (Satir 1972, 10-11). This "family atmosphere" does not disappear the moment we leave the family of origin, but accompanies us through the activity of the family field.

Salvador Minuchin and H. Charles Fishman assert that the therapist's behavior should be spontaneous and shaped by the context of the family he works with. They also use the concept of field:

> The therapist's spontaneity is constrained by the context of therapy. The therapist, an influencer and changer of people, is inside the field that he is observing and influencing. His actions, though regulated by the goals of therapy, are the product of his relationship with the client family. The therapist is like the continuo player in a Baroque suite. He is free to do whatever feels right, as long as he remains within the harmonic structure. [. . .] Because the therapist experiences the family reality, and because the rules of the family structure him from within the field, his interventions fall within a tolerable range. Interventions that are ineffective do not become chaotic or destructive; they are merely assimilated by the family without producing change. In a way, it is the constraints of the situation that give

> the therapist freedom. Because he is dependent on the field in which he is participating, his spontaneity is shaped by the field. (Minuchin and Fishman 1981, 3)

The constellator's approach is very similar—he too, already at the stage of listening to the client, lets the family field guide him. The difference is the range of the field that is taken into account, as the constellation therapist looks from a transgenerational perspective, and also at the victims, perpetrators, and excluded persons. Interventions of the constellation therapist, if he remains in harmony with the family field and respects the orders of love, are also absolutely safe for the client.

Bateson was the first to encounter the knowing field within his work with families and family studies. This is what Satir writes about it:

> The Bateson group, working in Palo Alto in 1954, came upon the notion that families are constrained by redundant behavioral patterns that occur over and over again outside of the family awareness. In attempting to demonstrate this by utilizing role-playing among the members of the group [. . .], they were surprised to find themselves developing strong feelings in relation to the behaviors they were merely acting out in the role of a particular "family" member. Further, they were able to show that, by following certain simple rules, they could simulate, for example, the family of a chronic schizophrenic patient to such a degree that the recording of these sessions sent for "blind" diagnosis to various other investigators in the country was considered to be a tape of a real schizophrenic family. Even the voices of the researches (who were well known to the other investigators) were not recognized, although no voice change had been intended by the so-called "role-players." (Satir 1983, 235–36)

And she describes her own experiences in this way:

> I have had experience now with utilizing "simulated family" techniques with hundreds of different audiences and with many different professional groups, from physicians to social workers, teachers, and nurses. [. . .] In all of my experience in using these games with many groups across the country, I have never encountered a person who did not, once involved in a game system, develop vivid "gut reactions" to the roles he played, particularly those roles which are contrary to his own self-image. It is very common for someone to say, after a particular game, "Now I know how Mrs. X feels and can sympathize with her ulcer problem! This sounds just like her. After five minutes of it, my own stomach is churning."
>
> On one memorable occasion, a young social worker played the identified-patient daughter in a particular simulated family, while a general physician, interested in family therapy, was her simulated father. At the end of about forty minutes

> of family interaction, the "daughter" stood up, threw her arms around the older man and stated, "I really love you!" and he, with tears streaming down his face, stated, "It's the first time I have ever really felt what I missed in not having a daughter." (Satir 1983, 236)

What Satir talks about is the experience of every constellation facilitator: we do not see people who do not display "organic" reactions during a properly conducted constellation. Note that Satir speaks of the phenomenon of representation as a discovery, emphasizing its fully repetitive nature. So Satir and the Bateson group are probably pioneers in using the phenomenon of the knowing field in therapy.

Satir used role-playing, knowing that it would not just be acting but that the player would be deeply moved. About the interview with the simulated family, Satir says:

> As far as I was concerned, this simulated family was as "real" to me as any family, in the sense that the people role-playing family members were real people doing real things. As you read the interview, you too will very quickly come to perceive them as a family. Recall for a moment what is involved in role-playing. Each person brings with him all of his knowledge and experience of how people feel and act in certain situations. Without coaching or rehearsing, this group of volunteers from the audience became a family system. (Satir, Stachowiak, and Taschman 1990, 163)

It is characteristic that the volunteers "become" a family without any training. Satir associates this with the knowledge we carry within ourselves. Thanks to constellations, we are sure that we do not carry this knowledge but it comes to us. Anyway, it is evident that these people—before they started playing roles—had no direct access to this knowledge. They would not be able to verbalize it and present it (otherwise every person would be a psychological genius, and they are not).

New information also appears when sculpting a family. The therapists describe the process of sculpting Joan's family, and the sculpture concerned the period when she was six years old:

> With the players in place, the monitor encouraged them to move and act, *without words*, in the patterns given them. In moments, an overall systemic pattern emerged. [. . .] More and more affect began to show as she [Joan] took in the stimuli of her own actions and others. The overall pattern was ritualized through the monitor's command to repeat it over and over. The ritualization locked the players into the feelings the players were experiencing. Suddenly Joan stopped. "God, I don't want to go into Father's room! . . . It's not that *he* kept me out. *I* don't want to go in. I want to be with Jack and Mother."

> Bu this time, Bill and Grace, caught up in the patterns, had moved closer to each other, revealing in action an intimacy not hinted at before. Joan had observed it, as had the monitor. To the monitor it was clear there was a "gray space," a family secret, emerging.
>
> The monitor suggested that Mother and Jack move closer. Suddenly, Joan blurted out: "Don't do that!" as if she were again 6 yr old. She regained her composure—"I used to wonder about that," she said. [. . .]
>
> The players' responses had begun to bring new information also, as they indicated to Joan what others in the family system might have been feeling or experiencing, although this had never been communicated or shared previously in the original family. (Duhl, Kantor, and Duhl 1973, 55–56)

Note that the players get "caught up in the patterns" and reveal the intimate relationship between the two family members, which Joan did not know about. The players' reactions are not understood as projections of their own mental states, but as information about the real family members and their experiences.

A similar technique, termed family portrait, is discussed by Wegscheider-Cruse, who notes that through the mere role-playing of strangers, the client (the "artist") begins to understand what is going on in his family:

> Even when the "family" is only being role-played, the players often experience strong feelings of fear, loneliness, frustration, and other emotions from having to occupy the positions assigned to them. This is enlightening for them, and as they voice their reactions, the "artist" can begin to sense what life may be like for other members of his family. (Wegscheider-Cruse 1981, 247)

And this is what the author and her colleagues write about family reconstruction:

> People working together in the reconstruction process somehow seem to do and say the right things to facilitate the process for the star [the client]. The business of acting in a reconstruction also enables the role-player to learn about another person. For example, someone playing an alcoholic parent might experience the shame, denial, and loneliness of being an alcoholic. This new perspective can be extremely valuable if he or she has ever lived with or loved an alcoholic because it can allow him or her to stand in that person's shoes, however briefly. (Wegscheider-Cruse et al. 1994, 6)

The authors note that the participants "somehow" manage to do the right things, do what corresponds to the situation and the problem of the client. They state that during the preparations for the reconstruction, when the client does not know certain facts from the life of the family, he should use his "hunches." If the guesses are accurate, people at the reconstruction "will generally know it" and if the guesses are inaccurate, "they'll likely know that, too" (Wegscheider-Cruse et al. 1994, 34). How could they detect what is a fact or what is not true in the client's history, if they did not receive the information in some way? The above-mentioned examples of acquiring new knowledge must be counted among the effects of the knowing field.

In the technique known as the empty chair, the therapist places a chair that symbolizes some absent family member (e.g., the father who left the family). The other family members can sit opposite or approach and express their feelings or thoughts toward this person (Kubitsky 2010, 162–63). This technique can activate strong emotions, which is not surprising given that the effect of representation in the form of feeling the presence of a person can also play a role in it. In another variant of this procedure, one member of the family sits on the chair and speaks for the absent person. And in the dubbing technique, the therapist, standing behind the chair on which the client is sitting, loudly expresses his alleged thoughts and feelings (Kubitsky 2010, 158).

When I work with the client's inner attitude during a constellation, I often use a similar technique, fully aware, of course, that I tune into his emotional field.

"The Spirit of the System"

Besides its purely cognitive effect, the knowing field has another dimension. Wegscheider-Cruse and her colleagues maintain that "it is virtually impossible to be in the room in which a reconstruction is taking place and not be engaged in the power of the process" (Wegscheider-Cruse et al. 1994, 6–7). Therefore, the nature of what happens during the reconstruction is not only cognitive but also energetic, which also affects the observers. We feel this in the same way during constellations. But that is not all. Experiences during family reconstruction have led the therapists working with this method to acknowledge the existence of the spiritual side of reality and a "Higher Power." This is how they write about it:

> The acknowledgment of the power of the human spirit as well as some divine kind of Higher Power are always part of a reconstruction. Virginia Satir referred to this Power as "the life force." The spiritual nature of all people is honored in a reconstruction. Those who have participated can attest to the mysterious, inexplicable coincidences that occur, as well as the beautiful moments of healing and change that are decidedly spiritual in nature. (Wegscheider-Cruse et al. 1994, 9)

We have a description here that fully corresponds to what we experience as a result of constellations. The combination of several elements, which include group work, family work, and role-playing, results in unexpected psychophysical ("beautiful moments of healing and change") and even material effects, we would say, synchronicities ("mysterious, inexplicable coincidences"). Therapy prompts to acknowledge the importance of the spiritual side of a man and the existence of a force that governs the whole of the observed processes ("life force," "Higher Power"). In constellations, we speak of the "family soul," and Hellinger speaks even of the Creative Spirit (German: *der schöpferische Geist*). Some family therapists, such as Satir and Wegscheider-Cruse, consider referring to a transcendence, something greater, as a healing factor. For example, in the case of an abortion or miscarriage, they consider the scene when a doll is held by the client in her arms and "turned over to some kind of Higher Power" to be an effective psychodramatic intervention (Wegscheider-Cruse et al. 1994, 118).

THE UNDERSTANDING OF DISORDERS AND THE PROCESS OF CHANGE

Relational Etiology

Family psychotherapy regards the problem of the "sick" person as a phenomenon that concerns the whole family. The early family therapists noticed that a child admitted to therapy is only an indicator of problems in his family, and the therapy of one of its members influences the behavior of others. Nathan Ackerman, a pioneer in family therapy, wrote:

> We were thus led to affirm once again the principle that emotion is shared experience, that illness is a contagious phenomenon, and that within the family, multiple members may be ill and these illnesses clash, complement, or otherwise influence one another. (Bloch and Simon 1982, 188)

The systemic approach emphasizes that interactions between family members take place all the time, creating a kind of communications network in which all members are immersed. These nonverbal messages modify their behaviors. According to Lederer and Jackson,

> The family is an interacting communications network in which every member from the day-old baby to seventy-year-old grandmother influences the nature of the entire system and in turn is influenced by it. For example, if someone in the family feels ill, another member may function more effectively than he usually

> does. The system tends, by nature, to keep itself in balance. An unusual action by one member invariably results in a compensating reaction by another member. If mother hates to take Sunday drives but hides it from her husband, the message is nevertheless somehow broadcast throughout the family communications network, and it may be Johnny, the four-year-old, who becomes "carsick" and ruins the Sunday drive. (Lederer and Jackson 1990, 14)

Some therapists try to see the family members' behaviors as resulting from their unconscious cooperation. The founders of the so-called Milanese model used the technique of "positive connotations," in which the patient's and other family members' behaviors are attributed with positive motives and objectives, such as preserving the cohesion of the family or helping someone in the family (Selvini Palazzoli et al. 1978, 55–56). Selvini Palazzoli also posits the causes of disturbed behaviors in the family altruism. For example, when the patient tries to help his brother in a difficult systemic situation:

> We point out that the identified patient is the only member of the family to have understood his sibling's true position and condition, which is far more alarming than his own, and that it has been his conviction that he alone can help them. [. . .] We say that we are impressed by the sensitivity and comprehension demonstrated by the identified patient and that, from the material we have gathered and the observations we have made during the session, we find ourselves in complete accord with him and are quite concerned about the supposedly "sane" sibling. [. . .] this unconscious attempt to obtain and maintain such a position of preference is very harmful to its author ["sane" sibling]: it prevents him from growing and becoming autonomous. Only the identified patient, thanks to his extraordinary sensitivity, has, for quite a while, understood the danger in which his sibling finds himself. The patient has developed his "illness," that is, his behavior, which in various ways limits his own existence and growth, thereby attracting the attention and preoccupation of his parents to himself. He implicitly urges his sibling to take advantage of this situation in order to free himself and become truly independent. (Selvini Palazzoli et al. 1978, 99–100)

Sometimes these processes are presented in such a way that the family "selects" one of its members to be the patient and it does not have to be the most disturbed person in the family (Satir, Stachowiak, and Taschman 1990, 27). Such a selected person (the so-called identified patient) is given the task of maintaining the family *status quo* in the face of problems that the family experiences as a whole. In the case of problems in children, therapists often focus on the parents, arguing that the child's problems may be an expression of the couple's hidden problems. Satir states:

> They inadvertently ask the child to deal with what they can't deal with themselves. Of course, the child cannot possibly do this in a constructive way, so the child often responds to this burden by becoming sick, bad, crazy, stupid or all of these things. (Satir 1972, 175)

Family therapists do not, however, only talk about the actions of parents, but also link the child's mental activity with the process of taking over problems, which is fully in line with the explanations given by Hellinger on this subject. We know that children "willingly" take on things that their parents cannot deal with. Strategic therapists—according to whom the child's symptoms may be a metaphor for the parents' problems—assume that the child may indirectly try to help the parents by developing symptomatic behavior (Górniak and Józefik 2003, 109). Satir asserts that the young patient's symptoms "are a message that he is distorting his own growth as a result of trying to alleviate and absorb his parents' pain" (Satir 1983, 2).

Ludewig observes that anorexia turns out to be "a readiness to sacrifice one's own development to prevent the loss of a loved one." If the therapist assumes the concept that the anorexic's "exhaustion is a problem related to love," he has to reject the assumption that "people suffering from anorexia are selfish, authoritarian, aggressive or regressive, or that they have simply become victims of a particular upbringing" (Ludewig 1995, 167).[1]

Minuchin studied the levels of biochemical indicators of emotional stress in parent-child interactions. When the interspouse conflict decreased after the spouses assumed parental functions, the children's stress levels increased, as if something was transfused to them. Minuchin said:

> The interdependence between the individual and his family—the flow between "inside" and "outside"—is poignantly demonstrated in the experimental situation, in which behavioral events among family members can be measured in the bloodstream of other family members. (Minuchin 1974, 9)

All these mechanisms indicate strong unconscious connections between the family members and being driven by love and consideration for others, which we observe during constellations. The family forms a whole, and one person expresses the problems of another. What family therapists tend to define as dysfunctions of the family, within systemic constellation therapy we identify as disruptions of the systemic orders. However, there is no fundamental difference between the two approaches.

Transgenerational Processes

The issue of transgenerational shaping of behaviors or problems in the family is addressed by many family therapists (Murray Bowen, James Framo, Carl Whitaker, Helm Stierlin, Mara Selvini Palazzoli). Ackerman wrote that family treatment:

> lends explicit emphasis to the principle of emotional contagion in family process, the transmission of pathogenic conflict and coping from one generation to the next. [. . .] the sphere of therapeutic intervention is not a single individual but the whole family. (Satir, Stachowiak, and Taschman 1990, 25–26)

Whitaker stated:

> I decided I didn't believe in individuals. They seemed more and more like fragments of a family. Then, as time went on, I heard the ghost of grandmother knocking on the door. (Whitaker 1976, 183)

Advocates of transgenerational approaches believe that "current family patterns are embedded in unresolved issues in the families of origin. That is not to say that these problems are caused by earlier generations, but rather that they tend to remain unsettled and thus persist" for several generations (Goldenberg and Goldenberg 2008, 175). The same view is shared by constellation therapists. The past generations, for example, the grandparents, did not cause our problems; they did not make any particular mistakes that we ourselves would never have made. Rather, they were, like us, driven by a wide network of factors. Problems result from unresolved issues (violated orders of love within belonging, bond, hierarchy, or balance) which affect us and which we try to unconsciously solve.

What is transmitted—according to family therapists—to later generations? Framo argued that intrapsychic conflicts of members of the family of origin are acted out in the current family (Namysłowska 1997, 49). Wegscheider-Cruse believes that "patterns from previous parenting, the compulsive diseases, family secrets, or shame" can be passed on to the next generation (Wegscheider-Cruse et al. 1994, 116–17). Bowen spoke of "family projection process," in which the parents become particularly preoccupied with one of the children (due to the lifestyle of the parents and the child or perinatal events related to the child; Roberto 1992, 11 et seq.).

As a consequence, the child is drawn into an overly strong relationship with one or both of the parents, which interferes with the child's individuation. Such a child will have a decreased self-differentiation, which means that he will be emotionally dependent in some way. As an adult, he will look for a partner with a similarly low degree of self-differentiation and as a parent, he will show the same intense focus on his own child. This process of multigenerational transmission will cause each successive generation to acquire a lower degree of self-differentiation. In the third generation, this can lead to problems such as schizophrenia, which is an extreme undifferentiation of self, or in fact the blurring of the boundaries between the self and the external world.

Many therapists stress that three or four generations are of importance. These include Whitaker (Whitaker 1976, 182 et seq.) or Wegscheider-Cruse, who maintains that sculptures should refer at least to the generation of the client's great-grandparents (Wegscheider-Cruse et al. 1994, 120). Selvini Palazzoli also takes a similar stance on the issue of the influence of three generations on the formation of psychotic behaviors (Selvini Palazzoli et al. 1978, 22). Considering three or four generations when solving the client's problems is a common practice in constellation work.

Family reconstruction uses the symbolic giving back to the past generations that part of the legacy that we do not want to transmit further. As a rule, this is the same act that we achieve in constellations through the words of strength such as "I leave what is yours with you." In family reconstruction, the deceased are "made alive" for a while—the person playing the deceased stands up from the floor, and the client can say something to him. We do the same in family constellations. We know that an unconscious and denied bond with someone who left or died is a common cause of problems. That is why we allow contact with the deceased.

Norman Paul, one of the pioneers in family therapy, saw these matters in a similar way. He maintained that therapy should deal with unresolved issues in the family of origin related to loss and death—he believed that dysfunctional behaviors are often the result of repression or inappropriate expression of grief over the death of a loved one (Goldenberg and Goldenberg 2008, 197). As constellation therapists, we know that the absence of grieving does indeed often correlate with a denial of the bond or exclusion, and these processes have a particularly strong intergenerational impact.

From the perspective of therapists using the reconstruction technique, it is important for the client to understand the family context and to forgive. This can be achieved by seeing the parents and grandparents as ordinary people and as children of their parents, affected by circumstances previously unknown to us or not considered. This aligns with the Hellingerian orders of love.

Quick but Profound Change

One of the phenomena we observe that goes beyond the dominant beliefs about therapy is that therapeutic change can happen quickly even in severe disorders.

Wegscheider-Cruse and her followers emphasize that family reconstruction is a strong psychophysical experience, engaging one's mind and emotions. Traditional therapy can take even several years and is unlikely to produce miraculous and sudden transformations. This is different with experiential therapeutic techniques, especially those that relate to the family. In the case of reconstruction, one speaks of a powerful tool and moments of miraculous resolutions. It lasts about twelve hours and is supposed to "totally change lives" (Wegscheider-Cruse et al. 1994, vii, 3). No doubt specific phenomena occur here, present only in this kind of methods.

To understand them at least a little, we can refer to the experiences of the Milan school. Therapists of this approach assert that the discovery and change of the "fundamental rule" of the system results in the quick disappearance of pathological behavior (Selvini Palazzoli et al. 1978, 4). The quickness of this change confirms the systemic assumption that the source of the problem is in a way "external" to the subject. The mind is to some extent free from pathology, and the disturbing factor comes as if from the outside. This is why a change within the system brings a radical improvement in the condition of the individual.

IVAN BOSZORMENYI-NAGY AND THE ETHICS OF RELATIONS

The achievements of the psychiatrist and psychoanalyst, founder of the so-called contextual therapy, Ivan Boszormenyi-Nagy, deserve special recognition in the context of the systemic constellation method. Boszormenyi-Nagy introduced a completely new dimension to family therapy, which he defined as ethical. He stated that deep interactions within the family are not governed by ordinary psychological factors such as sympathies, antipathies, drives, or needs, but by a particular sense of justice and a desire to balance what is given and taken. This landmark approach shows that it is conscience that determines behaviors on the primal and unconscious level. Boszormenyi-Nagy and Geraldine M. Spark noted in the book *Invisible Loyalties* that although "justice as an ethically grounded issue may sound alien to most current psychological and psychodynamic investigations, it seems to us to offer the advantage of an intrinsic structure of familial expectations and obligations" (Boszormenyi-Nagy and Spark 1984, xx).

In relational ethics, which refers to contextual therapy, the main role is played by balancing what is taken and given. There is an invisible "ledger" in the family, and its members feel an inner pressure to balance merits and obligations. This is ensured by the "intrafamilial intrinsic tribunal," and those who ignore its requirements are affected by negative consequences, which "may be psychosomatic and manifest themselves in insomnia, sexual inadequacy, self-destructive behavior, or patterns, guilt, and depression" (Boszormenyi-Nagy and Krasner 1986, 416–17).

Boszormenyi-Nagy maintains that the identity of a person with a large amount of merits

> is good, righteous, proud or like that of a lienholder who has a right to demand rather than pay. On the opposite end of the merit scale is the position that carries bad, worthless, or shameful identity as though belonging to a lienee who owes rather than demands. [. . .] A low state of merit corresponds to guilt feelings, while its counterpart characterizes the angrily indignant person. Bad conscience and indebtedness coincide with fear of retaliation or captively owed gratitude, while good conscience is consistent with freedom of action, even of vindictiveness and an awareness of deserved claims aimed at the partner. (Boszormenyi-Nagy and Spark 1984, 62)

The above citation could be a description of Hellinger's stance on conscience and how a "clear" and "guilty" conscience affects relationships and the inner attitude. A clear conscience gives a sense of superiority, freedom, and entitles to demands. It can also be the basis for vindictiveness and ruthlessness. An obligation burdens the conscience, enslaves, and causes fear of punishment. When it comes to the dynamics of interpersonal relations, Boszormenyi-Nagy—like Hellinger—states that "the paradigm of unrelieved, one-sided giving is an unrealistic and potentially destructive one that is fraught with the dangers of depletion and guilt-evoking control" (Boszormenyi-Nagy and Krasner 1986, 59). One-sided giving or taking, without exchange and without the possibility for balance, is destructive for relationships. It evokes feelings of guilt, anger, inadequacy, or inferiority in partners.

Boszormenyi-Nagy states that there is something automatic about the mechanism that maintains the balance of give and take, and this does not involve justice in the strict sense, but only—as he puts it—in the statistical sense, because it is not infrequent that there is a process of getting back at someone else. We have here a prefiguration of "group conscience," which, according to Hellinger, is not "just," because it burdens the descendants with the need to balance the transgressions of their ancestors. This is well visible in the case of Hellinger's "double shift" when, for example, the granddaughter expresses her grandmother's grievances toward her partner. According to Boszormenyi-Nagy, this type of behavior takes the form of compulsion, as every member of the family "is motivated to act out any significant revengeful (or grateful) impulse" and that is why "an ongoing seesaw process of retaliative justice can be counted on" (Boszormenyi-Nagy and Spark 1984, 81).

Interestingly, Boszormenyi-Nagy says that "emotional exploitation" that has not been balanced "is often beclouded by considerations of financial matters in the family" (Boszormenyi-Nagy and Spark 1984, 11), as evidenced by my own observations from systemic constellations.

Boszormeni-Nagy and Spark write:

> Certain families carry easily recognized multigenerational patterns of relationships. In one family we learned that for generations there were recurrent episodes of violent death of women caused by the men with whom they were sexually involved. In another family we saw a recurrent pattern of wives being allegedly martyred by their husbands through their obvious and constant involvements with mistresses. In another family three or four generations revealed the pattern of one daughter ending up as an outcast because of the "sin" of disloyally marrying outside the family's faith. We have seen families in which incest sequences occur for at least three or four generations. (Boszormenyi-Nagy and Spark 1984, 1)

The authors made similar observations to those we make in constellations. They pointed to behaviors resulting from motives such as loyalty, attempts at balancing, or penance, which produce intergenerational transmission of patterns.

So Boszormenyi-Nagy recognized much of what we call the orders of love in systemic constellation therapy. Among other things, he recognized that lifelong blood ties "have precedence over psychosocial determination," making children deeply indebted to their parents:

> My father will always remain my father, even though he is dead and his burial ground is thousands of miles away. He and I are two consecutive links in a genetic chain with a lifespan of millions of years. My existence is unthinkable without his. Secondarily or psychologically, his person imprinted an indelible mark on my personality during the critical stages of emotional growth. Even when I rebelled against all that he stood for, my emphatic "no" only further confirmed my emotional involvement with him. He was obligated to me, his son, and subsequently, I have become existentially indebted to him. (Boszormenyi-Nagy and Spark 1984, 3)

Our indebtedness to the parents is not just a response to their actions toward us:

> Even in cases of earliest adoption, the existential significance of the natural parents usually keeps the minds of adopted children occupied for a lifetime. They may surprise their adoptive family with their vehement desire for more knowledge of and contact with at least the memory of the natural parents. (Boszormenyi-Nagy and Spark 1984, 11)

The feeling of indebtedness is rooted in the fact that

> life is received from forbears and conveyed to posterity. Life is a chain of interlocking consequences linked to the interdependence of the parent and child generations. In human beings, relational ethics require people to assume responsibility for consequences. But consequences *per se* constitute unavoidable, existential reality. (Boszormenyi-Nagy and Krasner 1986, 420)

The author of *Invisible Loyalties*—just like Hellinger—departs from narrow psychologism and considers certain objective factors, whose meaning remains unchanged despite the variability of subjective attitudes. It is precisely the existential objectivity of merits and debts that creates relational ethics. Children's loyalty to their parents is something hidden; and external behaviors do not contradict it:

> Aggressive attacks, insulting neglect, physical departure, withdrawal of respect, etc., can all hurt the parents and yet not touch the basic question of loyalty. Overt roles and verbal attitudes rarely explain the status of underlying deep commitment. (Boszormenyi-Nagy and Spark 1984, 41)

The practice of family constellations fully corroborates Boszormenyi-Nagy's view that "no one ends up a winner" if one brings into one's life, for example, as a result of inadequate therapy, "a hopelessly incorrigible resentment and contempt towards one's parent" (Boszormenyi-Nagy and Spark 1984, 20). If such a person fails to transform his inner attitude toward the parent into an accepting one, the hidden bond and loyalty will continue within him, sabotaging his life. This is how Boszormeni-Nagy writes about it:

> Unless the person can struggle with his negative feelings and resolve them by acts based on positive, helpful attitudes towards his parent, he cannot really free himself of the intrinsic loyalty problem and has to "live" the conflict, even after the parent's death, through pathological defensive patterns. A suspicious rejection of

> the spouse or perhaps of the entire world may be one defensive attempt at resolving this sort of conflict. (Boszormenyi-Nagy and Spark 1984, 20)

Outwardly, invisible loyalties will manifest themselves as indifference, ambivalence, or avoidance, resulting in internal conflicts. It will be difficult for a man to respect and love his wife if he rejects his mother. According to Boszormenyi-Nagy, "This phenomenon can be understood as a covert attempt to balance vertical relationships through overt interference with horizontal [. . .] relationships" (Boszormenyi-Nagy and Krasner 1986, 417). By making his wife a scapegoat, projecting elements of his bad relationship with his parents onto her, the man actually "protects his parents by taking his revenge out on someone else. Unconsciously, he avoids blaming their memory while sacrificing his loyalty to his wife" (Boszormenyi-Nagy and Spark 1984, 25). One can only add that it will be no different for a woman, if she is internally cut off from her father, she will find it difficult to bear a relationship with a man or she will be difficult to bear for her own son. And these are only the most obvious consequences.

Boszormenyi-Nagy finds the same resolution of loyalty conflicts as Hellinger. He says that in therapy ways should be sought "to replace attitudes of invisible loyalty with acts of visible concern" (Boszormenyi-Nagy and Krasner 1986, 417). He introduces the notions of exoneration, which means no longer blaming someone, and acknowledgment (crediting) indicating that it is the right thing to recognize the objective caring merits of one person toward the other (the parent toward the child in particular). Boszormenyi-Nagy writes that exoneration

> differs from forgiveness. The act of forgiveness usually *retains* the assumption of guilt and extends the forgiver's generosity to the person who has injured her or him. Offering forgiveness, a person now refrains from holding the culprit accountable and from demanding punishment. In contrast, exoneration typically results from an adult reassessment of the failing parent's own past childhood victimization. It replaces a framework of blame with mature appreciation of a given person's (or situation's) past options, efforts and limits. (Boszormenyi-Nagy and Krasner 1986, 416)

"Exoneration" and "acknowledgment" build the exact equivalent of the Hellingerian concept of "accepting parents as parents." During a constellation, we can clearly feel how inappropriate—that is, how debilitating—it would be to *forgive* our parents instead of *accepting* them.

Boszormenyi-Nagy also observed that children try to take on their parents' problems and are unable to live their own lives when their parents suffer:

> Even very small children are sensitive barometers; they *know* when their parents are overburdened with anxiety, guilt and mistrust. Moreover, they want to do

> something about it. Clinical observation of families gives ample indications of how enormously giving and caring very young offspring want to be toward their massively needy parents. It is precisely this reality that lies at the core of later, adult-age loyalty conflict: "By what right can I enjoy other relationships if my parents are always suffering?" (Boszormenyi-Nagy and Krasner 1986, 15)

Both Boszormenyi-Nagy and Hellinger find that the process of give and take between parents and children is asymmetrical. The fundamental is what flows from parents to children, for which children can never compensate their parents. Boszormenyi-Nagy states that

> at one level, of course, the receipt of parenting is a debt that can never be repaid. [. . .] Parents deserve acknowledgement of their care and contributions. There are also times when they require their children's care and concern. At base, however, the direction of *repayment is forward* rather than backward. Parental investments are most fully repaid through an offspring's due contributions to posterity. Simply put, a person receives from his past and his parents, and gives through his children and his future. (Boszormenyi-Nagy and Krasner 1986, 100)

Boszormenyi-Nagy's clinical observations are identical to the conclusions emerging from constellations that the improvement of the child's state "often coincides with the renewed capacity of parents to exonerate their own seemingly failing parents" (Boszormenyi-Nagy and Krasner 1986, 416).

Merits and misconduct of one toward another constitute a kind of unwritten balance. The author obviously did not use the notion of orders of love, however, considering society as a whole, he wrote:

> It could be argued that there exists an invisible dynamic balance between all competing individual notions of justice. Such intrinsic consensus about the principles of subjective justice, i.e., how everyone's equity of benefits is to be measured, constitutes the basis of the "objective" judicial bookkeeping of the group. (Boszormenyi-Nagy and Spark 1984, 81)

EDWARD BRUCE BYNUM AND THE FAMILY UNCONSCIOUS

American clinical psychologist and family psychotherapist Edward Bruce Bynum put forth the concept of Family Unconscious, which classifies him as one of the explorers of the family field. He noted that family members share the content of dreams, emotions, attitudes, and behavioral patterns.

According to him, the family seems to be permeated by some information and energy field:

> After full sessions with families where all were present, *we* would work with parts or subsystems of the family. *Often* in these situations with siblings or parents "family secrets" would emerge. When the timing was right for these secrets to come out to the whole family, somehow everyone seemed to already have a vague image of the other's secret, *even though* these had never been openly mentioned. *Such* secrets often included the oddest of acts and the most intimate of fantasies. *There seemed to be a shared* central image, not fully located in any one person, but with each member having his or her own perception of it. I assumed that there must have been some nonverbal communication going on. [. . .] I had found many times that, though a particular problem was not spoken of in a family, nevertheless one family member somehow expressed the pain of another member. (Taub-Bynum 1984, 4–5)

Here we see the phenomenon known from systemic constellations that family members share problems, carry their pain together and possess unconscious knowledge about one another.

The Family Unconscious is a collective product of the family and consists of

> those personal motifs that have been repressed and also cultural and family-interactional styles that existed in some manifestation before the psyche's entrance into that system. [. . .] the Family Unconscious contains *shared* images, *experiences*, and roles held in common by the members of our family matrix. *It constitutes* a shared emotional field and matrix of consciousness. These shared images and affects are *active, intense*, and *immediate*. [. . .] At this level of family consciousness, intensity, energy, and affect are shared despite whatever distortions there may be in communication. The effects and affects of this level can be seen in the behavior, roles and dreams we create. (Taub-Bynum 1984, 11)

The matrix that is created by the Family Unconscious

> is to a large extent developed *before* the individual is even a breathing part of the family. We as individuals are born into a system with a significant part of the interactions already operative within the nexus. This is even stronger when there are already many siblings. These relations or energy patterns can exist overtly within the family's awareness but are generally unconscious in the family system. (Taub-Bynum 1984, 14)

As "energetic," the Family Unconscious influences the new family member on a nonverbal level, shaping his psyche probably as early as the fetal period. This is nothing other than the process I have termed systemic-psychodynamic transduction (Janus 2021, 233–35). For Bynum sees the Family Unconscious as the information and energy field that shapes our sensitivity, emotionality, ability to empathize and enter into relationships. The author writes:

> The Family Unconscious emerged within this study as a field of information and energy that enfolded the lives of any group of people with powerful affective connections, shared history, and recurrent transactions with each other. [. . .] this family is really the seed, the primal energy nexus from which almost all other relationships are later derived. Merely saying that each person is an "aspect" of this energy field is not enough. We *experience* this energy field as powerful emotion, imagery, the vortex from which many of our motivations spin out. [. . .]
>
> In its healthy form this field of the Family Unconscious is the taproot of compassion. It is the playground and laboratory of the Self, the place where the innate knowledge that all life is indeed One can be tangible reality, and we can act and expand accordingly.
>
> The family is where we learn to engage and disengage, where the sense of commitment and integrity spawns. In this context, psi [paranormal phenomenon] is simply another natural event that testifies to the interconnectedness of all beings and forces of nature. (Taub-Bynum 1984, 196)

Bynum also points to the existence of transgenerational processes. This "transmission" may be "discontinuous," for example, from the first generation to the third, bypassing the second. The author notes that the family system is built not only of current interactions between the living but also of "images" of the dead and the absent:

> This level of unconscious functioning also continues to exist after we are no longer an active member of the system. We note here the family mythology of persons who have died or left but whose images and example continue to influence others in the system who know of them. (Taub-Bynum 1984, 14)

Considering the features of the Family Unconscious, we can say that the presence of the deceased in the family system, as Bynum sees it, is not limited to the memory images of the family members but is active and dynamic.

The author also expresses the view that we are connected not only with the members of our family but also with all other families, and perhaps with all beings in general. On this basis, he seems to anticipate the existence of the knowing field in the form in which we use it during constellations, that is, as a channel allowing us to access the knowledge about others:

> If one had the correct way of decoding or transforming this deepest energy level (the correct Fourier transform), one would have access to this vast field of information. (Taub-Bynum 1984, 23)

It can be said that a way of "decoding" has been discovered—it is the technique of representation in systemic constellations.

Like Hellinger, Bynum sees the dangers of the illusion of autonomy and independence, also for our health:

> When we lose intimate connection with some kind of energy of the Family Unconscious and fall prey to the illusion of absolute autonomy or individuality, we run the risk of real illness and a loss of the sense of being grounded. Dynamic inter-connectedness or interdependence is vital to our well-being. (Taub-Bynum 1984, 22)

ATTITUDE OF THE THERAPIST

The role of the therapist has been reformulated many times in various schools of family therapy, so it is impossible to specify the generally prevailing standards. However, there are many similarities between the attitudes of family therapists and constellation therapists. First of all, it is necessary to point to the principle of impartiality or multipartiality, which involves adopting the point of view of each family member. Family therapist Karl Tomm argues that being neutral during an interview means avoiding any attachment or aversion to anything that the client says or does. The therapist should avoid taking a "for" or "against" position, and must be able to reconsider and change what he has imagined about the client. In this way, there is space for the intuitive, not always conscious, aspects of cognition to emerge (Górniak and Józefik 2003, 61). Similarly, Bandler, Grinder, and Satir write that the therapist "must become freely involved, with his eyes, ears, and body responding to the family members, while, at the same time, remaining outside their family system" (Bandler, Grinder, and Satir 1976, 157).

This is the same attitude as in constellations where we do not judge anyone or adopt anyone's perspective, respecting love and inner movement of everyone. We are free from attaching ourselves to our own perceptions and interpretations, especially those that arise before the constellation. Above all, we "secure the space" for the emergence of the unconscious aspects of the client's situation that are manifested through the knowing field.

Bateson believed that a too conscious goal adopted during therapy may limit the ability to see the variety of relationships (Górniak and Józefik 2003, 41). Many founders of family therapy accentuate the therapist's ability to reject old meanings and be free from ideas and intellectual assumptions, which is in line with the phenomenological attitude recommended by Bert Hellinger.

The therapists who are inspired by constructivism depart even further from imposing anything on the family and try to accept and understand everything that happens. That is why they will not consider events such as the family not coming to the session or not coming together to be resistance, but a systemic necessity. At the basis of this understanding of the family lies Humberto Maturana's concept of structural determinism, according to which living systems do what they have to do according to their structure, because this is the only thing they can do (Górniak and Józefik 2003, 49). It is similar to Hellinger's "Yes," acknowledging what is, because that is what it had to be.

In traditional family therapy, we can also find the recommendation to focus on the process rather than to infer from the content (Bandler, Grinder, and Satir 1976, 137–38). One must not delude oneself that the problem of the family can be solved "in the head" and by using words. This attitude should also be adopted by every constellation therapist, one should not try to solve the client's problem during the conversation, but be aware that only the constellation can provide a significant understanding and change.

FAMILY THERAPY AGAINST THE BACKGROUND OF SYSTEMIC CONSTELLATIONS

Regardless of the mentioned similarities between traditional family therapy and family constellations, it must be said that none of the classical schools has achieved the degree of theoretical clarity and coherence of practical conduct that characterize family constellations. Nor has the course and significance of certain processes been fully perceived, and for this reason the emphasis has been placed differently.

Family therapy sees an individual's mental problems primarily in the context of the influence that the family members who live and are in direct contact with one another have on that individual. Many therapists focus on the influence of the parents, whom Satir referred to as the architects of the family (Satir 1988, 27). Systemic constellation therapy broadens this context as the family, or rather clan, is more extensive than a conventionally understood family, even a multigenerational one. The family is not only the current interpersonal interactions but a kind of active record constantly affecting the psyche of the individual. It allows us to work effectively with adults, without involving their families. In constellations we take some of the burdens off the parents, seeing the importance of other persons too.

Traditional family therapy speaks of healthy and disturbed families, of dysfunctional marriages, and distinguishes between families that support and inhibit development. In constellation therapy, these categories are not used at all. Of course, we can see that something particularly bad is happening in a family, but we cannot define such a family as "dysfunctional." Its problems result from a wide background, including the living and the dead. It would be pointless to consider the whole multigenerational system to be disturbed, although we see that certain disorders cumulate or are transmitted from generation to generation.

Therapists such as Selvini Palazzoli are able to state, for example, that "the most prejudicial character in these families is the father" (Simon 1992, 154). He may be a "passive provoker" and his daughter may try to "punish the mother and revenge the father, who, in her opinion, is not capable of making himself respected by his wife" (Simon 1992, 150). These kinds of relationships and behaviors can obviously occur in families. The thing is, the therapist seems to believe that these dynamics are the ground of family problems. From the point of view of systemic constellations—or, in other words, if we were to conduct a constellation of this family—it would turn out that the relationships here are much more extensive and that the dynamics shown by Selvini Palazzoli are merely the result and the proverbial tip of the iceberg. And defining someone as the "source" of the family problems would turn out to be highly inadequate, completely unrealistic.

Without judging the clients or their families, we do not need to argue that all behaviors and relationship patterns are of equal value. Quite the contrary, as constellation therapists, we know very well that there are objective principles that lead to growth and health, and ones that always prove to be destructive. Recognizing that there are many individual stories about oneself or one's family, we do not impose anything on our clients. We know, however, that there is a deeper level which has the shape of a universal dynamic structure.

Although many developers of family therapy have recognized the function of love in the family, its importance has not been fully explored in traditional therapy, so there are therapists who bring chaos instead of order into the family. Ludewig states that "the therapists who need to assign blame to someone, take the side of the child or the father or mother, ignoring the phenomenon of love in the family," "intensify the fear of separation and the feeling of guilt." By adopting this attitude, they violate the principle of neutrality and "become overly involved in the family conflicts" (Ludewig 1995, 170). This attitude is not shared by those who understand the absolute power of bond and love in the family.

Walter Kempler, a Gestalt and family therapy practitioner, argued that no techniques are used in experiential family therapy and that the only "technique" is the therapist himself; Whitaker, and structural therapists thought in a similar way. In traditional therapy, the therapist's personality, creativity, and even his way of being seem to have a significant impact on its effects. The therapist's personality was also accentuated by Satir or Ackerman. In constellations, it is different. The therapist works primarily using the therapeutic technique. Of course, he works "himself" when he stands as a representative or contacts the client's field, but his personality traits, his style of being, or some particular personal sensitivity are not the essence of the practice and are kept in the background. What is needed to become a constellation therapist can normally be learned—no special talents or being charismatic are required.

Family therapists—as advised by Satir—take their emotions and associations into account during the session and even follow them (Kubitsky 2010, 137). It seems, however, that some of them may have a wider, and others a much narrower range of this kind of perception (this is probably why Satir uses the pronoun "I" so often in her works—she realizes that it is *her* who feels this way, who sees so much, who influences the family in this way, and not differently). In constellation therapy, by consciously focusing on the knowing field, we paradoxically avoid adopting the attitude of someone extremely sensitive. This kind of reception of information is available to everyone and one does not need to have any extraordinary abilities.

In properly conducted constellations, we follow the systemic orders and the client is protected against both the therapist's arbitrariness and against what can be directly hurting. In traditional family therapy, techniques such as provocation, destabilization, paradoxical interventions, manipulation, or persuasion are also acceptable (Kubitsky 2010, 83; Minuchin and Fishman 1981). In constellation therapy there are no such invasive moments, and thus risky for the therapist and client; we work within strict limits. We do not focus on people's life in all its richness and diversity, we do not refer to the palette of human dreams, drives, thoughts, goals, or judgments. We work on a different plane—the systemic orders, and that is why we gently disregard most of the personality "colorfulness" of our clients. This style of work offers a lot of comforts, because we do not get involved in people's natural differences of opinions and points of view. Traditional family therapists do not have this comfort because they constantly work in the field of family expectations, fantasies, and games. For this reason, it is much more difficult for them to define the area in which they should enter for the good of the client and separate it from the area which they should leave without interference.

The Goldenbergs specify the criteria useful in evaluating a given method of family psychotherapy. They ask:

- Is it *comprehensive*? Does it deal with understanding family functioning and avoid being trivial or oversimplified? Is it generalizable to all families as they behave in all situations [. . .]?
- Is it *parsimonious*? Does it make as few assumptions as necessary to account for the phenomena under study? If two competing theoretical systems both predict the same behavior, is the theory chosen the one with fewer assumptions and constructs?
- Is it *verifiable*? Does it generate predictions about behavior that can be confirmed when the relevant empirical data have been collected?
- Is it *precise*? Does it define concepts explicitly and relate them to each other and to data (avoiding relying solely on figurative, metaphorical, or analogical language)?
- Is it *empirically valid*? Do systematic empirical tests of the predictions made by the theory confirm the theory?
- Is it *stimulating*? Does it provoke response and further investigation to enhance the theory or even to demonstrate its inadequacies? (Goldenberg and Goldenberg 2008, 149)

How does the constellation method present itself in the face of the above questions? Systemic constellations speak of the principles that apply to each family and even refer to other human systems. Despite their simplicity, they are not trivial—many people have no knowledge of the orders of love, and discovering them seems to be an act of development. Hellinger's theory is also extremely parsimonious. With very few basic assumptions and terms (such as "bond," "balance," "belonging," "hierarchy," "knowing field," "family conscience") it explains all the phenomena that occur during constellations and allows for effective therapeutic interventions. Systemic constellations are a precise and logical method, in which I see no internal inconsistencies. They do not use analogies and images, but name very specific processes, and working with these processes always brings therapeutic effects. From Hellinger's theory, one can also make many empirical predictions about people's behaviors, problems, or quality of life (for instance, that if someone accepts his parents, he will be more able to improve relations with his own children, etc.).

NOTE

1. At the same time, Ludewig says that in anorexic families there is a problem of "how to deal with separations from the child (most often the daughter) or the parents (most often the mother)" (Ludewig 1995, 167). This is similar to the fear identified by Hellinger that the parent "will leave the family." In constellations we see that it is usually the father. This difference of opinion may result from the fact that positive feelings for the father are suppressed and the mother is brought to the fore.

Chapter 3

Family Constellations and Psychoanalysis

IN THE NETWORK OF UNCONSCIOUS RELATIONSHIPS

Psychoanalysis and systemic constellations are very different.[1] Constellations work fast, whereas psychoanalysis works slowly. Constellations lead the client to a kind of direct contact with the people important to him, while psychoanalysis is based on transference. Constellations are limited to a small number of general principles, and psychoanalysis is a vast set of ambiguous and sometimes contradictory concepts. There are many more differences, but there are also similarities between the two methods in terms of both understanding the causes of human problems and the ways of solving them. In different schools of psychoanalysis, we see common ideas that can be considered to be the core of this method. Much of them correspond to what we focus on in systemic constellations. The similarities I see in systemic constellations and psychoanalysis are as follows:

- working with the unconscious,
- orientation toward showing "what is,"
- importance of reconstructing the true story of life,
- restoring "good objects,"
- seeing the intergenerational connections,
- meaning attributed to gender and sexuality.

Although Sigmund Freud concentrated mainly on the world of the individual, he recognized that personality is formed in relationships, especially with the mother and father. He spoke of the Oedipus complex, that is, what emerges and remains in the human psyche as a result of the relationship between the child and his parents. Referring to this, Jacques Lacan wrote that

> man's individual behavior bears the mark of a certain number of typical psychical relations in which a certain social structure is expressed, at the very least the *constellation* within that structure that especially dominates the first years of his childhood.
>
> These fundamental psychical relations have been revealed in analytic experience and defined [. . .] with the term "complexes." (Lacan 2002, 72)

Post-Freudian psychoanalysts such as Melanie Klein and Donald Fairbairn developed a relational view of the psyche. However, they did not only mean external relationships with real people but also mean relationships with their mental representations. In this way, the term "internal object" was developed. In Klein's view, the "unconscious ego (self) lived in an inner world of internal objects with which it had various relationships" (Britton 2018, 93). This view of the psyche is close to the Hellingerian vision. We know that each of us is permanently connected to a certain system of people that affects our mood and motivation. The inner world is formed by the unconscious relationships with the mother, father, grandparents, siblings, and excluded people. The "unconscious ego" is indeed involved in these relationships, since we generally know neither about the power of their influence nor even about their existence (if we had no constellation, we would know nothing about being attached to our father's first wife or to a deceased sibling that we have never been told about).

For psychoanalysts, then, man is an aggregate of partially personified components that interact with one another—"internal objects," "complexes," "archetypes," or "mental instances," such as the ego or superego. Psychoanalyst Neville Symington writes: "An internalized mother, father, brother, sister, or whatever, these are internalized objects, and these objects act. They act within the personality. At certain points, they may even take over the personality" (Symington 1993, 20). Internal objects have such autonomy and power of influence as if they were separate persons. The precursor of such a view was Carl Gustav Jung, who even said that the archetypes have "a kind of consciousness" and "free will" (Jung 1960, 18).

So maybe they are more of real people than products of the psyche? Thanks to constellations, we can understand why. These objects remain "internal" because they affect the psyche regardless of the presence of the person they represent. The "internal mother" affects me also when I have lost contact with my real mother, and even when my mother is dead. However, they are also "external" because they are not products of my perception or memory. When they manifest themselves through a representative, they bring entirely true information about my mother, including what I could not possibly know.

DIFFERENT PERCEPTION, DIFFERENT HELPING

In *Recommendations to Physicians Practising Psycho-Analysis*, Freud states that the analyst "must turn his own unconscious like a receptive organ towards the transmitting unconscious of the patient" (Freud 2001, 115). This single sentence situates psychoanalysis in an area completely different from that of the therapies that we could define as rationalistic. If it is our unconscious that is the receptive organ, then we are far from simply perceiving and analyzing. In another article Freud writes:

> It is a very remarkable thing that the Ucs. [the unconscious] of one human being can react upon that of another, without passing through the Cs. [the consciousness]. This deserves closer investigation, especially with a view to finding out whether preconscious activity can be excluded as playing a part in it; but, descriptively speaking, the fact is incontestable. (Freud 2001a, 194)

The absence of mediation of preconscious activity would mean that people's psyches can contact one another at a very primal level. It is clear that this opens the way to all the "mysticism" of interpersonal contact and leads us far beyond the standard picture of communication. Symington wrote:

> Two inanimate objects, two stones on a beach, do not interpenetrate each other, but once we cross that great boundary between the inanimate and the animate world, the capacity for interpenetration of one living thing by another arises. (Symington 1993, 13)

Freud did not doubt the existence of telepathy, which he referred to as thought-transference (German: *Gedankenübertragung*).[2] He saw it as a primal way for organisms to communicate—replaced by language over time—which, however, continues to function in the background of our psyche. He noted that the material obtained through telepathy appears in dreams (Freud 1990, 38 et seq.). It is not possible to see it directly, and only the process of psychoanalytic interpretation of a dream brings out what telepathically reaches the dreamer.

Other early psychoanalysts, such as Wilhelm Stekel and Sándor Ferenczi, also observed the nonverbal and unconscious transmission of information. Psychiatrist and psychoanalyst Jule Eisenbud concludes:

> Stekel's main contribution was to show that "thought-transference," as telepathic phenomena were characteristically designated at that time, did not occur as the idle offshoot of a virtually accidental sensitization of the minds of the agent and percipient, but that it proceeded along the lines of strongly charged emotional relationships. The content of the materials that was conveyed and picked up, he showed, was apt to reflect the conflictful affects of love, hate, jealousy, etc., in terms of which the participants in a telepathic episode related to each other. (Bychowski and Despert 1952, 46)

Franco De Masi, psychiatrist and psychoanalyst, states that much of the works on the analytical relationship are based on the assumption of the existence of unconscious communication or even dialogue between two unconsciouses (De Masi 2018, 58). Not only does the analyst identify in this way the hidden aspects of the patient, but the patient also has a kind of access to the analyst's interior, as indicated, for instance, by Hanna Segal (Segal 1990, 85). Helena Deutsch described a patient who somehow knew that her wedding anniversary was nearing, and Michael Balit said that his patient's abilities seemed to be telepathy or clairvoyance (Brottman 2011, 37). Similarly, Eisenbud maintained that his patients had telepathic access to his repressed psychic material and that telepathic perception was a normal part of human personality (Eisenbud 1970). Almost the same view was held by the psychiatrist Jan Ehrewald, who believed that many of his schizophrenic patients expressed his own secrets about guilt, anxiety, and other states that preoccupied him (Brottman 2011, 32).

Many other psychoanalysts, such as Hanna Segal and Jean-Michel Quinodoz, also acknowledge the existence of telepathy (Quinodoz 2008, 53–54).

An analysis is a long-lasting contact with another person, and the analyst's mind is employed in a different way than in a normal conversation. Although most psychoanalysts do not use the concept of telepathy in their work, the processes they consider are not far from this phenomenon and sometimes appear to be telepathy, but with a different name. Theodor Reik spoke of "listening with the third ear," that is, listening to what the unconscious says beyond words (Reik 1948, 144–56). This was supposed to allow him to discover not only the things the patient did not say but also the things he did not know about. Karen Horney emphasizes the role of intuition in arriving at conclusions and interpretations. She speaks of thoughts coming without any conscious analysis that explain the patient's situation, of associations that metaphorically depict it, of emotions that give the analyst data about the patient, and finally, of intuitive putting together a multitude of information that could not be put together intellectually (Horney 1991, 65 et seq.).

Two important phenomena that are mentioned in psychoanalysis—countertransference and projective identification—seem to have telepathic aspects. Countertransference is the analyst's response to the patient's transference, that is, to his internal situation and unconscious messages toward the analyst. As psychoanalysts argue, countertransference can be a source of information about the patient. Initially, it was treated as a simple disturbance of the analyst's attitude toward the patient, that is, bringing one's own problems into the therapy, but later it was observed to be informative. Countertransference provided clues probably from the early days of psychoanalysis, although it was not officially recognized, as pointed out by Paula Heimann, the author of a pioneering article on the informative meaning of countertransference (Heimann 1989, 73–79). She found that the notion of resistance, so important in psychoanalysis, was born out of Freud's feeling that in trying to elicit from his female patients their repressed memories, he encountered almost physical resistance.

Projective identification is a concept developed by Klein. The patient projects elements of his own self onto the analyst in order to gain a sense of control over these parts and the analyst. Wilfred Bion, Herbert Rosenfeld, and other analysts noticed that these projections have a real impact on the psychoanalyst's sensations. They have thus become information about the patient. Segal's description of the treatment of a psychotic patient can be used as an example:

> After his sessions, I would go and have the soles of my feet massaged in order to get back in touch with actual sensations—I had the impression that I was slipping into a smooth and flat world in which there was no room for any kind of sensation. [. . .] I could then understand that the patient was conveying "something about himself" to me—a state in which he had no sensations at all. I was able to relate that to what I knew of his childhood—he had often been left all alone in his cot, which was all white, in a world in which sensations no longer existed. That was what he was communicating to me unconsciously; I was able, thanks to my counter-transference experience, to let him understand that. (Quinodoz 2008, 58)

Ronald Britton writes:

> In a consultation when a woman patient who had initially been sombre in style had on a return visit provoked in me an unexpected awareness of her sexuality, I made a private prediction that somewhere along the line an erotic transference would appear. In fact, before the session was over she told me with some embarrassment of an unambiguous sexual dream of the night before that she herself related to the transference. (Britton 2018, 46)

Willy and Madeleine Baranger say that each analyst "responds with his or her own body to the patient's unconscious communication," which they describe as "corporeal projective counteridentification" (Harris, Kalb, and Klebanoff 2017, 32).

So there are manifestations of mutual mental influence between the analyst and the patient, basically a kind of transfer of psychic content. One can say that the patient's states get out and can have a strong influence on the analyst, as was the case with Margery Kalb, who describes her sessions in the following way:

> Cumulatively and over time, the fearsome unmetabolized affect in the room became overpowering. One day, I stood up at the end of a typically nightmarish, nameless dread-filled session with Charlie—simply stood up—and felt a sudden migraine-like pain behind my eyes, followed by excruciating dizziness. I yelped involuntarily, but single-mindedly managed to get Charlie out the door. And then, I fainted. (Harris, Kalb, and Klebanoff 2017, 20)

Experiences in psychoanalysis suggest that human minds are not closed systems, but they "radiate" and "absorb" information. In this way, the communication between members of the family, known from constellations, becomes a little less amazing. The fact that the analyst absorbs some of the patient's mental states and uses feelings as a source of information is similar to representing and getting information from the knowing field in constellations when the therapist, without words, finds out about the client's inner problems and relationships.

In this purely internal sphere, processes of fundamental importance to therapy may take place. This is illustrated by the example given by Symington. He treated a female patient who had had two partners suffering from impotence and her new boyfriend also lost his potency. When working with this patient, Symington noticed that whenever he was about to give her an interpretation, he forgot what he meant:

> I then made the connection between her boyfriend's impotence and what was happening in my mind, and I felt fairly certain that there was a connection between the two. I saw it then as my task, the next time something began to crystalize, to be able to maintain it mentally and give expression to it to her. Later on in that session something did become clear, and I concentrated all my psychic attention on it and made an interpretation. I put it into words, and there was silence. I sensed that what I had said had been received by her.
>
> She came back the following week with a smile on her face and said to me, "A funny thing happened when I got home. Michael came round, and we made love, and he was able to penetrate me. There was no problem. I have a feeling

that it had something to do with the session you and I had." I have no doubt that through my own psychic attention to what was happening, the interpretation I made, and the interaction between the two of us, a change occurred in her, which affected her boyfriend's capacity to make love to her.

She did not know what the change was, but her psychic activity altered, and that changed her circumstances. Psychic choices and actions affect people in the environment, especially those in the intimate environment. (Symington 1993, 14–15)

There is no doubt that the described processes—the cognitive and healing one—have nothing to do with conventional methods. Instead, they resemble the effects we experience in systemic constellations. The psychoanalyst read the patient's internal world, then, provided an impulse for internal change through interpretation, and finally concluded that this purely psychic change had a corrective effect on another person, emotionally connected with the patient.

TRANSGENERATIONAL PROCESSES AND SPIRITS OF ANCESTORS

In his work *Totem and Taboo*—in which he reflects on the beginnings of religion, morality, and society—Freud wrote:

> We base everything upon the assumption of a psyche of the mass in which psychic processes occur as in the psychic life of the individual. Moreover, we let the sense of guilt for a deed survive for thousands of years, remaining effective in generations which could not have known anything of this deed. [. . .] no generation is capable of concealing its more important psychic processes from the next. For psychoanalysis has taught us that in his unconscious psychic activity every person possesses an apparatus which enables him to interpret the reactions of others, that is to say, to straighten out the distortions which the other person has affected in the expression of his feelings. (Freud 1946, 203–204)

In constellations, we do not observe the sense of guilt that lasts for thousands of years (which does not mean that such a process does not exist), but Freud's general opinion is confirmed—psychological influences are transmitted from one generation to the next. This happens unconsciously and involves a specific process, which is the ability of children to read their parents' internal states.

Psychoanalysts have observed that in patients' psychopathology the psychic material that has been taken over from ancestors plays a role. The discoveries of Nicolas Abraham and Maria Torok deserve special mention. Nicholas T. Rand writes about Abraham's concepts in this way:

> The concept of the phantom moves the focus of psychoanalytic inquiry beyond the individual being analyzed because it postulates that some people unwittingly inherit the secret psychic substance of their ancestors' lives. The "phantom" represents a radical reorientation of Freudian and post-Freudian theories of psychopathology, since here symptoms do not spring from the individual's own life experiences but from someone else's psychic conflicts, traumas, or secrets. [. . .] Abraham's theory of the phantom enlarges upon Freud's metapsychology by suggesting that the unsettling disruptions in the psychic life of one person can adversely and unconsciously affect someone else. [. . .] The concept of the phantom redraws the boundaries of psychopathology and extends the realm of possibilities for its cure by suggesting the existence within an individual of a collective psychology comprised of several generations, so that the analyst must listen for the voices of one generation in the unconscious of another. (Abraham and Torok 1994, 166)

Although the phenomenon of the phantom manifests itself in the psyche of one person, it "eventually leads to the psychoanalysis *in absentia* of several generations (parents, grandparents, uncles, et al.) through the symptoms of the descendant" (Abraham and Torok 1994, 168). According to Rand, the concept of the phantom is the basis for the assertion that the transmission of secret family history acts like the "hidden motivating force," it also makes it possible to understand how the "falsification, ignorance, or disregard of the past," institutionalized or practiced by parents and grandparents, "is the breeding ground of the phantomatic return of shameful secrets on the level of individuals, families, the community, and possibly even entire nations" (Abraham and Torok 1994, 169). This is, of course, an independent discovery of what we know so well from constellations—the disregard of the past, secrets, and exclusions that follow them have great power, affecting the demeanor of the descendants.

Psychoanalysts have observed the process of identification with the ancestors and assuming their qualities. This phenomenon is part of the foundation of family constellations. French psychoanalyst Alberto Eiguer stated that adolescents, for unclear reasons, take on the characteristics of their ancestors and become like them without even knowing them (Walewska 2007, 108).[3]

It is not easy to understand unconscious identifications within the family without knowing about the existence of the information field; so there is puzzlement and reference to unclear causes of these identifications.

Lacanian psychoanalysts also recognize transgenerational processes. In reference to the case of the Rat Man described by Freud, Lacan wrote:

> The original constellation that presided over the birth of the subject, over his destiny, and I would almost say his prehistory, specifically the fundamental family relationships which structured his parents' union, happens to have a very precise relation, perhaps definable by a transformational formula, with what appears to be the most contingent, the most phantasmatic, the most paradoxically morbid in his case. (Lacan 1979, 410)

Lacan states that there is a structure of family relationships that the child encounters when he is born. This structure, completely independent of the subject, turns out to be the factor that shapes the most individual and seemingly random elements of his neurosis. The difference between Lacan's vision and family constellations is that Lacan recognizes only one medium of transgenerational transmission—speech. He states that the constellation is shaped "by a narration of a certain number of traits which characterize the parents' union" (Lacan 1979, 410). He notes, however, that transgenerational succession exists and, moreover, is governed by certain laws:

> Everything happens as if the impasses inherent in the original situation [related to the patient's father] moved to another point in the mythic network, as if what was not resolved here always turned up over there. (Lacan 1979, 414)

In the context of intergenerational relationships, some psychoanalysts—for example, Abraham and Torok—speak of "revenants," "ghosts," "phantoms," "hauntings," and even "demons" and "vampires," whose influence on the patient is manifested during a psychoanalysis. They do not understand the term "spirit" literally, but I get the impression that they do not use it merely metaphorically either. The fact is that terms such as "internal objects," "dissociation," and "repression" are insufficient for them to describe what they observe. A group of American psychoanalysts state in their publication that they use the term "ghost" to "capture the sense of objects that are neither internal nor external solely, that may disturb the atmosphere, the soma, the mind, temporality, and the surrounding fields" (Harris, Kalb, and Klebanoff 2016, 1). This kind of reality is known to constellators—it is a systemic reality that is closely connected to the mind of the individual, but irreducible to it.

Psychoanalyst Hans W. Loewald states that in the psychoanalytic process

> the old ghosts may reawaken to life. Those who know ghosts tell us that they long to be released from their ghost-life and led to rest as ancestors. As ancestors

> they live forth in the present generation, while as ghosts they are compelled to haunt the present generation with their shadow-life. Transference is pathological in so far as the unconscious is a crowd of ghosts, and this is the beginning of the transference neurosis in analysis: ghosts of the unconscious, imprisoned by defences but haunting the patient in the dark of his defences and symptoms, are allowed to taste blood, are let loose. In the daylight of analysis the ghosts of the unconscious are laid and led to rest as ancestors whose power is taken over and transformed into the newer intensity of present life. (Loewald 1960, 29)

What we can easily understand from this text is that when ghosts are transformed into ancestors, we obtain their power and greater ability to cope with our lives. This process takes place during a constellation, when we face someone who until now was represented in our life only by a physical symptom, anxiety, or unclear emotions. This is also how psychoanalysts see ghosts—as something that is undefined, of unspecified origin, yet troublesome and constantly accompanying us. But when, through a constellation, the mystery is resolved and we deal not with a ghost, but with a person from the past, then the "spell breaks" and we gain strength. Rand writes:

> One could say metaphorically that Abraham calls for a psychoanalytic cult of ancestors and a psychoanalytic form of honoring the dead with rightful burial. But in the psychoanalytic realm, laying the dead to rest and cultivating our ancestors implies uncovering their shameful secrets, understanding their nameless and undisclosed suffering. We should engage in this unveiling and understanding of the former existence of the dead not because we may want to appease them or prevent them from perpetrating their nocturnal pranks, but because, unsuspected, the dead continue to lead a devastating psychic half-life in us. (Abraham and Torok 1994, 167)

The dead lead a "half-life" in us. We intuitively feel that the deceased are more than just a state of our memory, and psychoanalysts, during their sessions, feel it also more directly. Susan Klebanoff describes a meeting with one of her female patients:

> It was as if I had offered her deceased mother a seat at the table. I told her we could speak of both her mother's life and her death and promised I would be there to help hold her overwhelming affects for as long as she needed.
>
> This invitation had a calming effect on Sophie and the treatment and allowed us symbolically to hold her mother's ghost together in a shared experience [. . .]. At times, these early sessions had the feeling of a séance. There could have been a sign on the door: ghosts welcome here. Because, for Sophie, this

> haunting was the opposite of unwanted; her ghost world was familiar, a source of identity and continuity, a place of comfort. (Harris, Kalb, and Klebanoff 2016, 22)

Many psychoanalysts say that in the family system, certain persons have an impact through their absence, being forgotten and kept secret. This may be the mother's former lover, the biological father, the deceased siblings (Walewska 2007, 114). These "present absences" "can be emotionally, viscerally, or even unconsciously felt in the patient, in the analyst, and in their interaction" (Harris, Kalb, and Klebanoff 2016, 2).

Some psychoanalysts argue that the sexual identity of girls is shaped differently from that of boys, because girls tend to build a generational identity, which means that a little girl places herself between her mother and her future child (Welldon 2018, 45). This corresponds to my reflection on the generational sequence of women and the specificity of the female transgenerational transmission. Women focus more than men on certain biological aspects of life, on cycles, sexual organs, and time pressure. The factors related to giving birth and caring for a newborn, almost unchanged for millennia, play a role in their lives. Psychiatrist Estela V. Welldon states that

> from the moment a baby girl is born, her mother sees a miniature version of herself, a woman, as she mothers her daughter. [. . .] problems arise from the reenactment of motherhood. The mother's attitude towards the development of her little girl is influenced by how she feels towards her own mother, the body her mother provided her with, and the way she felt accepted or rejected by her mother as a child in her own gender. Thus, the birth of a girl might evoke in the mother the same response her own birth created in her own mother. (Welldon 2018, 52–53)

She continues:

> A woman's conflicts about her own gender can result in perverse or perverting attitudes which may well be traceable across at least three generations. (Welldon 2018, 53)

Psychoanalysts observe that a woman who becomes a mother activates her attitude toward her mother and the memories of her childhood relationship with her. In constellations, I observe the same phenomenon, and even the correlation between the mother-newborn relationship and the relationship the mother had as a newborn with her own mother.

According to psychoanalysts, the multigenerational transmission of problems is caused by the phenomenon of receiving of psychic material (emotions and content) by children from their parents. Although the exact mechanisms remain unknown, the transmission undoubtedly takes place outside the conventional channels. Psychoanalysts relate it to projection or projective identification as a result of which the child becomes a "reservoir" for the unbearable emotions and memories of his parents. He begins to feel and behave as if his parents' experiences were his own. Autism researcher June Felton referred to the unconscious processes between mothers and their autistic children as "osmotic pressure," concluding that in such a woman's mind there were areas "which she was intensely disturbed and embarrassed about, and which she had made brave efforts to exclude from consciousness. But it appears that the pregnancy activates these hidden processes which were never supposed to be known but which nevertheless in a mysterious way seemed to have seeped into the child" (Rosenfeld 1990, 276). Psychoanalyst Piera Aulagnier states that what the parent has failed to repress returns as a delusion in the child's psychosis (Green and Kohon 2005, 71). The child is a sensitive receiver of the parents' internal world, as we know from constellations. His soul goes where his parents go. The child unconsciously looks at what they look at.

It seems that most of these processes result in some kind of identification. This is what Freud writes about this psychic mechanism:

> The basis of the process is what is called an "identification"—that is to say, the assimilation of one ego to another one, as a result of which the first ego behaves like the second in certain respects, imitates it and in a sense takes it up into itself. [. . .] It is a very important form of attachment to someone else, probably the very first, and not the same thing as the choice of an object. (Freud 1990, 78–79)

Freud refers here to the same characteristics of identification that we observe in entanglement, which, according to Hellinger, "means that someone in the family unconsciously takes on the fate of an earlier person and lives it again" (Hellinger and Hövel 2007, 15). In constellations, we see how, in different ways, the ego of one person imitates the ego of another, in a way taking it into itself. Freud says that identification is "the earliest expression of an emotional tie with another person" (Freud 1975, 37). This is confirmed by constellations, as entanglement appears to be a truly archaic process. It can be so strong that the entangled person in a way abandons himself in order to become someone completely other, usually someone who had a difficult lot and is not alive. This is a manifestation of an extreme bond that goes beyond even the strongest relationship with a living person. The same was observed by French psychoanalyst

Alain de Mijolla, who stated that "ghosts" can manifest themselves in such a way that those they haunt begin to live as if they became strangers to themselves. This can cause giving up one's own identity, "being condemned to live and sometimes die in the name of someone else" (Mijolla 2003, 17, 33).

Psychoanalysts noticed that the children of Jews who survived the Holocaust, identifying with their grandparents, try to substitute for the lost parents of their own parents, as they seek to stop their suffering (Coles 2011, chap. 4). Also, this interpretation is consistent with the systemic dynamics in which we observe that children try to take on themselves the suffering of their parents and become their saviors (although identification with grandparents is probably motivated also by another process, as they are usually excluded to some extent because of a burden of trauma). According to Hellinger, this kind of magical thinking can determine psychopathological problems—someone trusts that through his own suffering he will save his parent from death, someone else believes that he can take over his guilt or die in his place.[4]

Also observations of psychosis indicate points of convergence with the perspective provided by constellations. De Masi argues that "the psychotic experience frequently includes an identification with destructive figures or objects" (De Masi 2018, 277), which in part confirms Hellinger's observation that the underlying cause of psychoses issome past murder in the family and identification with the killer.[5]

BOND, LOVE, AND FORMATION OF DISORDERS

Love-Bond

Psychoanalysts pay much attention to negative emotions such as aggression, envy, and guilt. However, they do not neglect the issues of love and bond that they associate with the concept of libido. Klein considers love to be a fundamental emotion:

> One of the great problems about criminals, which has always made them incomprehensible to the rest of the world, is their lack of natural human good feelings; but this lack is only apparent. When in analysis one reaches the deepest conflicts from which hate and anxiety spring, one also finds there the love as well. Love is not absent in the criminal, but it is hidden and buried in such a way that nothing but analysis can bring it to light [. . .]. Hate is often used as the most effective cover for love. (Klein 1975, 260)

According to Klein, those who hate—like criminals—actually persecute the object that was originally loved by them and is now perceived as threatening. Here we have a parallel to Hellinger's concept of primary and secondary feelings—hateful behaviors can in fact be motivated by frustrated love. Klein also sees that the child's love is not merely a "selfish" response to care, but contains a genuine urge to make sacrifices:

> Even in the small child one can observe a concern for the loved one which is not, as one might think, merely a sign of dependence upon a friendly and helpful person. Side by side with the destructive impulses in the unconscious mind both of the child and of the adult, there exists a profound urge to make sacrifices, in order to help and to put right loved people who in phantasy have been harmed or destroyed. In the depths of the mind, the urge to make people happy is linked up with a strong feeling of responsibility and concern for them, which manifests itself in genuine sympathy with other people and in the ability to understand them, as they are and as they feel. (Klein 1975, 311)

Donald Winnicott describes the development of a "false self" in a child to support the depressed mother, which corresponds with the fundamental observation of Hellinger and other constellation therapists of the power of the child's love that transcends concern for oneself (Trowell and Etchegoyen 2002, 29). Essentially the same processes, albeit in a completely different form, are articulated by Lacan, according to whom the child "offers himself or offers his body as a symptom for what is symptomatic in the family structure" (Lacadée 2019, 64). The psychopathological symptom in the child appears as a response to what is problematic in the family and represents the truth of the parental couple. Thus, by virtue of the existence of the bond, the child unconsciously devotes himself to the affairs of the family.

The emergence of the symptom enables something related to the family structure that cannot normally be said or articulated to be brought to light (Lacadée 2019, 67). In addressing this issue, Lacan uses the category of the lack of symbolic representation, but this—as he puts it—"hole in knowledge" does not necessarily result from the structural impossibility of articulation. It may result from, as we well know from constellations, family secrets. This content is hidden because of its traumatic nature or because of the ancestor's inability to confront it but it is generally possible to articulate it to a degree sufficient for the "hole in knowledge" to be filled.

Often the child offers himself primarily to the mother—then his symptom depends on the mother's subjectivity and, as Lacan puts it, manifests the truth of her phantasm (Lacadée 2019, 70). In an extreme case, such a child will become psychotic. Interestingly, when the child—as we could put it—takes upon himself what is his mother's affair, then, according to Lacan, he "alienates in himself all possible access by the mother to her own truth" (Lacan 2018,

14). It seems that this is what we observe during family constellations when the child (client) gives back to the mother what is hers, her responsibility, and the mother's representative gains a sense of strength and dignity. It is as if the mother gains access to the truth about herself and thus her own strength.

John Bowlby, in psychoanalysis, and Harry F. Harlow, in ethology, formulated concepts of child-mother attachment as a primary and unlearned reaction. The observations and conclusions of these authors show that attachment is independent of, and even stronger than, the sexual drive and hunger. Bowlby stated that an infant develops certain "mental models" of the world around him and of himself from the first months of life. He found these "models" to be fairly accurate reflections of interactions with the mother, containing far fewer phantasms than many analysts claimed. They affect the individual even in adulthood, when the conditions of his life are radically changed. They can impose upon him forms of behavior that are sharply contrary to his own interests (Zazzo 1978, 227). Thus Bolwby emphasizes the meaning of the bond. For the child is so strongly attached to the parent that he transcends his fear of death and his need for self-preservation.

The Interrupted Movement toward the Mother

The works of Donald Fairbairn and Donald Winnicott address the question of the child withdrawing into his inner world as a consequence of the mother's unavailability, which resembles a disorder referred to in constellations as the interrupted movement toward the mother. Winnicott quotes his female patient:

> I was about two. The family was on the beach. I wandered away from mother and began to make discoveries. I found seashells. One seashell led me on to another and there was an unlimited number. Suddenly I became frightened and I can see now that what had happened was that I had become interested in discovering the world and had forgotten mother. This carried with it, as I see now, the idea that mother had forgotten me. I therefore turned round and rushed back to mother, perhaps only a few yards. Mother took me up and a process started up of re-establishment of my relationship with her. I probably seemed uninterested in her because of this fact that time is required for me to feel re-established and to lose the sense of panic. Then suddenly mother put me down. (Winnicott 1986, 135–36)

Based on the work done during her analysis, the patient could add:

> Now I know what happened. I have been waiting all my life till now to be able to reach the next stage because if mother had not put me down I would have thrown my arms round her neck and have burst into a flood of tears, tears of

> joy and happiness. As it was, I never found my mother again. (Winnicott 1986, 136)

According to Winnicott, who emphasized the subject's relative passivity toward the caring environment, this woman could only realize her problem and take a more distanced position toward it. In systemic constellations, the patient would be able to move on to the next stage and restore the broken bond with her mother (I leave aside the fact that the bond was almost definitely not broken during the situation on the beach described above—it is just a "screen-memory" with another, really important incident behind it).

Constellations shift the emphasis to the child's internal activity—ultimately it is the child who, although influenced by external experiences, turns away from his mother. In psychoanalysis, Symington proposed a very similar approach. Reflecting on the causes of narcissism, he introduced the concept of the "lifegiver"—an internal object, related to the mother figure, but somehow beyond her. The existence of such an object results from the fact that in order to survive—biologically and emotionally—we all have to turn to the outside of ourselves, to others. Symington stresses that at the root of narcissism lies the intentional act that can already be done by an infant—turning away from the lifegiver, which happens as a consequence of a trauma experienced in the relationship with the mother:

> If one accepts the idea of the *lifegiver* being the source of emotional life and also the source of biological survival—that the two are linked—then the self can never effect a total repudiation, and so a split takes place, with one part of the self turning against the *lifegiver*. As the *lifegiver* is incorporated into the self, a division and a repudiation of the self's own nature occurs, resulting in an anti-relational position being taken. It is somewhat like a prisoner saying, "I am going to have nothing to do with these prison warders," but having to have something to do with them in order to receive meals and so on, or he will die. (Symington 1993, 39)

This is a description of the interruption of the movement toward the mother, in which the author highlights the internal activity of the subject, intentionally turning away from the mother. This results in turning away from relationality, the disappearance of creativity, and waiting for the environment to act, to define, and to change our situation. I could add that the situation is often that on the surface level, the individual proves to himself that he does not need anything and that he can provide everything for himself, and on the deep level, his own activity is completely blocked, and he expects, in resentment, that it is the world (mother) that will come to him.

In constellations, we are aware that accepting the parents is not limited to them—through the parents life and vital energy comes to us, and in this sense they are its donors. Interruption of the primal movement of love and depression are closely related. Freud compared depression (melancholy) to the process of mourning (Freud 1957, 124–40). He stated that, just like in mourning, melancholy involves the loss of a person, although in the latter case the person is unaware that he has lost someone. So the feeling of loss is the essence of depression and we can assume that it often refers to the mother. Interestingly, this sense of loss may be conscious, although its source remains unknown. William Styron, a writer suffering from depression, noted:

> At a later date I would gradually be persuaded that devastating loss in childhood as a probable genesis of my own disorder; meanwhile, as I monitored my retrograde condition, I felt loss at every hand. (Styron 1992, 56)

The further mechanism, according to Freud, is that the ego becomes identified with the lost object of love. In this way, the accusations and grievances against the lost person are directed toward one's own ego. This builds a picture of depression with an accompanying low self-esteem, moral inferiority, apathy, and dark thoughts about the future. Styron writes:

> The loss of self-esteem is a celebrated symptom, and my own sense of self had all but disappeared, along with any self-reliance. This loss can quickly degenerate into dependence, and from dependence into infantile dread. One dreads the loss of all things, all people close and dear. (Styron 1992, 56)

Alexander Lowen wrote that a child who was prematurely separated from his mother has the inclination "to get back to the mother in order to complete the aborted maturation process" and "all his available energy is invested in this attempt" (Lowen 1993, 57). He is also prone to depression. In constellations, we initiate this halted internal movement, allow the client to connect with his mother, and in this way complete the maturation process and overcome his depression.

Psychoanalyst André Green coined the concept of the "dead mother" complex (Kohon 1999). It refers to the situation of an early emotional absence of the mother, where this absence remains unrecognized—the child consciously knows nothing about it and cannot name it. This condition may be due to the mother's involvement in an affair or to her mourning for someone close to her, such as a miscarried child. In such cases, the patient suffers from a kind of hidden depression that does not appear in his narration, but manifests itself as a psychic void, a kind of lifelessness of a certain area in the self. In constellations, this kind of process is associated with the interrupted movement toward the mother. The thesis that we speak of the same phenomenon is additionally supported by the fact that the dead mother complex can entail problems with giving and taking, namely an inability to take "without the immediate need to settle accounts so as not to feel guilty" (Walewska 2007, 142). And, as we know from constellations, such problems are often due to a disturbed relationship with the mother.

The internal "dead mother" may also result from the actual death of the mother. Constellations show that a small child is incapable of mourning and accepting the mother into his heart, as her death is an event impossible for him to assimilate. The child turns away from the memory of the mother, but harbors a suppressed grudge and anger against her.

In adulthood, an incapacity to accept the mother into the heart may occur if she is associated with the dead body, for example, if the child accompanied her dying in some way. Only by acknowledging the mother's "spiritual" existence and seeing something more than her dead body—which can happen during systemic constellations or psychoanalysis—is a step toward renewing the internal relationship with her. Quinodoz, referring to Segal's views, writes:

> For as long as the dead person is felt concretely to be a dead body, normal mourning is not possible. "It is only if the dead person is symbolically represented in the mind that the symbolic internal reparation can be done." (Quinodoz 2008, 71)

Hellinger says that we look for our mother also in our partner. This corresponds to the conclusions of some psychoanalysts. For example, Otto Fenichel said that

> superficially, no sexual attachment is completely attractive because the partner is never the mother; in a deeper layer, every sexual attachment has to be inhibited because every person represents the mother. (Lowen 2003, 33)[6]

But does the individual have to be sexually blocked by this? If, as in constellations, he accepts the mother as a mother, then he has a chance to detach everything else, and leave the mother's sexuality with the mother, and take his own sexuality. Then he no longer has to look for his mother in his partner, because he has her in his heart. The fact remains, however, that this is usually a long process.

Father, Mother, and Their Child

Family constellations make us realize again and again that every child has both a mother and a father. The child's movement toward the mother triggers the need to move toward the father, and vice versa, moving toward the father opens up the possibility to move toward the mother. In other words, loving the father makes mature love for the mother possible. All of this translates into both how the individual feels and how he functions in the world. Psychoanalysts Mary Target and Peter Fonagy observed something similar. Namely, that the existence of the child's relationship with the other parent helps the child to have a constructive relationship with the first parent. They write that

> in benign circumstances, mother and father both become established as object representations within the child's mind, independent and separate from the child's self-representation. In pathological cases, one or other of the primary objects may not be represented sufficiently separately and may become part of the child's self-representation, which is inevitably distorted. (Target and Fonagy 2002, 59)

In other words, thanks to the relationship with the mother, the child can, so to say, "face" the father, and thanks to the relationship with the father, the child can "face" the mother. The latter is of particular significance, since symbiosis threatens the child in the relationship with the mother rather than with the father. The child who, because of the lack of a relationship with the father, has introjected "the mother's image into the self" cannot have an undisturbed relationship with her (Target and Fonagy 2002, 60). It is not so much that such a child "loves the mother" as that he "becomes the mother." So the authors describe, albeit in a somewhat convoluted way, the processes that we constantly observe in constellations—those who are overly attached to their mothers, who have not turned to their fathers, despite their apparent attachment to the mothers, are unable to truly love them.

Segal remembered that psychoanalyst John Rickman reiterated that if the patient keeps talking about just one parent or has a transference of just one parent, the analyst should always ask himself: "Where is the other parent?" (Quinodoz 2012, 18). The importance of having both parents has been recognized by many psychoanalysts, and Britton states directly:

> For psychic balance, we need two internal parents: whatever the case for single parenthood in the outside world, I believe that there is no case for it in the internal world. (Britton 2018, 70)

Today, the figure and role of the father is often forgotten, as if it were difficult to perceive or define. Freud stated that the very concept of reality is inseparably related to the father figure. One of the factors determining psychoses is, according to psychoanalysis, the absence of the paternal function. Lacanian psychoanalyst Bruce Fink writes about it in this way:

> The father who embodies the paternal function in a nuclear family generally comes between mother and child, stopping the child from being drawn altogether to or into the mother and stopping the mother from engulfing her child. Lacan does not claim that *all* mothers have a tendency to smother or devour their children (though some do); rather, he says that children "perceive" their mother's desire as dangerous or threatening. [. . .] the father keeps the child at a certain distance from its mother, thwarting the child's attempt to become one or remain forever one with the mother, or forbidding the mother from achieving certain satisfactions with her child [. . .]. The father protects the child from the mother as desire (as desiring or as desired), setting himself up as the one who prohibits, forbids, thwarts, and protects. (Fink 1997, 80)

The picture of the mother and father that psychoanalysis draws here is fully in line with what constellation therapists argue. The power of mothers is enormous and the father is necessary to balance it; to show the child that the mother is only human, that she is not omnipotent and unerring. Without this guidance from the father, many children cannot realistically look at their mothers. Therefore, they cannot fully accept them—their mothers are too terrifying for them with their power over life and death. Loewald argued that a boy needs an "exquisitely masculine" identification with his father that gives him support against "the danger of the womb" of the mother (Target and Fonagy 2002, 49).

Psychotic persons are often attached to the mother in a deeply symbiotic and destructive way; the father is in some way dwarfed and does not give protection. Another Lacanian psychoanalyst, Moustafa Safouan, writes on this subject, stating that in the mother-child relationship everything

> depends upon the degree to which the mother herself succeeded in integrating the symbolic order, that is, the degree to which she herself has a certain respect, not so much for the person of the father as to the name of the father inasmuch as it signifies the prohibition of a perverse relation with her child. [. . .] So if a child finds herself in front of this entire *toute puissance* [omnipotence], in front of some creature who can do anything she likes without any limit to what she can or can't do, this will have the most devastating effect. (Safouan 2004, 39)

Safouan refers here to the situation where the mother, in the relationship with the child, excludes the father. The pathogenic impact of this situation is undisputable, as confirmed by the observations of constellation therapists. Safouan points out that it is important for the child's destiny that the mother has respect for the "name of the father." There is a considerable correspondence here to the theory and practice of systemic constellations. It is part of the orders of love that the mother respects the father of the child, and in doing so respects the part of the child himself that is related to the father. The mother does not have to respect the father as a person, but the "name of the father." After all, it may be that the father is an alcoholic or a member of the mafia who is difficult to respect, but this does not change the orders of love. The point is that the mother should respect the very "fatherhood of the father," for instance, through the ability to feel grateful that it is thanks to him that the child she loves exists. If she does not respect the father and rejects him, then she truly binds the child to herself and commands him to tolerate all her caprices and perversions (these are not necessarily strictly sexual, the point is that the mother does not take into account the fate and "what is," organizing the child's life according to her own ideas).

Constellations attest to the existence of feelings and processes related to the Oedipus complex, although they do not, as psychoanalysis does, attest to its fundamental role in the development of the psyche (Janus 2021, 121 et seq.). One can see, among other things, that while having both parents is an imperative of the child's soul, it may be difficult for the child to recognize the parents as a couple, especially when, for various reasons, one of the parents was absent in his mind. Britton writes that "the oedipal encounter [. . .] involves recognition of the difference between the relationship between the parents as distinct from the relationship between parent and child: the parents' relationship is genital and procreative; the parent-child relationship is not. This recognition produces a sense of loss and envy, which, if not tolerated, may become a sense of grievance and self denigration" (Britton 1989, 84–85). However, when the child establishes this couple in himself, when he accepts the couple—to which we lead the client in a constellation—he becomes internally strengthened and gains better orientation in life. For, as Britton says, "the acknowledgement by the child of the parental relationship with each other unites his psychic world, limiting it to one world shared with his two parents in which different object relationships can exist" (Britton 1989, 86).

A person who has never seen his parents together or pushed such an image out of his consciousness can regain the right view of them during a constellation. This sometimes evokes resistance in the beginning—if someone shaped his personality based on the idea that "the parents are strangers to each other," "they've never had anything in common" and the like, he feels threatened when confronted with the reality of his parents' relationship. In the end, however, he regains them, which also means having each parent "equally." If, for example, the child witnessed his mother's perpetual complaining about his father, he can now see that on the soul level they understand each other perfectly. Their union is no coincidence. This gives space for one's own development, and it allows one to detach oneself from the mother, who until now has been the center of the child's universe.

The Meaning of Siblings

The meaning of the internal representations of brothers and sisters for the psychological life of an individual is rather underestimated by psychoanalysts; only some see the role of siblings in the formation of psychopathological problems as well as in the process of freeing oneself from these problems. Vamik D. Volkan and Gabriele Ast write about it:

> Our own clinical experiences and our work with those we have supervised has shown us that analyzing internalized childhood sibling experiences often provides a key to patients' symptoms or personality organizations. (Volkan and Ast 2018, 157)

One must also consider deceased siblings, the memory of whom is consciously or unconsciously transmitted to the child by the parents. Françoise Dolto, a French psychoanalyst, answering the question of what to say to the eight-month-old child about the death of his older brother whom he has not known, says:

> First of all, the child who is present in their hearts, who was loved, should still have his place there, and it will be good if the family and friends still talk about him when the little one is around. Second, whenever he is mentioned—and one can start when the little one is eight months old, although the parents could have done so even earlier—he should be told, "We are talking about your older brother, whom you do not know." Please note the word "older brother." For there is nothing more harmful to children whose older brother died as a baby than to tell them about their "little brother." The mother tends to say, "My dead little baby"; and I think the opposite, one should say, "Your older brother," "You are the second one." It is important for the child to always hear that he is second to his brother, and that he is the joy of his parents, because luckily, fate has allowed him to exceed the age that is still the reference point for the parents when they think of the oldest one. (Dolto 2002, 203)

In the above statement, Dolto points to the importance of preserving the bond with the deceased, to talking about him and remembering him. She also advises the parents to keep the hierarchy among siblings. This is nothing but the orders of love.

Otto Rank observed the identification with the deceased siblings that leads to neurotic problems:

> The marked impressions, which the premature death of a brother or sister leaves in the Unconscious of the survivors, who later often become neurotic, clearly show the strange aftereffects of this identification with the dead. This not

> seldom expresses itself in the fact that the person in question spends his life, as it were, in perpetual mourning, that is, in a state which is adapted in a bewildering way to the dead person's supposed place of abode. Many neuroses, taken as a whole, can be understood as such an embryonal continuance of the prematurely cut-off existence of a brother or sister. (Rank 2014, 25–26)[7]

Psychoanalysts stress the role of rivalry and envy in sibling relationships, especially in the early years of life. In constellations, we can sometimes see how envy and grudge against siblings stand in the way of accepting one's lives with gratitude and thanking the parents. But we see something else too. When the older siblings have murderous feelings and fantasies about eliminating ("disappearing") their younger rival, this younger brother or sister starts to want to die. For the love for his or her older siblings, he or she wants to die to make room for them. At an older age, these people have suicidal fantasies or talk about their imminent death.

HEALING PROCESSES IN PSYCHOANALYSIS AND FAMILY CONSTELLATIONS

In a psychoanalysis, the goal is to make the patient more self-aware, which is undoubtedly also a result of a family constellation. Some schools of psychoanalysis aim to provide a corrective experience, and other schools see the healing effect rather—as Carlo Strenger says—in taking responsibility for what kind of person one turns out to really be. In psychoanalysis, the two approaches compete with each other to some extent. It is different in systemic constellations. The client can, for example, experience the period just after his birth, when due to his mother's immaturity, he experienced a lack of care from her. This process goes from the clear feeling and realization of this experience to the reconstruction of the relationship with the mother. So it takes the form of a "repeated" birth, which we can consider to be a kind of corrective experience. At the same time, however, in the same process, the client agrees to this mother, to these parents, and to the life he has received from them, and thus, ultimately, to everything as it is. As can be seen, constellations combine the processes that seem contradictory, namely, the acceptance of the existing context of one's own life with a radical change in this regard, which looks even like a "change of the past."

Arguably, it is Klein's view that is closest to how constellations understand the importance of the bond with parents and the child's own role in establishing it. Klein saw children's inherent love for their parents, perhaps mainly for the mother, but also that the child creates images of them in which "in every case" they are "of an unreal and terrifying character" (Klein 1975, 251).

The task of the child, but also of the patient in his analysis, is to make "reparation" of the internal images of the parents so that they become less persecutory or indifferent and more supportive. Since they are always to some extent unrealistic and colored by the child's aggressive projections, understanding this enables the patient to build inside himself a better relationship with better parents.

Klein states that patients "are enabled to revise their relation to their parents—whether they be dead or alive—and to rehabilitate them to some extent even if they have grounds for actual grievances. This greater tolerance makes it possible for them to set up 'good' parent-figures more securely in their minds, alongside the 'bad' internal objects" (Klein 1975, 369). The existence of these "good" internal parents is one of the basic conditions for successful functioning and coping with reality, which is completely in line with what constellations say about this issue. Segal states that a part of reparation is "learning to give up omnipotent control" of the object and "accept it as it really is" (Segal 2018, 93). In constellations, we refer to this as "accepting the mother as a mother" or "the father as a father," as they are, without trying to force a change on them.

Accepting parents makes autonomy possible, as Klein knew well when she wrote that only if one has been able "gradually to detach oneself from as well as remain attached to the parents, is one capable of transferring these wishes to other people, who then stand for desired objects of the past" (Klein 1975, 317).

Accepting one's parents leads to the capacity for gratitude that Klein emphasized so much. She gives the example of a little girl who said that she "loved her mother most of all people, because what would she have done if her mother had not given birth to her and had not fed her?" At the same time, she notes that this "strong feeling of gratitude was linked with her capacity for enjoyment and showed itself in her character and relations to other people, particularly in generosity and consideration" (Klein 1977, 254). The spontaneous attitude of the aforementioned girl is something we lead clients to during constellations—a fundamental gratitude, a gratitude for life that changes one's mood, that heals, and that improves one's relationships with others.

In a common-sense perspective, it is possible to accept parents when we can "forget" the hurting situations or "forgive" them. It turns out, however, that the opposite process is possible and effective—accepting parents gives us a chance to go beyond the tormenting memories or narrations. This is like the process of psychoanalysis in the Lacanian approach, which is a way of distancing oneself from the "signifiers," that is, words that in a way automatically affect our lives. As children we were, as analysts put it, struck by certain "signifiers" and shaped by them, which made each of us adopt a unique relation to language and reality. However, to become more free, also from neurotic symptoms, we need to distance ourselves from these words. Constellations show that the act of accepting a person increases our ability to forget the negative stories associated with that person. In this way, we detach ourselves from the mass of words that previously determined the shape of our lives.

The analyst becomes a recollection and embodiment of objects from the patient's past, which we define as transference. It is for this reason that most analysts focus on observing their relationship with the patient and his reaction to them. But will the analytical relationship "reflect" all the patient's important relationships that have left their mark on him? Some analysts point out that in therapy there is a need to directly refer to concrete persons and related events. This corresponds with the concept of reconstruction ("construction in analysis") introduced by Freud. Constructions are hypotheses about childhood, early conflicts, and even family relations. Eric Brenman writes:

> It can be argued that if the past is relived in the transference and the patient enabled to face the truth in his current life, he is equipped with an object (the introjected analyst) which strengthens his ego. Although I believe this to be essential, I do not believe it to be sufficient. To face guilt and make reparation to past objects, to mourn what is lost and irreparable, to come to terms with the limitations of past objects [. . .] is important to work and requires reconstructions. Also, of course, the recapturing of good aspects of past objects and the past self is invaluable in rebuilding. (Brenman 2006, 12–13)

Brenman emphasizes that what happens in transference is insufficient for the success of psychoanalytical work, and points to the value of investigating the true history of the relationships with the persons close to the patient. The systemic constellation method makes it possible to take a giant step toward objectifying such constructions and get closer to the true knowledge about the client's life history. And, as Brenman writes, man has an inherent need to discover the truth and it seems important for him

> to pursue enquiry about his origins, to find his roots; he needs roots and objects, he cannot function alone. To my mind, knowing his background provides him with a sense of continuity and meaning. Only if he feels he belongs can he achieve his own identity. Reconstruction is of value as a means of rediscovering roots, past objects and lost parts of the self. (Brenman 2006, 11)

Prophecy Coles, a psychoanalytic therapist, is of a similar opinion. She believes that knowledge of ancestral history is an important part of our self-knowledge, although many psychotherapists think that life history is not something important because this "dead" past has no impact on the psyche

(Coles 2011). However, as family constellations show, the past is by no means dead and passive, because it contains an area that actively affects us—the domain of our ancestors and the events related to them.

THE THERAPIST'S ATTITUDE

The proper therapeutic attitude in family constellations is similar to that of a psychoanalyst. Freud often stressed that nothing hinders a psychoanalysis as much as "therapeutic zeal" (Segal 1990, 69). He thought that a psychoanalyst should not focus too much on therapeutic objectives, as this could make it impossible to learn about the patient. Hellinger recommended a similar attitude, which he referred to as "phenomenological." The point of constellations is not to simply eliminate the problem, regardless of everything that is behind it, but to give voice to what the problem results from. We take an open approach, ready to let ourselves be surprised. In psychoanalysis, the assumptions are similar. Lacan stated that "what the psychoanalyst must know: how to ignore what he knows," which means that he should be open to the new that appears with every session. A similar opinion was held by Bion, who said that during a session the psychoanalyst should get rid of "memory and desire."

Patients want to see the psychoanalyst—as Lacan recognized—as "the one who knows" and assume that he has a solution to their unawareness and failures. The psychoanalyst, however, shows them that the solution is nowhere else but in themselves. He does not stick to the stories the analysand tells, but rather tries to see something beyond what he wants to tell him. This something is independent of the analysand's conscious intentions and should be maximally independent of the analyst's subjective interpretations. The psychoanalyst does not focus on the content of the narration, aiming to discover what is still unknown to both him and the patient. Similarly, the constellation therapist should not discuss, oppose, or impose interpretations on the client, but should refer to the reality beyond their control—to the constellation process. The constellation therapist stays in the "last row" and is, like the analyst, frugal with words. He knows that his role must be limited to enabling the client to confront what is in his system and his unconscious. He must withdraw immediately afterward.

In constellations, we try to capture the client's situation from a wide perspective without focusing on the details of his problem. A similar aim is behind the psychoanalytic recommendation that the analyst should use "evenly suspended attention," that is, not choose any line of understanding and getting to know the patient, but look at the whole of his words and functioning. Neither the psychoanalyst nor the constellation therapist trusts the superficial, and they do not believe that the essence of the problem lies in the stories told by their clients. They always go deeper, toward what is unconscious at this moment. This causes a kind of distance toward the clients' ideas about the source of their problems and ways of solving them. Externally, this is reflected in the attitude of "benevolent neutrality," which is the term used by psychoanalysts to describe the proper attitude of a psychoanalyst.

Hellinger often stressed that the therapist must not retreat from what he sees because "a therapist who is afraid to confront a client's reality, for example, the fact that the client does not have long to live, is not up to dealing with the client's reality and is appropriately mistrusted or even feared by his client" (Hellinger 2001, 3). Freud also spoke of "education to reality"—in a very similar sense—as an ability to abandon infantile illusions (Freud 1989a, 63). The common feature of constellations and psychoanalysis is humbleness. Their role is not to equip a person with additional skills, to make him think positively, or to confirm his self-esteem. Psychoanalysis and systemic constellations show "what is." Their healing effect involves giving up the false omnipotence of our ego.

FAMILY CONSTELLATIONS AND PSYCHOANALSIS—MAJOR DIFFERENCES

The psychoanalyst and the analysand come to knowledge through a long process of gradual approximations, often meeting several times a week for several years. Still, the psychoanalyst's interpretations are much more likely to be subjective than the conclusions that arise during a constellation. When facilitating a constellation, we also often just guess at something and communicate it to the client, but we can base on what is certain. For example, that there is someone else in the system who is forgotten but important; that the mother is internally attached to someone; that the father is internally going toward death; that the hierarchy is violated; that the bond is broken; and so on. We do not have to say that "the grandmother was raped during the war by a soldier," though such images may come to us; it is enough to say that "the grandmother suffered some trauma related to aggression and sex." The psychoanalyst has a more difficult task, as he has to decide whether a given statement and behavior of the patient is the result of resistance, of unconscious activity, an element of the current transference in the analytic situation, or—if he takes such factors into consideration—something nonbiographical, related to the patient's family past. What is essential for treatment? When and what to interpret?

All schools of psychoanalysis focus on parental figures as the most important elements in the child's development and his potential psychological pathologies. In the contemporary Kleinian approach, "it is the nature of the parental couple that the infant and young child internalizes that is central to successful psychological development" (Barrows 2008, 171). We will notice some confusion in the psychoanalysts' writings: sometimes they speak of the "objective" relationship of the parents, and at other times they emphasize the "quality" of its representation in the child's mind. The relationship that the parents form "stays with them." It is the child who establishes the relationship with the mother and the father and with the parents as a couple. All parents have a strong enough and "right" relationship with each other, as evidenced by the child's existence. One only needs to find this reality within oneself.

One author states that "infants begin life by relating to many different people, rather than just to one, the mother, followed by a gradual extension of their circle" (Barrows 2008, 172). While this is true, it remains more within the realm of hypotheses than what direct or psychoanalytical observation suggests. Only family constellations are able to strongly confirm this, I think, semi-intuitive statement. The infant, and even the fetus, develops in the field of his family and from the beginning enters into relationships with his mother, father, grandparents, and siblings, as well as with their deficits and traumas. This is what Selma Fraiberg spoke of in the work *Ghosts in the Nursery*, stating that "in every nursery there are ghosts. They are the visitors from the unremembered past of the parents, the uninvited guests at the christening" (Fraiberg 1987, 100). Children encounter the "ghosts of their parents," with unfinished business from their childhood and past.

There is a particular problem that psychoanalytical practice faces, the importance of which was repeatedly stressed by Freud. He referred to it as the "economic problem of masochism." It boils down to the question of how it is possible that people can actively direct themselves toward what brings them suffering (humiliation, failure, illness). This problem is also related to such issues as "negative therapeutic reaction," that is, a worsening of the patient's condition precisely when the therapy seems to solve some of his problems, as well as an "unconscious sense of guilt" and a "need for punishment." With regard to these issues, Freud commented that

> the battle with the obstacle of an unconscious sense of guilt is not made easy for the analyst. Nothing can be done against it directly, and nothing indirectly but the slow procedure of unmasking its unconscious repressed roots, and of thus gradually changing it into a *conscious* sense of guilt. One has a special opportunity for influencing it when this *Ucs.* sense of guilt is a "borrowed" one—when it is the product of an identification with some other person who was once the object of an erotic cathexis. A sense of guilt that has been adopted in this way is often the sole remaining trace of the abandoned love-relation and not at all easy

> to recognize as such. [. . .] If one can unmask this former object-cathexis behind the *Ucs.* sense of guilt, the therapeutic success is often brilliant, but otherwise the outcome of one's efforts is by no means certain. It depends principally on the intensity of the sense of guilt; there is often no counteracting force of a similar order of strength which the treatment can oppose to it. (Freud 1989b, 50–51)

In the above passage, as in many other parts of his work, Freud is driven by perspicacity and honesty. He points to the great difficulty that the patient's unconscious sense of guilt (unconscious need for punishment), which can be stronger than any of the analyst's efforts, is for the progress of therapy. At the same time, however, he discovers an astonishing fact: a "brilliant success" in solving the patient's problems can be achieved under certain conditions, namely, when the person with whom he subconsciously identified himself is discovered.

What Freud put in a footnote, as if not knowing what to do about it, systemic constellations show clearly and completely. It is obvious to us that only if the patient is confronted with the person whose emotions he has taken on himself, which is done in the face of the representative in a constellation, can he get out of the entanglement. The results are then instantaneous and the intervention looks "brilliant." From constellations, however, we know more than that, and taking a sense of guilt on oneself is just one kind of identification with another member of the family. One can "take on" also other feelings or experience one's own feelings but triggered by the fate of someone else, someone one has not even met.. So the object of identification does not have to be an old object of the "erotic cathexis" that has been repressed.

Psychoanalysts recognize transgenerational influences but have not developed consistent theories of this experience and clear guidelines on how to identify and integrate them into the process of therapy. Psychoanalysis, considering the psychogenesis of disorders, uses linear causality—when psychoanalysts talk about transgenerational transmission, they mean direct succession, which is always mediated by parents.

Those psychoanalysts who recognize that the individual's identity is built on a multigenerational foundation tend to see ancestors as "haunting ghosts." Without conceptual tools for understanding the ancestor-related aspects of their patients' lives, they sometimes adopt an attitude that demonizes their figures and impact. They say, for example, that the deceased ancestor "does not give the living peace of mind," as if "demanding that certain dues be repaid," that he "does not tolerate the joy of life" that the living enjoy, and each family member internally feels his "animosity" (Walewska 2007, 105). Of course, such phrases function as metaphors rather than strict terms, but thereby show the theoretical difficulties of psychoanalysis in the face of this subject.

Within the framework of constellations, we approach the impacts of the deceased in a more unequivocal and calm manner. We know that the nature of their impact is primarily connected with the conscious and unconscious attitude of the living toward them. The assertion that it results from the "animosity" of the dead toward the living is incorrect even as a metaphor. We also have greater clarity about the nature of their existence—the dead exist to the living members of the family, given the psychological realm, just as the living do.

Although—as I demonstrated above—some psychoanalysts explore the issue of more distant ancestors and broad family ties, the mainstream of psychoanalysis is far from this. In general, psychoanalysts concentrate on one's mother, father, rarely on siblings, and basically only on the living ones. In considering only the persons in the patient's immediate environment, psychoanalysts are unable to link the numerous manifestations of the patient's psyche to any particular person. This explains why psychoanalysis has not noticed that "internal objects" reflect the existence of real people and their fates, and instead claims that they are the result of phantasmatic processes.

Things look quite different when the members of past generations, the unborn children, or the parents' ex-partners enter the pool of people to be considered. Then much of what seemed unrelated to reality and strange becomes clear.

When psychoanalysts observe a strong identification with, for example, a deceased brother or sister, they consider it to be "hypercathexis," a kind of pathological attachment. They do not notice that it stems from something fundamental and universal, from the bond that prevails in families. Freud erroneously derived this bond from the sexual libido, "inhibited in its aim" (German: *zielgehemmt*), whereas constellations show quite clearly that it is not of an erotic nature.

NOTES

1. When we want to compare any method with psychoanalysis, we encounter a significant difficulty, because there are basically many psychoanalyses. There is Freud's psychoanalysis, Klein's psychoanalysis, ego psychology, analysis of self, Lacanianism, Reich's and Lowen's bioenergetics, and analytical psychology developed by Jung. There are various paradigms within which psychoanalysis is practiced (such as interpersonal paradigm or analytic field theory). The concepts of the most influential psychoanalysts, even those from one school, differ and contradict each other. Here I am addressing psychoanalysis *en bloc*, that is, all these schools together, considering psychoanalysis to be one for the purpose of my investigation.

2. Probably because he recognized the gravity of this type of phenomena, he stated in a letter to the parapsychologist Hereford Carrington: "If I had to live my life

over again, I should devote myself to psychical research, rather than psychoanalysis" (Brottman 2011, 1). Note that Freud was one of the greatest critics of people' illusions, magical thinking, and infantile wishful thinking. However, he considered telepathy a fact.

3. The researchers who analyzed the children from families affected by the Holocaust noted that some of them, born after the war, reported nightmares about the camps and the Nazis, which depict the scenes from their parents' past, even though their parents did not talk about these events and their children have no conscious knowledge of them (Coles 2011). A well-known trauma therapist Peter A. Levine recalls:

> From my own clinical work with children and grandchildren of Holocaust survivors, I have frequently noticed and tracked symptoms of generalized anxiety and depression. I have also noted that these individuals frequently describe surprisingly specific and often horrific images, sensations, and emotions about events that seemed quite real but could not possibly have happened to them. I was able to confirm that many of these specific events had actually happened to the patients' parents, and could not have possibly happened to their children. However, the children were clearly experiencing their parents' traumatic memories as if they were their own. Significantly, most of the parents and grandparents had not initially shared these memories with their children. (Levine 2015)

4. Sabina Spielrein, Jung's patient and lover, and later a psychoanalyst, was particularly interested in the issue of the death drive in her work (Britton 2018, 27 et seq.). She believed that in the psyche, there are tendencies to regression, death, and connection with ancestors through it. She also wrote, "Since in the beloved, one seeks the parental resemblance, it is conceivable that one may seek to experience in reality the destiny of the ancestor, specifically the parents" (Britton 2018, 42).

5. Gregorio Kohon states that "confusion between birth and death seems to be particularly evident [. . .] in the case of genuinely schizophrenic patients" (Green and Kohon 2005, 52). This is in line with my observation based on constellations that psychosis may involve a "stillbirth," a kind of not taking one's life on a deep level (Janus 2021, 168–70).

6. Probably, the "inhibition" mentioned by the author can manifest itself in men in various types of decrease of interest in the partner or impotence, and in women even in anorgasmia. The way to reduce this inhibition will be a more complete acceptance of the mother, and thus, at least partial ceasing to project her image onto the partner.

7. Rank sees the desire to symbolically return to the mother's womb rather than the direct relationship with the deceased as the reason for the identification with the deceased. However, he points to the same phenomena as we know from constellations.

Chapter 4

Other Therapeutic and Para-Therapeutic Methods

TRANSGENERATIONAL PHENOMENA AND "SOULS" OF ANCESTORS

Genealogy and Psychogenealogy

Genealogy is not psychotherapy, but it has something in common with the orders discovered by Bert Hellinger, for the interest in our own past reflects our understanding of the importance of ancestors in our lives:

> Amateur genealogists associate historical dates with dates in their genealogy. They no longer think, "That was before Napoleon marched on Moscow," but: "Great-great-grandmother Marianne was two years old then." [. . .] When I learned that one of my maternal grandfather's uncles had emigrated to America, for the first time in my life I tried to imagine how he got from Huta Połoniecka to Chicago: what the route was, how far he walked, whether he drove by carriage. I also have purely practical questions: "What did the chimneyless hut look like where my serf ancestors lived?" and psychological and emotional questions: "How did my great-great-grandmother feel when her child died as an infant in the same year that her older son died?" or: "What was the seventeen-year-old bride thinking of when she was marrying the forty-year-old widower who had five little children at home waiting for her care?" Underlying such an emotionally charged approach to genealogical work is the simple fact that these are our ancestors. Perhaps it is a feeling of gratitude that they survived, and that we exist thanks to them. Perhaps it is a belief that our ancestors live in us and will live in our descendants. (Nowaczyk 2015, 239)

As one can see, genealogy can lead to similar reflections as constellations. We start to perceive the ancestors as concrete people and gain understanding and empathy for them. We begin to see our own fate in a broader context. Daniel Foor, a practitioner of ancestral medicine, writes that "any effort to understand family history or research your genealogy can help awaken your relationship with ancestors, both known and unknown" (Foor 2017, 34).

A psychotherapeutic method similar to genealogy is working with genograms. Genograms became popular after Bowen's speech at the family therapy congress in 1967. Bowen presented his own "journey into the past," visits to closer and further family members and the information he received from them. He believed that transgenerational influences are the basic determinants of the nuclear family and therefore developed a graphical way of studying the origin of the problem in the form of diagrams covering at least three generations. This work gave birth to the contemporary genogram.

Genograms made it possible to look at the line from a bird's-eye view and thus identify relationships not otherwise detected. Monica McGoldrick writes that clinicians should look in a genogram for negative behavioral patterns, relationships, and family structures that repeated themselves over several generations. Knowing them can help the family avoid repeating them or passing them on to future generations (McGoldrick, Gerson, and Shellenberger 1999, 13).

Repeating patterns are probably most evident in the so-called anniversary reaction. This phenomenon was discovered by psychologist Joséphine Hilgard in the early 1950s. Based on the analysis of hospital archives and patient observations, the researcher discovered that illnesses such as psychosis break out when the context of the past is repeated, for example, a given person is the same age as his parent when he got mentally ill, or the person's children are as old as he was when it happened. Based on family constellations, one can say that he identifies with someone with whom he not only has a bond, but who was probably excluded (as is usually the case with the mentally ill), which intensifies the tendency to repeat the fate.

The anniversary syndrome and the patterns that repeat themselves across generations were studied extensively by Anne Ancelin Schützenberger. She observed the frequent correlation between the dates of death or birth of ancestors and descendants, as well as events such as weddings, christenings, and promotions. She said that a child can be born, for instance, on an anniversary of the grandfather's death or on the day of the great-grandmother's birthday, as if he "honored" the memory and bond with the family member. The author also observed that accidents are "inherited" (with injuries often affecting the same part of the body), that incest is repeated within the family, and that family structure is also "inherited" (number and age of children, partners, miscarriages, and abortions).

Schützenberger's genosociogram is "a kind of family tree drawn from memory, without researching information or documents, and annotated with important life events" (Schützenberger 1998, 70). This technique "sheds light on sociometric relations, context, and important facts and events. In addition, it makes use of the experience and unconscious of both the therapist and the client (his or her dreams, slip-ups or errors, free associations)" (Schützenberger 1998, 64). The therapist sees the causes of problems, accidents, or illnesses as transgenerational influences of lack of mourning, family secrets, unfinished important tasks, and identification with ancestors resulting from love and loyalty. The latter may result in diseases with similar symptoms to those experienced by grandparents or great-grandparents (e.g., someone's dyspnea may be connected with the death of his ancestor suffocated with war gas). In order to stop the repetition of destructive patterns and events, one must get to know the past of one's own family and accept one's own ancestors with their deeds, because—as Schützenberger notes—we do not choose our family, but we can accept that we were born into it and consciously become part of it. She says that we must stop living someone else's life, suffering and striving for what our ancestors lacked. All this, of course, is very much in line with family constellations.

Intergenerational Healing

Intergenerational phenomena were already known to the ancients. Greek tragedies, such as *Oedipus the King* by Sophocles or *The Oresteia* by Aeschylus, refer to matters that continued or escalated from generation to generation. Plato wrote in the *Phaedrus* dialogue that

> madness can provide relief from the greatest plagues of trouble that beset certain families because of their guilt for ancient crimes: it turns up among those who need a way out; it gives prophecies and take refuge in prayers to the gods and in worship, discovering mystic rites and purifications that bring the man in touches through to safety for this and all time to come. So it is that the right sort of madness finds relief from present hardships for a man it has possessed. (Plato 1995, 28)

As one can see, it was obvious to Plato that the descendants' illnesses and misfortunes could result from their ancestors' deeds (madness is an attempt to deal with this difficult legacy, leading to rituals that have a healing function).

In the womb of Christianity, the practice of so-called intergenerational healing was developed. The doctrine of original sin already assumes that the consequences of sin are inherited from generation to generation.[1] This is how John Paul II explains it:

> Because of the bond which unites us to one another in the Mystical Body, all of us, though not personally responsible and without encroaching on the judgment of God who alone knows every heart, bear the burden of the errors and faults of those who have gone before us. (Healy 2015, 202)

Let us look at the above not as religious ideas, but as a discovery of certain psychological facts, that is, as a bond that connects us with others through time and space. Father Robert DeGrandis writes:

> Intergenerational healing is, for the Christian, an opportunity to recognize and bring healing to the family influences from the past, with implications for the future. Intergenerational healing suggests the possibility that negative acts and deeds of ancestors can somehow enter into our "bloodstream" and take a toll on future generations. Transforming the connection with these troublesome roots is what intergenerational healing is all about. (DeGrandis and Schubert 1989, Preface)

The Christian practice of intergenerational healing is based on the findings of psychiatrist Kenneth McAll, who developed the method known as "Healing the Family Tree." McAll, a devout Christian, had long contact with Chinese culture, where he was greatly moved by the case of the a "possessed by the devil" who was healed by prayer. He wrote:

> An increasing number of the patients sent to me admitted that they suffered from the presence of "spirits" or the intrusion of "voices" from another world which were apparent and audible only to themselves and which psychiatry dismissed as madness. [. . .] Some seemed to be evil and often came as a result of occult practices, while others seemed to be neutral, harmless voices begging for help. Sometimes the patient could identify the voices as belonging to a recently dead relative but often there was no known connection in the patient's mind. (McAll 1986, 5–6)

McAll stated that many of his patients were living their lives "to a greater or lesser extent under the influence of someone else who might be alive or dead, known to the patient or unknown" (McAll 1986, 6). They were in bondage to their "ancestors, to those not related, to stillborn, aborted or miscarried babies, or to those who once inhabited a particular place now occupied by the living" (McAll 1986, 7). McAll also observed the power of the effect of the twin who died in the womb on the the survivor.

The practice of intergenerational healing stemmed from McAll's encounter with the same processes that constellation therapists work with. This proves the universality and importance of these processes. Focusing on the family, ancestors and problems associated with them brought to light the relationship between someone's life and past situations. It should be noted, however, that McAll and others (Kurt Koch, Robert DeGrandis) did not identify intergenerational influences as clearly as Hellinger. They consider "intergenerational sins" and inherited bondage to be the basic transgenerational burden. These concepts assume that the "sins" committed by ancestors, such as practicing the occult, produce multigenerational effects in the form of heritable "demonic bondage." The essential therapeutic techniques here are prayer, confession of sins, renunciation of Satan, surrender to Jesus, but also such specific actions as putting one's family tree on the altar.

The author saw the possibility of immediate healing if the therapeutic work is done by someone related to the sick person, which we know also from constellations, for example, when a session with the mother leads to the healing of the child.

In his service, McAll is guided by the "visions" that appear when he prays for a person and for his problem to be solved. These visions are not uncommon for a constellation therapist who makes use of the resonance with the knowing field. McAll says he had hundreds of visions about children who had been aborted and their age matched the age they would have been if they had lived. This seems to make sense—Hellinger sometimes recommended that the mother imagine that the unborn child was alive, growing, and accompanying her. This allowed her to get rid of her guilty feeling or rejecting attitude toward the child.

McAll also cites other examples that are consistent with the orders of love, he speaks, for instance, of an adopted boy whose functioning improved when his adoptive parents gave a name to their child who had died at birth, whom the boy was expected to replace; of a mother who heard Jesus say that she must first give a name to her deceased child and "show him that he has a mother's love" and only then commit the child to Him; of illnesses that seem to be caused by disrespecting or excluding a person, such as an aborted child. McAll also observes the characteristic phenomenon that when we free ourselves from a destructive attachment to some living or dead person, a void appears in us (which can be filled by commiting ourselves to the care of Christ). We encounter the same in constellations—giving up an entanglement is often initially associated with a feeling of emptiness.[2]

A similar phenomenon is prayers for healing, where family and intergenerational issues are also addressed. Mary Healy, involved in the movement of Catholic Charismatic Renewal, writes:

> When evidence of such a generational pattern comes to light during prayer for healing, we can ask the Lord to break the unhealthy cycle and heal the wounds caused by it. For example, I recently prayed over a woman who suffered from severe depression. When I asked if anyone else in her family had depression, she affirmed that her mother and grandmother and several other relatives had suffered from it. I asked her to pray a simple prayer, renouncing a spirit of depression in the name of Jesus. I prayed that this generational pattern would be broken and that she would be released from all spiritual bondage related to it. There were also abusive behaviors in her family that probably contributed to the depression. I led her in a prayer forgiving each family member who had hurt her or failed her in some way. (Healy 2015, 103)

"Renouncing a spirit of depression" can be understood as an act of leaving what I unconsciously carry and what does not belong to me, because it is a business of someone older in the family. Similarly, DeGrandis finds that "after a miscarriage or abortion, the next child who is born and lives, can sometimes carry the mother's guilt and fear," which corroborates our observations on the unconscious perception of children and their taking on the problems of their parents (DeGrandis and Schubert 1989, 40).

What does the healing process look like? As in constellations, it consists of a diagnostic part in which the Holy Spirit gives insights into the client's present and past (the so-called visualization prayer), and a therapeutic part in which problems are entrusted to Jesus Christ. One of the priests wrote:

> Prayer for intergenerational healing often bears good fruit. Many people felt great relief experienced not only in their soul or psyche, but also physically. Many people begun to understand where their personal and family problems could come from. It is important in this prayer to find the source of the wound, but it is even more important to trust God, because it is not always possible to find out where our problems come from. (Różański in: Guzowski et al. 2015, 60–61)

"Guiding the Spirits"

Psychiatrist Carl Wickland maintained that mental disorders were the result of the influence of spirits of the dead and that a significant number of his patients were possessed by those spirits. He used electric shocks, among other methods, get rid of the possessing spirits.

Psychologist Edith Fiore argues that many mental disorders may be due to the client being possessed by spirits of the dead. She assumes that what patients say under hypnosis are the voices of spirits (although she admits that she is not certain about this). Her observations have several elements that converge with constellations to some degree, such as the idea that gender identity problems or homosexuality may result from possession by a spirit of the opposite sex. Fiore writes:

> When the therapy is lengthy and the spirits do not leave after a few sessions, I generally find that the possessor and the possessed have been together in past lifetimes! The motivations for the possession may be found in events from the previous times they have been together. There may be a burning desire for revenge on one or both parts. [. . .] On the other hand, there may be a powerful attachment between the two based on mutual love and/or dependency. For example, the spirit may have been the mother of the person in another incarnation and possessed him or her in childhood. In most instances, neither is aware of the subconscious memories of the previous lives they have shared—or the real reasons for the possession.
>
> I find that in every case that is investigated, the possessee has possessed another in an earlier lifetime—deliberately or unwittingly. (Fiore 2006, 156)

The concept of spirits possessing, "entering," a person may seem nonsensical. Looking from the perspective of family constellations, we are able to introduce more logic here. First of all, we can reduce the whole menagerie of spirits, among which some are "malevolent," other ones "lustful," "lost," or "friendly," to the systemic influence of the dead and transgressions of the orders of love. In this view, ghosts cease to be otherworldly visitors, and our interactions with them no longer assume the most fanciful forms, but fall within repetitive patterns. Ghosts become simply our systemic heritage, in which there is nothing scary or supernatural. Based on constellations, we can surmise that the spirits Fiore discovers are, in many cases, persons from the system processed by the patients' imagination.

Neoshamanism and Ancestral Medicine

Contemporary North American shaman Medicine Grizzlybear Lake treated a Vietnamese immigrant who was in a coma. The shaman learned from the "spirits" that the woman's soul had left her body "out of fear and bewilderment" and gone to Vietnam, wanting to be with her relatives, in a familiar place. The treatment consisted in persuading the woman's soul to return to her body (Lake 2006, 121–23).

The shamanic view of reality is not far from the systemic one—even if souls really do not travel, a person's mental states can still be expressed by distant representatives, as if his "soul" could really move from place to place. From a systemic point of view, in the above example, we see the connection of the child with the family, which is stronger than the fear of death, and the desire to die in order to "go" to the deceased relatives. We do not employ such a realistic understanding of the soul as in shamanism, but we know that there is magical thinking that through death it is possible to "go" to the dead. It is more than a passing fantasy—in a sense, it is a real mental attachment to it.

The shaman Tela Starhawk Lake treated an autistic girl who did not speak or make contact with her mother or anyone else around her. The shaman said that the girl had imaginary playmates with whom she talked in her mind. They were the so-called "Little People," according to Indian beliefs—real spiritual beings. Lake and I share the view that pathological states can intensify paranormal perception, the effects of which then contribute to the psychopathological picture. In this case, the girl's paranormal abilities were thought to enable her to perceive the invisible "Little People" who, as the shaman says, "were in complete control of the child's mind and soul" (Lake 2006, 139). Psychologists of the prevailing paradigm would classify the "Little People" as products of the child's mind, that is, as hallucinations. Since we know systemic constellations, we can adopt a different stance. We can assume that the origin of the "Little People" lies "outside" the child's mind. They may have resulted from the child's imagination processing her unconscious knowledge about certain people in the family. Possibly about deceased children.

The concept of "losing one's soul" is interesting in the context of constellations. Shamans maintain that many ailments may be caused by the fact that the soul has left the person or has been stolen. As neochaman Arvick Baghramian argues, the concept of soul loss is similar to the psychological term of dissociation (Baghramian 2015, 155). Dissociation, generally speaking, consists in the fact that the psyche (memory, personality) "splits" into relatively independent and isolated parts, many of which remain below the threshold of consciousness. However, while according to psychology, dissociated (split) fragments of the psyche belong to the inner world of the subject, in shamanism they are understood as being in another dimension of reality (lost). From the perspective of systemic constellations, the two concepts are not mutually exclusive—the dissociated part can be so strongly attached to someone or something from the past (e.g., to a trauma that occurred generations ago) as if it lived really there and not here and now.

"Ancestral medicine" assumes that relationships with ancestors are of fundamental meaning when it comes to our health and well-being. Foor writes:

> Practitioners of ancestor reverence generally assume that the ancestors influence us to a degree that truly matters and that we also affect them in important ways [. . .]. What *is* an option is whether the influence will be conscious or unconscious, beneficial or harmful. Many rituals focus on maintaining positive relations between the living and the dead precisely to ensure that their influence is beneficial rather than harmful. [. . .] The ancestors can confer blessings of health and longevity, or they can send us to an early grave. (Foor 2017, 28–29)

And further:

> In my experience, the ancestors who are strong and bright in spirit are also the best guides and allies for living family members who seek to transform and end difficult intergenerational burdens. [. . .] In brief, when we enjoy the active support of our loving ancestors, life tends to go more smoothly, with higher levels of luck, ease, and vitality. (Foor 2017, 29)

Foor also says that when we "forget our origins, we're more likely to enact and reinforce unhelpful intergenerational patterns" (Foor 2017, 31). This is in line with the basic principle of systemic constellations, that it is including the excluded (forgotten) and realizing the bond with the ancestors that allows negative patterns to be left behind. The bond is also a source of life energy, which flows through several generations. This is why it is so strengthening in constellations when the male or female client stands in his male or her female "line of the family" or in the "pyramid of the family." Foor observes this phenomenon and concludes that when the spirit of the youngest of the ancestors "merges with the greater lineage," for the descendant this can be a source of the feeling of "being in the presence of a larger energy" (Foor 2017, 40).

The Psychomanteum and the IADC Method

A significant percentage of people who have lost a loved one experience the phenomenon of contact with the dead. Apparitions of the deceased or feelings of presence are important in the process of mourning and help to maintain emotional balance (Moody and Perry 1993, x). Japanese widows, for example, who have a "continuing bond with the presence of their deceased spouses," are psychologically stronger than their American counterparts (Pearson 2015, 113).

So psychiatrist Raymond Moody used the old technique of looking into the mirror to enable people to contact their departed relatives for therapeutic purposes. He arranged a darkened room with a large mirror and armchair (the so-called psychomanteum) and developed a procedure to develop visions of the dead. It turned out that this technique allowed most people to "see the spirits of departed relatives *virtually anytime they want*" (Moody and Perry 1993, xviii). These visions are very realistic and, according to the accounts, in many cases, they are almost no different from an ordinary encounter:

> Many of the people I have worked with say that these visions result in an alleviation or even resolution of their grief. In the people I have helped to have apparitions, the event is primarily one of the healing, in which the relationship with the deceased is improved. (Moody and Perry 1993, 9)

Note the interesting statement about improving the relationship with the deceased. From the point of view of systemic constellations—although the issue of life after death remains a mystery to us—it is quite understandable.

The Induced After-Death Communication (IADC) method, developed by psychologist Allan Botkin while counseling war veterans, brings very similar results (Botkin and Hogan 2014). He used the method developed by Francine Shapiro for treating post-traumatic stress disorder, known as EMDR (Eye Movement Desensitization and Reprocessing). In EMDR, the patient reaches his trauma memory while simultaneously experiencing sensorimotor stimulation in the form of rhythmic eye movements. It turns out that this quite simple method yields huge positive effects. Botkin used his own version of this method, which he referred to as CoreFocused EMDR, assuming that the core and primary emotion in post-traumatic disorder is deep sadness. Reaching it through secondary emotions, such as rage or guilt, the patient experienced significant improvement. However, when Botkin modified the procedure again and asked the patients to sit with their eyes closed at the end of the session, it turned out that most of them experienced realistic "encounters" with the deceased, the same people whose loss caused their pain or pathological mourning. Importantly, these meetings were radically transformative—feelings of guilt, pain, or grief that had sometimes lasted for decades disappeared in a single session.

Stanislav Grof, a pioneer of transpersonal psychology, also encountered ancestral experiences during his research on the therapeutic effects of LSD-25 and the so-called holotropic breathwork (supposed to produce similar effects as hallucinogens). He found that these complex experiences sometimes

> take the form of the actual reliving of short episodes or entire sequences from the life of one's ancestors that are concrete, specific, and rich in detail. They can involve full experiential identification with the ancestors, including the body, image, facial expression, gestures, emotional reactions, and thought processes. [. . .] Some subjects have reported in this context that as a result of such experiences they have developed a new understanding of some of their personal

problems and conflicts that did not make sense before. [. . .] objective investigation, if it can be carried out, typically brings results that are congruent with the subject's experience. (Grof 1988, 79–80)

THE EFFECT OF FORGIVENESS, GRATITUDE, AND SELF-RESPONSIBILITY

Forgiveness and gratitude are important issues of positive psychology, created by Martin Seligman. Robert Enright found that as readiness for forgiveness increases, the rates of depression and anxiety decrease, hope and self-esteem increase, physiological parameters improve (e.g., cortisol and blood pressure levels), and the immune system functions better. In contrast, holding a grudge causes that "there is an imbalance in the body, resistance to sickness is reduced, minor dysfunctions become more troublesome (blood pressure problems, colon diseases, etc.), and can even lead to serious illnesses such as cancer" (Lemoine 2016, 103).

Many studies show that practicing gratitude contributes to lowering blood pressure, reduces susceptibility to addictions and the risk of falling ill with depression and anxiety disorders, and increases the level of happiness. Psychologist Robert Emmons states that gratefulness "is the understanding that life owes me nothing and all the good I have is a gift" (Emmons 2016, 11). This is the same approach as the one we suggest during constellations—recognizing what we have received, gratitude and abandoning accusations and unconstructive demands (especially toward the parents).

In systemic constellations, we do not speak of forgiveness, but of acceptance and reconciliation, because forgiving could mean some degree of self-aggrandizement. However, forgiveness, present in various help systems, refers to processes similar to those that heal in constellations. This is particularly evident in Colin Tipping's Radical Forgiveness and in Ho'oponopono, a Hawaiian ritual of healing and resolving conflict (Vitale 2013; Karwat 2015; Dupreé 2012).

Tipping's method is based on the assumption that people are connected into an invisible system, which causes life events—also the unpleasant ones—to acquire a meaning which is unseen at first glance. The basis of the capacity for forgiveness is to see these hidden connections and our part in the conflict situation. Even negative situations are necessary, and people who harm us actually provide opportunities for our growth. If we look at the wrongs that have happened to us in this way, then instead of anger, we can even feel grateful to the people who, through their "bad" deeds, have given us the opportunity to develop.

"Radical" forgiveness is different from traditionally understood forgiveness in that we perceive that there is actually nothing to forgive because everything is as it should be. Tipping also recognizes the possibility that our mental change, forgiveness, directly and remotely affects the other person. He argues that on the spiritual plane souls work in agreement, including the souls of people who are in conflict on an everyday level. What is very important in Radical Forgiveness is, as Tipping puts it, to transcend the victim archetype. For here, as in constellations, we are aware that being a victim leads to judgments and getting stuck all our lives in one emotion and the same pattern of functioning. Radical Forgiveness, like the constellation method, transcends judging others. Tipping writes:

> Traditional forgiveness depends entirely upon our own capacity to feel compassion, so it is limited in this regard. No matter how much compassion or tolerance in this regard. No matter how much compassion or tolerance we muster for someone like Hitler, and no matter how much we empathize with the pain of his upbringing, nothing enables us to forgive him (using traditional forgiveness) for the mass murder of over 13 million people.
>
> Radical Forgiveness has no limits whatsoever and is completely unconditional. If Radical Forgiveness cannot forgive Hitler, it can forgive nobody. Like unconditional love, it's all or nothing. (Tipping 2009, 60)

Note that Tipping, like Hellinger, speaks of unconditional love. He gives as an example the person of Hitler, to whom Hellinger referred in a similar vein, for which he was roundly condemned. Society keeps the guilty and the victims in their places, separates the "beasts" from the "decent people," but Radical Forgiveness and systemic constellations transcend judgment. Some might object and claim that this is a moral relativization or condoning of evil. However, inner forgiveness does not bring evil, it brings good.

It is quite similar in Ho'oponopono—the idea behind it is to stop judging, to stop, for example, considering oneself a victim and someone else a perpetrator—and to take full responsibility for the presence of the problem in our lives and the people who, we think, cause it. This is possible when we see the problem not as something random and unnecessary, but as an opportunity for growth. In the exercises of this method, there is the tuning into the person for whom we hold a grudge and through this, finding union with him. Four sentences are used having the nature of sentences of strength: "I'm sorry," "Please forgive me," "I love you," "Thank you."

Forgiveness is also found in Christian counseling methods because it is grounded in the text of the Bible (e.g., Mt. 5:23–24: "If therefore thou art offering thy gift at the altar, and there rememberest that thy brother hath aught against thee, leave there thy gift before the altar, and go thy way, first be reconciled to thy brother, and then come and offer thy gift."). Pastor and counselor David Augsburger states that "forgiveness is release, release from a whole spectrum of negative emotions like fear, anger, suspicion, loneliness, alienation, mistrust" (Augsburger 1981, 68). Augsburger recommends forgiveness that restores love, leads to reconciliation, and separates the person from his actions, which allows to see his human value. He says that "true forgiveness restores the other's freedom with no questions asked, no demands imposed, no repentance required" (Augsburger 1981, 67). At the same time, he warns against false forgiveness:

> One-up-forgiveness is an emotion which exists solely in connection with judgment and condemnation.
>
> To say, "I forgive you," is to say, "I have examined, weighed, judged you and your behavior and found you sorely lacking in qualities that are worthy of my respect. [. . .] We will henceforth have a relationship based on the recognition of my benevolence in the hour of your neediness, my generosity in the face of your guilt. You will find some suitable way to be dutifully grateful from this day forward." (Augsburger 1981, 10–11)

The author states that the guilty party realizes, consciously or not, that he should submit to the other party, and this causes resistance in him and leads to conflicts. The position of being inferior and permanently judged is unbearable for most people, especially when the partner feels good in such an arrangement and does not intend to change it.

So Augsburger addresses the same psychological dynamics that Hellinger referred to as balance. When we forgive feeling superior, there is no balance—the other person feels overly indebted, it will be unbearable for him and the relationship will have to end. Augsburger says: "When 'forgiveness' ends open relationship, leaves people estranged, don't rush to it" (Augsburger 1981, 70). He suggests that when forgiveness is to conceal true emotions, conflicts, and avoid efforts to understand what separates one person from the other, then it "impoverishes both, and the moment of growth is lost" (Augsburger 1981, 86). This also corresponds to Hellinger's standpoint that teaches how to develop mutual relations, even at the price of temporary unforgiveness. Sometimes we have to hurt someone a little less for the wrong they have done to us, otherwise the relationship will die—neither our own nor their psyche can bear the injustice.

Christian authors also speak of forgiving parents and respecting them. The basis here is the fourth commandment of the Decalogue: "Honor thy father and thy mother, as Jehovah thy God commanded thee; that thy days may be long, and that it may go well with thee, in the land which Jehovah thy God giveth thee" (Deuteronomy 5:16). As St. Paul notes, this is the first commandment "with promise." Is it not interesting? In my opinion, the commandment describes a psychophysical truth—our body functions better when we are reconciled with our parents. The absence of this reconciliation is one of the strongest chronic stressors, and this can undoubtedly translate into the length of our lives.

We find an interesting phrase also in Sirach's Wisdom, which links the attitude toward one's mother with success and prosperity: "Those who honor their father atone for sins; they store up riches who respect their mother" (Sir. 3:3–4). It corresponds to Hellinger's statement: "Success has the face of the mother."

The absence of forgiveness entails costs. The Christian author Leslie Leyland Fields writes:

> Often we think the cost of forgiving is too high. But we do not consider the cost of not forgiving. We do not see who we're becoming. We're so busy trying to extract our debt from our parents that we do not see what it has done to us. (Fields and Hubbard 2014, 68)

As one of the ways to forgive our parents and reconcile with them, Fields suggests that we see the parents' problems, their difficulties with their own parents, or possible mental disorders. The author, referring to the biblical parable of the merciful Samaritan, writes:

> We are not the only ones who started out on that road and were jumped from behind. Our mothers—our fathers too—started off in hope. They, too, were unprepared for the dangers that lay ahead. They, too, were unsuspecting, not knowing they were entering such danger. When we begin to look at them again, even if we can only lift our heads, we can see they are there as well, bleeding, weak. They are as human, as fully human, and likely as wounded as we are. (Fields and Hubbard 2014, 47)

> We are training our spirits in compassion. When we do this, we discover or remember again the frailty of our parents, the burdens they bore, the weight of their own parents' sins upon them. And we'll find something much larger happening. When we truly see others in all their humanness, we become more alive, more awake, more fully human ourselves. (Fields and Hubbard 2014, 57)

During constellations, we see, sometimes with surprise, the pain and load that our parents carried. With this emotionally moving knowledge, reconciliation becomes much easier:

> we're called to respect our parents not because of their character but because of their position. Somehow, for reasons we'll never fully know, God chose *them*,

> those very particular women, those very particular men, to give us life. [. . .] Even when a father tears his own family apart, we are enjoyed to treat that parent not on the basis of his sin but on the basis of his God-given place in our lives. How does this bless us? How will "things go well with us" when we do this? We get a small taste of a perfect world when we extend grace and goodness to our renegade parents, reminding us of what is coming: a new world where all divisions are restored, all wounds are healed. The kingdom of God comes among us. (Fields and Hubbard 2014, 118–19)

In constellations, too, we do not focus on the parents' character, not even on their behavior. What is important is the position they have in our lives—they are the beginning and the foundation for us. It is impossible not to respect them without hurting ourselves. Some people, thinking they are rational, say, "I don't owe anything to my parents, they just gave me life." The contradiction in this sentence will hit them with real force. Fields says that reconciliation with the parents is a small taste of a world without divisions or wounds. During a constellation, when there is reconciliation and harmonization within the family, we have a similar feeling of the "better" side of reality without judgments or exclusions.

A DIFFERENT PERCEPTION

Knowledge from the Field

In Gestalt psychotherapy developed by Fritz Perls, an exercise called the "empty chair" or "two-chair dialogue" is often used (Houston 2003, 65–66; Rogers 2012, 195). It is considered to be the most effective technique of Gestalt. The chairs represent some polarity in the client's life; and he sits alternately on one chair or the other, confronting his feelings and uttering the words that come to his mind. This technique was developed in NLP, in the form of the so-called "perceptual positions" or "meta-mirror." Co-creator of NLP John Grinder and his student Judith DeLozier, emphasize that systematic changing of perceptual positions helps to obtain knowledge about specific contexts, which would normally be unavailable (Bavister and Vickers 2010, 173). The meta-mirror is used primarily to work on a relationship that is important for the client. Jenny Rogers describes it this way:

> The meta-mirror asks a client to enter into a state of maximum empathy with another person and then to identify and draw on their own insight and resourcefulness. By physically moving around, the client "breaks state"—that is, changes both the physical and mental dynamic—and gains new insights and

> energy. The physical movement of the exercise also enables the client to see the relationships from different perspectives—literally looking at them from another point of view. (Rogers 2012, 196)

She continues:

> This is a potent activity. I have used it many times with clients and there has never been an occasion where the client has failed to enter an intense and concentrated state. There is a stillness and deep absorption, which is quite unlike the usual run of coach-client conversations. Of course, there is no way of verifying the accuracy of our perceptions of what the imagined other person in the chair is feeling unless we check with them later—which some clients do—but my sense is that the insights from the perspective of the other chair are often spookily close. Most of us *can* actually access the cues others give us about their feelings towards us in the right circumstances, and this is what empty chair activities can provide. (Rogers 2012, 196)

We see the—familiar—astonishment at the accuracy of the information obtained in the process of imagining the other person as well as an observation about the easiness of reaching this effect. In another passage, Rogers mentions the connection between the client and the coach, which she refers to as "radio-field listening"—when the coach intuits the emotions, choices, and risks the client faces. She says that "these are moments of real connection—of a kind that few of us ever reach in a 'normal' conversation with a friend" (Rogers 2012, 68). I experience it the same way during constellations.

Through constellations, the process of therapy supervision can be deepened. Supervision is an analysis of the therapeutic process, the therapist's behaviors, and the client's problems, which the therapist conducts together with a supervisor, that is, typically a more advanced therapist, or in a group of people, usually therapists. Systemic supervision—that consists, for example, in representing the client and the therapist by other people—can be applied to virtually any type of therapy (psychodynamic, family, Gestalt, and many other approaches). It provides an insight into the aspects of the therapeutic relationship and the client's problems that the therapist cannot see.

Constellations, systemic supervision in particular, and so-called Balint groups are similar. Balint groups are a method of group meetings developed by Michael Balint for practicing physicians, and now used also by other helping professionals. Their aim is to emotionally unburden the professional and to improve his contact with his patients. In a Balint group, one person first describes a difficulty in his relationship with a given patient, provides information about the patient as well as about his own actions and emotions, and then the others share their thoughts, reflections, and associations, from which, under the guidance of the group leader, a broader picture of that relationship is built. Here is what Balint leaders write about this second stage:

> The next stage of group work, initiated by the leader, is a temporary identification with the partners of the subject relationship, that is, putting oneself in the shoes of each of them, both in the shoes of the patient and of the specialist who presents the problem with the patient. Associations, fantasies, and words emerging at this stage, in which one avoids intellectualizing and judging, and prefers descriptions of personal feelings and imaginings as well as personal tone of speech, provide much valuable material that enables one to better understand the nature of difficulties that occur in the discussed relationship. (Wasilewski and Engel 2011, 95)

The recommendations like "Put yourself in his shoes and speak as him," "Speak on his (her) behalf" are characteristic of the Balint technique (Wasilewski and Engel 2011, 94). The members of the group empathize and fantasize about the emotional and mental world of the patient and the therapist. This leads to insights that broaden the understanding of the therapeutic relationship and the physician's or therapist's own reactions. We often get the impression that the insights into the emotional state of the patient or the nature of the physician-patient relationship go beyond the information provided. This state of affairs in Balint groups is considered normal, and yet it should astound. Part of the information is probably achieved through connecting with the knowing field. It is precisely the instructions such as "Put yourself in the patient's shoes," as well as psychodramatic elements used sometimes in this practice (playing the patient and the therapist), that make the connection with this field possible.

Psychophanie

Rosemary Crossley developed the so-called facilitated communication method based on pointing to letters and building sentences or typing on a keyboard with the help of another person (Biklen 1993). Thanks to this method, mute people—for example, those with autism—started to communicate their feelings and needs. Moreover, it turned out that people considered mentally handicapped were not only able to write—which they had never been taught—but also had logical and moving reflections. The method is that the facilitator holds the handicapped person's hand over a letter board or keyboard, trying to sense what letters he wants to point to. Sometimes the action of the disabled person is strong and evident, sometimes weaker. When the answers concern feelings or are otherwise difficult for the subject, even someone with a disability who uses the keyboard well may get blocked and need help to clearly indicate the answer. Sometimes it is enough to simply have a kind person behind them.

Speech therapist Anne-Marguerite Vexiau developed this method and termed it *psychophanie*—"revelation of the soul." She observed the same relationships that were identified in constellations. This method enabled Vexiau to bring to light family dramas, fetal experiences, as well as the child's feelings such as the feeling that he is responsible for the tragic events that sometimes took place several generations earlier (Brune 2011, 274). She also reached the same conclusions as Hellinger about ties—they must never be broken, the aim is to harmonize them, as, for example, in the case of adopted children and their unknown parents, whose constant influence was brought to light by the *psychophanie* method.

Vexiau observed a strong influence of the excluded and deceased, for instance, the unborn children. Bringing them back to memory resulted in healing. She also observed that perpetrators and victims tend to reconcile—which is well known from constellations. The therapist saw interpersonal connections going far beyond what is visible from the outside and showed the extended spiritual life of the deeply disabled, which is fully in line with what we see in systemic constellations.

The Cognizing Body

During constellations, our body helps us. If my contact with the client is reduced to mere conversation, I am unable to see or understand many important things. For instance, when the client tells me about his relationship with his father, I can infer its nature, taking literally what he said, I can try to extract the hidden meanings of his words, and finally, I can count on my feelings and intuitions. But I can also go further, stand up, and "as the father" let my body show me this relationship more fully. Then the information that is most important from a therapeutic point of view arrives.

Bodily sensations as a source of cognition are used in the focusing method developed by the philosopher Eugene T. Gendlin (2003). He found that the body has a kind of wisdom that can be accessed through simple procedures. The body is like a powerful computer that has a connection to the surrounding environment. As a result, it usually "knows" more about our situation than the conscious mind, because it accumulates millions of bits of information in one feeling. By focusing on bodily sensations, we can obtain a comprehensive understanding of the problem and achieve inner change. Gendlin refers to this ability as our "felt sense."

Focusing is similar to constellations in many ways. We do not try to find meaning or analyze, but rely on the autonomous bodily process. One should accept what emerges and what is sometimes surprising and goes beyond logical reasoning. Gendlin proposes that the original and still unclear feeling concerning the analyzed problem be connected by the client with a word, sentence, or image. This resembles Hellinger connecting to the client's field and extracting a meaningful word that describes his inner world. We find that the client has been internally moved based on the same indications that we pay attention to in constellations. These include a deep sigh, a relaxed posture, and a feeling of getting rid of the burden. An inner change, an intrapsychic shift from one feeling to another, from one image to another, initiates life changes, as when working with the inner attitude in constellations.

The concept of "cognizing body" is consistent with the somatic marker theory formulated by Antonio R. Damasio (2006). He argues that the body provides the brain with more than just physiological support. In fact, it is essential for the proper functioning of the mind. As in the focusing technique, it is considered a kind of cognizing organ. Its special role is revealed in the process of making decisions and reacting to events or people. When we consider alternative decisions, and for a fraction of second negative effects of a choice come to our minds, then we do not even consciously capture this thought; however, the visceral or postural reaction sends the right signal to the brain. This causes that we reject the given choice without even considering why.

Damasio says that somatic markers increase the accuracy and efficiency of decision-making processes. In case of impaired reception and processing of bodily impulses, our life choices, from minor to major ones, become irrational or decision-making becomes inhibited. Thus, the whole body takes part in the cognitive functioning of the brain, contributing substantially to its performance. Interestingly, Damasio emphasizes our urge to "approach" or "withdraw" in the process of somatic marker activity, which can be understood as the primary ways of reacting to the objects of the world. In constellations, the movement "from" and "to" is very important, not to say fundamental. The body and its processes are therefore an essential medium thanks to which the mind does not get lost in the inundation of stimuli.[3]

NOTES

1. Intergenerational healing in the biblical dimension is generally based on several quotations: "I Jehovah thy God am a jealous God, visiting the iniquity of the fathers upon the children, upon the third and upon the fourth generation of them that hate me and showing lovingkindness unto thousands of them that love me and keep my

commandments" (Exodus 20:5–6). The Lord "visiting the iniquity of the fathers upon the children, and upon the children's children, upon the third and upon the fourth generation" but "merciful and gracious, slow to anger, and abundant in lovingkindness and truth, keeping lovingkindness for thousands" (see Exodus 34:6–7). The Lord "visiting the iniquity of the fathers upon the children, upon the third and upon the fourth generation" but "abundant in lovingkindness, forgiving iniquity and transgression," "pardon, I pray thee, the iniquity of this people according unto the greatness of thy lovingkindness" (see Numbers 14:18–19). "I, Jehovah, thy God, am a jealous God, visiting the iniquity of the fathers upon the children, and upon the third and upon the fourth generation [. . .] and showing lovingkindness unto thousands of them that love me" (Deuteronomy 5:9–10). Note that the quotations refer to four generations, which, as we know, is an essential systemic fact. At the same time, God says that He shows lovingkindness to the thousandth generation of those who "love" Him. We can understand this in terms of an act of transgression of generational determinants. Note also that the Apostle Paul, in his Epistle to the Romans, referring to his contemporaries as "the enemies" of God, adds: "they are beloved for the fathers' sake" and says that "the gifts" are passed on to later generations, which also points to the positive influence of the ancestors (Romans 11:28–29).

2. In Christianity, there are also masses intended to heal the genealogical tree. There should be thirty such masses, each for one of the ancestors, in four generations.

3. In the San Francisco Bay Area, "intuitive diagnosis" was taught (Heinze 1999, 162). The physician who conducts the training puts his intern at the foot of the patient's bed and invites him to "tune into the patient." He then asks the intern how he feels, expecting that he "absorbed" the patient's condition. This procedure makes it possible to detect even the imbalances not yet diagnosed by conventional methods.

Part II

TOWARD A NEW PARADIGM IN HUMAN SCIENCES

Chapter 5

Family and Parenting Revisited

ALICE MILLER—HER THEORY AND TRAUMA

The importance of parenting and the role of parents (caregivers) are the basic issues addressed by developmental psychology, guides for parents, many schools of psychotherapy, and common psychological knowledge. We all know that life problems "start in childhood" and it is the parents who are responsible for what it looks like. These beliefs gave rise to concepts that ascribe all the evil in the world to our homes and our parents' behaviors.

An icon of the concept that "bad" parents have a destructive influence on a child's future was the Swiss therapist and writer Alice Miller. Thousands of people have found their own traumas and problems in her works—which, as she admitted, were in many cases autobiographical in nature. Many of those people are grateful to her for having encouraged them to look at their childhood without fear and confront the pain that was then born in them.

However, Miller's concepts have such fundamental weaknesses that they can barely be considered a first step toward the correct understanding of childhood, the role of parents, the essence of trauma, and the ways to deal with it. In this chapter, with reason, I will address not only Alice Miller's views but also some facts about her life.

Miller believed that most adults have a traumatized child in them, and we should give it an opportunity to express its hatred toward the parents. By judging them and naming the wrongs we have suffered from them, we will be able to live happily and not hurt others. And if traumas remain repressed, they will manifest themselves in the form of emotional and physical problems or will lead to psychopathic behaviors. The therapist opposed all concepts that involve forgiveness, claiming that it is never healing. Generalizing Miller's views, one can say that the emotion responsible for any pathology is suppressed hatred, resulting from childhood wounds, and the transition from victim to persecutor is the main mechanism of destructive behaviors. The force that keeps this hatred in the unconscious is the cultural obligation to respect parents.

Thanks to Alice Miller's son, Martin Miller, also a psychotherapist, we can better understand her life and work. Miller started her career with psychoanalysis, but she began to see this practice as a kind of blaming the child and protecting the parents. Miller writes:

> The therapist's efforts are often directed toward reconciling patients with their parents because he has been taught—and is also convinced on a conscious level—that only forgiveness and understanding bring inner peace (which in the child's world is actually the case!). Possibly it is the therapist's unconscious fear of his repressed anger against his own parents that leads him to recommend reconciliation to his patients. In this way he is really rescuing (in the therapeutic process) *his* parents from his own anger, which he imagines to have a fatal effect, because he was never allowed to find out that feelings do not kill. If the therapist is able to relinquish entirely his unconscious identification with the parents and their methods of child-rearing and identify instead with the suffering child, serving as his advocate, in a short time his understanding, freed from anxiety, will set in motion processes that at one time were considered miraculous, because their dynamics had not yet been conceptualized. (Miller 1998, 14)

This quotation demonstrates Miller's way of thinking an the essence of her approach as a therapist. According to the author, any therapist who pursues reconciliation is overcome by repressed hatred, and in order to improve his therapeutic effectiveness, he should abandon his identification with his own parents. Only then will he be able to become an "advocate" of the harmed child in the patient.

Did Miller's recommendations help her patients? How did they work in her own life? Based on what her son Martin revealed, we must conclude that Miller's theory was not so much a result of her work with her patients as a way to prove to herself that her attitude of rejecting her own parents and ancestors was right. After she quit psychoanalysis, Miller wrote rather than practiced therapy, although she implied to her readers that she continued to be a therapist. Her son says:

> My mother would have certainly revised her radical stance if she had tried to validate her ideas in practice. She herself became a victim of her radical feelings of hatred for her parents. She never succeeded in escaping these feelings of hate. (Miller 2018, 153)

Martin Miller wrote that his mother had told him about her childhood in a manner which made it impossible for me to form an emotional connection with my own Jewish heritage, or with my relatives and ancestors. They remained strangers. My mother stressed entirely different matters in her account of her Jewish upbringing. She portrayed Judaism as an authoritarian religion, and her parents as stupid, mentally dull people, who against better judgment held on to all sorts of meaningless rules and laws. (Miller 2018, 27)

In a letter to her son, Alice Miller writes:

> Why did I need sixty years to see how cruel, destructive, exploitative, thoroughly mendacious and loveless my mother was? That she systematically destroyed love and life within me, and later did the same with my sister and my nephew? (Miller 2018, 5)

While it is difficult to say what Miller's mother was actually like, the Swiss therapist's method failed because it did not help its author (although she recognized the value of self-therapy) to cope with the emotions that were difficult for her. Instead, as her son stated, she "ranted about" her parents' behavior all her life and her memories were full of "embitterment and rage" (Miller 2018, 28).[1] Martin Miller wrote:

> She effectively made me feel like a monster she wanted to destroy. [. . .] To be sure, her books were a great success, and in them many readers saw themselves understood, and above all felt accepted in their emotional suffering. However, the books were worlds apart from the real life of Alice Miller and the way she treated her son. It was not a good experience to be the son of Alice Miller—quite the contrary. (Miller 2018, 19)

In the letter to her son, she compares herself to a child who is attacked by him (which her son signals in several other places in his book). This kind of role reversal could not be constructive for Martin, but it is typical of those who do not accept their own parents—they need to find a substitute parent for their inner child. It is also common for people who in their childhood experienced parentification themselves, and put themselves in the adult position toward their parents. And this also was the case in Miller's life. In her books, the author argued that it was best if those who held a grudge against their parents found a better person to understand them in their place. During her stay in France, she stayed with her friend and her family. Martin Miller wrote: "It was not until after my mother's death that I realized how closely she had bound herself to that family" (Miller 2018, 21). This situation is not surprising—if we reject our own roots, we can "bind ourselves" this way, looking for a substitute family (it is often the spouse's family).

The author of *The Drama of the Gifted Child* also had episodes of severe pain in her entire body, which had no medical justification. She tried to find their cause in the relationship with her son, which, in my opinion, is rather another manifestation of the reversal of roles between her and Martin. The actual cause could have been the radical rejection of her parents and ancestors.[2]

Martin Miller's mother tried to control him and got angry when he displayed his own initiative. At the same time, she avoided him, treated him as an enemy, and when there were letters or personal interactions, she tried to analyze his, in her opinion, crazy behavior. However, the factors that she took into account in these ad hoc theories could not be sufficient to explain anything. For she did not consider not only the importance of her relationship with her ancestors, but also even the early abandonment that her son had suffered.[3] It was only in her old age that she admitted in a letter that she had made mistakes in her conduct toward him and that she had avoided admitting this fact all the time. She also stated in this letter:

> I had to see that I had treated my first child almost like my mother had treated me. Despite my training I did not succeed in escaping this fate. (Miller 2018, 133)

This cannot come as a surprise either. If Miller's mother was indeed unsupportive in some sense, it would have been very difficult for Miller herself not to repeat the fundamental elements of her own fate without taking her mother into her heart. However, Miller chose a completely different solution: internal isolation, blaming the mother, and even formulating a theory whose core was "holding the parents accountable."

Pointing out that children are sometimes victims of their parents' withdrawal, indifference, aggressiveness, and unhealthy sexuality is important, and parents should not be protected by denying that they have done something wrong or suppressing awareness, but what Miller proposed works counterproductively. It strengthens unconscious identification, ruins relationships with one's own children, and binds them to the pain of the past.

Alice Miller despised her mother, hated her, and did not want to identify with her:

> I did not want to become like my mother since forever, under any circumstances. Any, even the slightest similarity drove me to despair when I recognized it. (Miller 2018, 6)

However, identification with the parent is a normal and involuntary process, and if we deliberately oppose it, if it arouses our fury, the only effect will be an increase in our internal conflict. The more we reject the parent, the wider we open the back door to him and assume his negative qualities and behaviors, such as malice and alcoholism, instead of accepting him. Not only did Miller, in her writings, oppose identification with the parents, she also blamed her son for "imitating" his father "more and more" and thus losing his chances to develop. Why, then, was she so affected by all the things she wanted to escape from and "save" others from?

Miller wrote to her son: "If at all possible, I want to save your children from also having to suffer because of the curse of your and my childhood" (Miller 2018, 10). Would such "saving" be possible at all? The saving we can give to our child is that we become reconciled with our own parents, his grandparents. Besides, we have the fundamental respect for the other parent, knowing that the child is as strongly connected to him as if he is a part of him. Instead, Miller attacked her son for his relationship with his father. In constellations, we see that almost automatic processes work here—when the parent gets closer to his own parents, the child is instantly freed and strengthened. Acknowledging the other parent results in a breath of relief and an inflow of strength.

Martin Miller speculates that the mother felt affronted because he did not want to drink her milk as an infant and that this affected her attitude toward him. For Alice Miller, who imagined that what happened to the baby had its roots solely in his parent-child relationship, the fact that she had a problem with her son from the very beginning must have been particularly difficult. From the point of view of family constellations, the occurrence of such problems seems to be predictable—Miller rejected her mother along with the entire female line of the family, which extremely weakens subtle maternal competencies. In such a situation, the child also turns away from the mother very easily.

Martin Miller is much closer to the orders of love. He does not judge his mother ruthlessly, but when talking about his suffering, he tries to understand her. He also rebuilds his inner ties with his Jewish ancestors. Only this kind of approach can be free of aporias. Miller instructed her readers to enter into an open dispute with their parents and to not hesitate to describe their activities as criminal, and at the same time she rejected all her own son's objections, being unable to tolerate the slightest criticism. So she violated Kant's principle that one's own maxim can at the same time become a general law: I reject my parents, but I do not want to be rejected by my own child. So I do not follow the general law, but I create my own for my own use. Of course, I will argue that my parents "deserve it" and that I am "better." But what if—as in Miller's case—the child starts to judge me negatively? Will I admit his childlike feelings that I value so highly in a different situation? Miller did not do it for a long time, and her later confessions do not give the impression that she was truly sorry and more aware of the events.

Interestingly, the author stated at some point of her work that if someone's "anger is followed by grief over having been a victim, then they can also mourn the fact that their parents were victims too, and they will no longer have to persecute their children" (Miller 1998, 273). So why did she not express compassion for her own parents? Her works are filled with contempt for parents as such, and she became a persecutor of her son.

There is yet another aspect of Alice Miller's views that a family constellation therapist must address, namely her statements about unwanted children and abortion. Commenting on the reminder that bells rang in Germany in 1989 to make the faithful realize that abortion is a sin, Miller writes:

> Do they not know that mistreatment is a parent's way of taking revenge on the children they never wanted? Shouldn't the authorities do everything in their power, in the light of this information, to see to it that the only children who are born are wanted, planned for, and loved? If they did, then we could put an end to the creation and continuation of evil in our world. To force the role of a mother on a woman who does not wish to be a mother is an offense not just against her, but against the whole human community, because the child she brings into the world is likely to take criminal revenge for its birth, as do many (mis)leaders threatening our lives. [. . .] The injunction against abortion goes even further: Consciously or unconsciously, it represents support for cruelty against children and active complicity in the creation of unwanted existences, existences that can easily become a liability for the community at large. (Miller 1997, 142–43)

Isn't the above quote shocking? The author asks the authorities to do "everything in their power" to kill children who are "unwanted." Note that the person who was supposed to help us free ourselves from the power of our parents basically suggests that we have no meaning other than that attributed to us by our parents. If their attitude toward us is not acceptable, we had better not be born. There is no rescue for us; we will become a "liability for the community." Could there be a clearer declaration of therapeutic helplessness?[4]

Miller does not see not only the life of unborn children but also the whole psychological complexity of the situation where a woman or a man, for various reasons, fear having a child, feel negative emotions related to the child, and are entangled in their own families and external situation. She considers abortion to be one of the techniques to fight against child murder and mistreatment, which has been "part of our 'traditions'" for thousands of years (Miller 1997, 77).

There is something insane about proposing to cope with someone's potential hatred through his early elimination. We see here a specific lack of logic (characteristic also of other authors who accuse parents, as I will show later). Miller considers herself to be an "unwanted" child and her mother to be inappropriate. Should she have been "aborted?" Did she take revenge for her traumas in her life? If she had a different opinion of it, she contradicted her own theories. To follow Miller's peculiar logic—if we were not "wanted," we will be marked forever. In her method, there is no such thing as in the constellation method—a chance for everyone to live a good life, just because they are alive (by the way, how many "wanted" and even "dreamed of" or "craved for" would we find, who now have a grudge against their parents and their lives are a series of failures?). In constellations we lead people to a completely different solution—we lead them to accept their lives with gratitude.

Alice Miller's ideas may have been formed as a result of her experiences in childhood and the unconscious attitude adopted at the time. One of my clients, Lucia, said during a constellation, that in her childhood she was surprised that people got so emotional when a child died in a car accident. She said, "Do they not think that the child might have been unloved by his parents?" She believed she was unwanted herself. Sometimes she thought that it might have been better if her parents had died. The constellation showed that this "unloving" in her family had begun with the death of her grandmother's parents, when she had been a child, with grief and anger she had not experienced. Interestingly, Lucia gave the impression of being warm, open, and ready to develop. She agreed that certain things in her mind—as she put it—got "twisted."

One of the German editions of Martin Miller's book about his mother is subtitled "The tragedy of Alice Miller: How repressed war trauma affects the family" (*Die Tragödie Alice Millers—Wie verdrängte Kriegstraumata in der Familie wirken*). This trauma explains Alice Miller's many behaviors, her style of raising children, and the main theses of her work. Alicija Englard, which was her real first and maiden name, was a Polish Jew who survived the bombing of her hometown Piotrków Trybunalski in September 1939, hid in Warsaw until the Warsaw Uprising—during which the Germans destroyed the capital of Poland, killing about 150,000 people—and finally escaped across the Vistula river, which was the front line, to the Russians. At that time, she saw death and cruelty, and a large part of her family died—her father in the ghetto, the others—in gas chambers in the camps. She never referred to these matters.

Miller was interested in the roots of tyranny and genocide and found them in the social problem of parental maltreatment of children. She also authored analyses of Adolf Hitler's childhood. However, she disregarded the impact of his actions on her own family and on herself. She never linked the injury of children to external and random events, and she always considered parents to be the ones who caused traumas. Underlying the evil of Nazism were Hitler's parents; underlying her personal misery were her parents. The role of war experiences as such remained taboo for her. Wasn't discovering "painful truths" about her own parents and patients' parents a defense against a far greater trauma?

Miller fell victim to the process I described in the book *Systemic Constellations: Theory, Practice, and Applications*—she attributed the consequences of externally determined traumas to the parents' indifference, stupidity, and meanness. She directed her fury primarily at her mother (and her sister). Much seems to indicate, however, that it was caused or magnified by war events. The life of a Jew in Warsaw under German occupation was extremely dangerous and exhausting emotionally. Alicija Englard felt, as she said herself, threatened by the demeanor of her mother, who did not renounce her Jewish identity. She was also threatened by the necessity to take care of her younger sister, who she managed to hide in the convent. Miller confessed to her son: "For fear of death I could no longer know at all who I was. I had to impose total self-control upon myself" (Miller 2018, 45). She stated that she was afraid of her "own liveliness," that she "had to erase" her "whole biography" and "construct a new person" out of herself, "a false identity" (Miller 2018, 45–46).[5]

Because of her negation of the war trauma, some of Miller's arguments sound bizarre. While she advocates considering real circumstances rather than drives and fantasies, she completely ignores the reality of war. For example, she writes that when people describe their "childhood experiences that were free of conflict," these usually "concern experiences with nature,"

> which they could enjoy without hurting the mother or making her feel insecure, without reducing her power or endangering her equilibrium. But it is remarkable how these attentive, lively, and sensitive children who can, for example, remember exactly how they discovered the sunlight in bright grass at the age of four [. . .] at the age of two, one of them could be left alone while soldiers forced their way into the house and searched it, and she had "been good," suffering this quietly and without crying. They have all developed the art of not experiencing feelings, for a child can only experience his feelings when there is somebody there who accepts him fully, understands and supports him. (Miller 1981, 9–10)

It is hard to say what psychodynamics lies behind this kind of repression of feelings—we all lose part of our childlike sensitiveness. Something else is important in this case. Miller refers to the reality of occupation as if parenthetically, as to any other ordinary situation that could be given as an example. The child was calm when "soldiers forced their way into the house and searched it," because earlier—this is Miller's perspective—the child had suffered harm from her parents who had not understood her and had not accepted her feelings. Even if one were to agree that in the case of a child such as the one described, the parents' behavior played a decisive role in shaping her cutting off from deeper feelings, the simplest clinical honesty requires considering the circumstances of war and how it shaped the parents' actions. We can guess that Miller writes about herself, about the fact that during the war—as she said—she had to "kill herself" to survive (Miller 2018, 46).

TOXIC PARENTS?

In her book *Toxic Parents*, Susan Forward presents an approach similar to that of Alice Miller. The basic assumptions of Forward's therapy seem to be as follows: many of our problems are caused by our parents; patients are extremely resistant to noticing—as she often refers to it—the "inadequacy" of their parents; overcoming this resistance is necessary to improve the patient's functioning, which causes that the patient becomes independent, distances himself, and sometimes separates himself from the parents; it is also important for the patient to find other, supportive and loving persons.

To give an example of Forward's thinking and style of work, let us use fragments of sessions with the patient named Sandy. Sandy's parents, practicing Christians, opposed her decision to terminate her pregnancy when she was a teenager. Her father criticized her for seeing boys and even allegedly called her a "whore." The patient's parents were described by the author as "cruel and emotionally abusive" (Forward and Buck 2002, 20), although it is difficult to find evidence for such an extreme assessment in the text. Sandy terminated her pregnancy at the age of under sixteen, and when she was twenty-eight she unsuccessfully tried for a child. She said:

> This whole pregnancy has become a real obsession with me. When I had lunch with my mom I told her how disappointed I was. She said to me, "I'll bet it's that abortion you had. The Lord works in mysterious ways." I haven't been able to stop crying since. She never lets me forget. (Forward and Buck 2002, 18)

Sandy's only problem that Forward raises is her dependence on her parents. The therapist sees neither her potential guilt, the possible weight of the abortion and marital problems, nor the patient's possible personality problems (the threat to commit suicide). Forward sees Sandy's words that she wants to make it up to her parents "for hurting them so bad" with her "sins" as a mere resistance to accepting the brutal truth: the parents "have failed," they are "cruel," they are not "loving enough," and so on. The therapist ignores the fact that a sixteen-year-old person who is allegedly so dependent forced her decision to have an abortion.

Forward writes that most societies "glorify mothers, as if the mere act of giving birth makes them inherently capable of nurturing" (Forward and Frazier-Glynn 2013, 13). Even if mothers were "glorified," the path of solution does not lead "from" the mother, and it still leads "to" the mother. If we focus on "nurture" and its deficiencies, and completely lose sight of the bond with the mother as the source of life, we will turn away from our own life. This will affect every sphere of life, from health to relationships. For a child, the fact that he was born by this and not another woman is essential. That is why we never consider "parenting incompetence" to be essential. It is not here that the most important determinants of the child's life stem from.

The therapist tries to direct her patients toward independence and maturity, and toward liberation from the dependence on their parents that is destructive for their lives. We do the same in constellations. However, Forward does not acknowledge the existence of deep bonds between children and parents. She does not know that improving the relationship with parents (above all accepting them as parents internally) is a healing factor in itself. According to Forward, a person's parents are nobody special. Their existence does not affect the inner world of a healthy person; it only affects a person who is dependent and abused by his parents.

Forward writes, "No matter how toxic your parents might be, you still have a need to deify them. Even if you understand, on one level, that your father was wrong to beat you, you may still believe he was justified" (Forward and Buck 2002, 17). I see it quite differently. A lot of people do not "deify" their parents, and at the same time often reject them. However, if there is a need to defend or protect a parent in patients, we must not see it as a mere manifestation of social modeling. Behind the fact that patients defend their parents—including what they do not have to or should not defend in them—there is an irreducible bond. If this bond is not addressed or if it is attacked by the therapist, his patients will not free themselves from indeed "toxic" loyalties, but will plunge into them, only on an unconscious level.

When Sandy says—using religious language—that her parents were simply trying to "save her soul" and adds "If they didn't love me so much, they wouldn't care," the therapist goes on to intervene in a bizarre way:

Susan: Let's look at this from a different perspective. What if you hadn't had that abortion? And you had a little girl. She'd be about sixteen now, right?

Sandy nodded, trying to figure out where I was headed.

Susan: Suppose she got pregnant? Would you treat her like your parents treated you?

Sandy: Not in a million years!

Sandy realized the implications of what she'd said.

Susan: You'd be more loving. And your parents should have been more loving. That's their failure, not yours. (Forward and Buck 2002, 20)

The above reasoning is quite twisted. To see it better, let us go further and imagine that Sandy is talking to her sixteen-year-old daughter Sandra, who she did give birth to:

Sandy: When I was your age, it all looked different. My parents were absolutely against my idea to have an abortion. They threatened me, said that if I did this, they didn't want to see me anymore. I was under such pressure (crying). It's hard to describe it. I didn't want to give birth to you at all, but I couldn't resist them, I gave in. So now I know what it's like when parents are so cruel. I would never let you experience what I've experienced. You can terminate this pregnancy, my child.
Sandra: Thank you, mom, for being different from my grandparents. If I had parents like you have, it would be hard for me to endure.

My goal was not to ironize, but to highlight the illogicality of Forward's reasoning. As one can see, to save the thesis about the total role of the parents' attitude in Sandy's problems, Forward does not refrain from idealizing the patient and fantasizing about her alleged parental qualities.

The main objectives of therapy that we can find in Forward's works, that is, emotional separation from negative influences from parents, strengthening one's independence, and detaching oneself from the parents' judgments, are in line with what happens during constellations. Also ending the struggle to change parents and allowing them to be as they are is in line with the aims of family constellation therapy. However, Forward's ways to reach these goals are completely different from the actions of the constellation therapist who is aware of the loyalty processes that exist between children and parents.

Nevertheless, the therapist's following statement is almost Hellingerian:

> Emotional independence doesn't mean that you have to cut yourself off from your parents. It means that you can be part of the family while at the same time being a separate individual. It means you can be who you are and let your parents be who they are. (Forward and Buck 2002, 194)

Forward invited Sandy's parents, and her father said, "You don't know what a bad kid she was, Doctor. She went nuts over boys and kept leading them on. All of her problems today are because of that damned abortion"

(Forward and Buck 2002, 23). The therapist immediately—as she wrote herself—"rushed to defend" Sandy. She considered abortion to be an irrelevant event and was not interested in the attitude of the parents, whom she treated as enemies.[6] After this session, the patient tried to defend her parents, said that they "really loved her" and asked Forward to "give them some time," but she seemed to ignore all of this, stating in the book that the session proved that Sandy's parents were "closed-minded" to "anything that challenged their perception of Sandy's problems."[7]

So Forward believes that it is possible and necessary to "defend" the patient against his parents. As a constellation therapist, I see this quite differently. In some extreme cases—if we are social workers or police officers—we can rescue people from their parents. As psychotherapists, we are obliged to see and respect the depth of the child's relationship with them. Some therapists think that they can take the place between the parent and the child and manage it as they wish. They argue that there is "no bond" between the individual and his parents, or that the parents "do not love" the individual. They think that there is nothing in the psyche that connects the person to those from whom he was born. In their opinion, one can free oneself from negative emotions, memories, or loyalty to his parents, and become someone completely unrelated to them. But these are just usurpations and fantasies. In fact, one can only become free from unnecessary loyalties and tormenting memories by acknowledging one's bond with one's parents.

In constellations, we leave grief and painful history behind by putting it in a broader multigenerational context, and by connecting with our parents, we gain strength that flows from the family. According to Forward, our losses are obvious and lasting, and the source of strength can only be other people. She writes:

> Once you understand what love is, you may come to the realization that your parents couldn't or didn't know how to be loving. This is one of the saddest truths you will ever have to accept. But when you clearly define and acknowledge your parents' limitations, and the losses you suffered because of them, you open a door in your life for people who will love you the way you deserve to be loved—the real way. (Forward and Buck 2002, 305)

For many, it will be a path toward a permanent sense of deficiency and own incompleteness along with a futile search for "love," always associated with failures. For, the absence of reconciliation with one's parents will always lead to a deficit, which will affect many areas of one's life. If we do as the author of the book about "toxic" parents recommends, we will open a door not to people but to illusions. The love we give and receive in relationships with men and women is not the same love that is desired by the part of us connected to our parents. Reaching maturity and autonomy without reconstructing our bond with our parents, without accepting this profound bond, will leave a permanent deficit in our psyche. It will subject us to any manipulation of our own psyche and of other people who we want to see as "truly" loving.

Accepting or rejecting one's parents, especially the mother, is not only associated with a better or worse mood. Sometimes life or death is at stake. Internal rejection of the mother may result in serious illnesses. This was the case with Xenia.[8] She came to me with a whole bunch of problems, ranging from her relationship with her ex-husband, through problems with her son and longing for her current partner, to the issue of cancerous tumors in her internal organs. I started with her health, asking her to stand in front of the sheet of paper that represented her illness. Then I stood on this sheet and "followed my movement"—I spread my arms out, and a word addressed to the client came to my mind: "Child!" I asked Xenia what she felt and she replied: "fear." With the word "child" in my mind, I asked if she was afraid of her father. She said she was not. "And the mother?" "I've never been close with my mother, she's had constant resentment . . . and when she talks about her diseases . . . compared to what's happening to me"—Xenia changed her face as if she were going to cry. To test the hypothesis that her mother mattered here, I wrote "Mother" on another piece of paper, put it on the floor, and stood on it "as the mother." I immediately felt the same as before and spread my arms to the sides as if to embrace. It does not matter what Xenia's mother was like, whether she was hard to bear or not. Xenia compensated herself for the lack of a close bond with her through the reactions of her body. Her tumors represented her mother, or actually the missing bond with her mother.

What can we do to change our situation? Forward tells us to accept the fact that we will not get what we needed as children from our parents, and states:

> The striving child within you probably still clings to the hope that someday your parents—no matter how limited they are—will see how wonderful you are and give you their love. [. . .] but when you go back to your toxic parents for the nourishment and validation that you missed as a child, it's a lot like going back to an empty well for water. Your bucket is going to come up dry. (Forward and Buck 2002, 302)

We should stop waiting for our parents' move. And we often have to accept that our parents will not change. And yet, it turns out that if we want it, our bucket will not come up dry. Hellinger expressed this in the words: "The move is up to the child." This surprising discovery breaks with the whole tradition of psychology according to which "what's done cannot be undone" and "what we didn't get" is already gone. We can take from our parents what we wanted as children and what we still want deep inside. It turns out that there is a process that enables us to control whether we will let the emotional deficit remain within us or will sooner or later—sometimes just in one session—leave it behind. Working at this level has far more profound consequences than dealing with the emotional level in a conventional sense. When our childlike part opens up to the source of its life, which are the parents, the pain and reproach for them begin to suddenly fade.

Forward opposes forgiveness because she believes it would be a form of denial: "If I forgive you, we can pretend that what happened wasn't so terrible" (Forward and Buck 2002, 178). The question arises, however, why stress that "it was so terrible." Do we have to prove with our lives that our parents made mistakes? Or would it be better to give it up? Some people are trapped by a grudge against their parents that prevents them from being fully independent and enjoying life. They believe that all they have is "evidence" in the form of their memories and pain, which they treat as internal anti-capital. These people live in infantile pain and in a demand for compensation from their parents. As we work with them, we lead them to connect with their parents as parents, although initially they want to focus solely on their "evidence." As if something in them were saying: "You can't forget." In such cases, the conflict between love and justice is clearly revealed during a constellation. A sense of justice turns out to be a life-destroyer. To live a better life, one must go beyond it, toward love that does not judge. Even in the case of great trauma and a great demand for redress, only a step toward one's parents brings true relief and life energy. However, Forward states that instead of forgiving, one should get rid of one's responsibility and put it on one's parents' shoulders. In constellations, we also work with similar processes, which we refer to as "leaving what belongs to the parents with them," "leaving the past in the past," and so on. However, we always do this with respect, so that this is not a way for someone to revenge or accuse the parents. Then he would not be able to truly give these burdens back. They would become a substitute for the broken bond with the parents and the son or daughter would cling to them even more. This is how the unconscious conscience works, the conscience that Forward underestimates, seeing only a social convention ("Love your parents!") in its manifestations.

In constellations, we do not speak of "forgiving." Something similar happens in them, but in a completely different way than the one we usually associate with forgiving: despite the pain, I let go of something, I stop blaming someone, holding a grudge against them, and so on. In constellations, the pain disappears, and in its place comes gratitude. If we spoke of "forgiving" in constellations, we would position ourselves and the client in the sphere of judgments, that is, of classifying the others as good or bad, of exalting and humiliating. If we encouraged the client to "forgive" his parents, we would put him above them and thus violate the system hierarchy. This would have a destructive effect on the client. He would have to pay for elevating himself above his parents and become "small" in other areas—health, work, or other relationships. By giving up judgments, the client has a chance to open up to what the parent still has to give him and what he has not yet taken. The child, by isolating himself from the pain, blocks the power flowing from the parents and the power flowing through them from previous generations.

The arbitrary judgments about who was and who was not loved and who could and could not love are Forward's biggest psychological misconception. Forward assumes the position of someone who knows perfectly well what love is, she assures her readers: "And I'll help you gain an understanding, perhaps for the first time, of what real love from a parent, or anyone, looks and feels like" (Forward and Frazier-Glynn 2013, 6). It is a huge usurpation and psychological naivety. Forward uses a kind of questionnaire to "separate" loving mothers from unloving mothers (Forward and Frazier-Glynn 2013, 7). The therapist knows nothing about the family histories of her patients or the lives of their parents. What truth can be said about, for example, the love of a mother who did not notice her second child because she remained by the first one who had died? That she is an "unloving" mother? And if it were a twin sister who died in the womb, for whom unconscious longing made the mother unable to truly engage in any emotional relationship, even with her own child? Can this be judged at all?

That is why we move with each client toward "accepting the parents as parents." What are "parents as parents?" They are all that "remains" of parents when we leave aside their character, their words, events related to them, and the suffering they have caused us. Then, for the conventional therapist, there is little or nothing left. As is the case for many people who say, for example, about their father: "He only made my mother pregnant," or about their mother: "She only gave birth to me." Thanks to family constellations, we discovered how much such words are inappropriate here. When we manage to put stories and grievances aside, we can feel how much it means that this man and this woman are our parents. Accepting parents as the only beginning of our existence is of great importance to our health and well-being. Any judgment of our parents will stop us on this path, so the label "toxic parents" introduced by Forward may have a strong anti-therapeutic effect.

THE NURTURE ASSUMPTION

Parents are Unimportant?

For Alice Miller or Susan Forward, finding the causes of a child's difficulties in his parents' behavior was easy. Their conclusions came down to simple schemes. Forward's patient, Sandy, suffers due to her parents' intransigence. Eli, a multimillionaire unable to enjoy his life, whose suspicion of women "bordered on paranoia" and who was constantly afraid of bankruptcy, owes this to his father, who told him that he should save every penny. According to Miller, the Nuremberg Laws against Jews were related to the fact that Hitler had been beaten by his father, and the order to murder the mentally ill was related to the fact he had had to endure the company of his mentally ill aunt (Miller 1990). Some of these kinds of cause-and-effect connections may seem to be convincing. It turns out, however, that they are generally not so. When we work with family constellations, we discover that the causes are much more complex and simple connections often serve as a kind of rationalization. Despite the apparent obviousness, such relationships do not explain human behavior, but may rather be a kind of illusion. Our behaviors and moods are also influenced by persons other than our parents, by those we do not even think about. A psychologist analyzing our biography will not think about them all the more.

It is not surprising, then, that scientific research also fails to confirm simple relationships between the behavior of parents and the personality and behavior of their children. In the 1990s, an independent researcher, Judith Rich Harris, challenged traditional psychology by claiming that the way a child is reared is not essential when it comes to the development of his personality (Harris 1995). She referred to the belief that it is parents who form their children's traits, being the most important part of the children's life environment, as "nurture assumption" (Harris 1998, 2). Everyone believes in this assumption, from professors of psychology to uneducated parents. Everyone knows that one should "give children plenty of love and approval, set limits and enforce them firmly but fairly," that one should not use "physical punishment or make belittling remarks, be consistent, et cetera" (Harris 1998, 17). Then we have a big chance that our child will grow into a valuable and happy person. Harris said there was no evidence of this.

The assertion that parents do not have much influence on their child's traits aroused negative reactions, and some psychologists called it absurd. According to the author, parents are only important as the first teachers and caregivers who, by providing material resources, make the child's development and education possible. However, the kind of person their child will become is essentially beyond the significant influence of the parents. Such a perspective on the parents' function and role undermines the idea—cultivated for decades—that their meaning in the child's life is fundamental. Harris concludes that differences in the form of care provided by parents are irrelevant "as long as the kind of care the parents provide is within the normal range for our species" (Harris 2007, 61). At the same time, she concludes based on many studies that this normal range is very wide (Harris 2007, 61).

From the point of view of systemic constellations, the author's conclusions do not shock. Constellations confirm the thesis of limited parental influence on the child's personality for the following reasons:

- Children's psyche (personality) is determined not only by their parents but by the whole family system. Parents are an important element of this system, but only an element. Children are influenced by their grandparents, some former parents' partners, siblings, excluded persons, also those from the third or fourth generation. It should be stressed, however, that these people are important because of their very existence (especially if they were forgotten or unknown) and because of their fates (especially if these were dramatic), and not because of the influence of their personality traits (which we do not observe in constellations).
- The future behavior or emotionality and personality of children is primarily influenced by factors independent of what verbally or even by "own example" is transmitted by parents to their child. These factors are related to the structure of the family, past events, exclusions, and traumas. Parents often do not know about them themselves, have no possibility to control them, or are not interested in them. This also includes personal histories and internal attitudes of parents (e.g., repressed grudge against one's own mother, reluctance to take responsibility for an abortion, putting oneself above one's parents or older siblings, and many more). Parents "transmit" to their child affective states associated with these attitudes, but this transmission has nothing to do with what they consciously want to communicate. To give just one example, a parent who focuses on fun and humor may as well "transmit" his own hidden depression to his child.
- The child is an active participant in the events and ultimately it is the child who creates and sustains his individual "response" to what he encounters. Therefore, referring to the above, it is more accurate to say that the child himself "takes from the parent" than that the parent "transmits" something to the child. Of course, this happens quite unconsciously.
- There is a very early prenatal and perinatal influence, which is generally not taken into account neither by parents nor researchers. Of course, it has nothing to do with the personality of the parents, let alone their child-rearing methods.

- Children are affected not so much by how we treat them, but by how we treat other people. First of all, our own parents—what our internal attitude toward them is. Also, how we treated our previous partners and—if we had them—children from previous relationships. Of course, it includes unborn children. Researchers always focus on the present family completely without seeing the foundation from which it stems.

If we take the above factors into account, the apparently absurd research results seem to be fully possible. Harris writes that "most of the things that were believed to have important effects on children turn out not to have important effects on them" (Harris 1998, 39). As a systemic constellation therapist, I have observed the same: most of the events that clients see as determining their lives are not. The father's alcoholism, the mother's favoring the other child, or the parents' "constant quarrels" do not turn out to be what is behind the client's problems.

Harris shows that much of what was considered to be the effect of nurture is in fact due to heredity. The similarities between children and parents, or between siblings, cannot be explained by the fact that they live together. Actually, there are the same similarities between biological parents and their children given up for adoption, and between siblings who were raised separately. The children of "peaceful parents" are "peaceful" not due to upbringing, but because they are genetically related to "peaceful" people. In other words, because of the genes.[9]

But do we really deal here with material genes studied by biochemists, or do the studies simply show heredity? In constellation therapy, for example, we may encounter clients suffering from a variety of anxieties, whose mothers or fathers were also full of anxiety. It is not infrequent that the grandmother or grandfather also experienced anxiety. Harris and behavioral geneticists cited by the author would probably consider it an effect of genes. However, children become similar to their parents not only because they are biologically similar but also because they may be subject to similar intergenerational influences, or unconsciously take on the burden of their parents. If we look at inheritance in this way, we introduce the factors that have not been taken into account so far, which are not "environmental" in the usual sense, and are not "genetic" either, they are contained in the family field.

Parents Are Important, Upbringing Is Less Important

Harris writes that she did not try to "argue that parents don't matter but to answer a question about *differences* in parenting: Are differences in the kind of care parents provide, or in the way they provide it, responsible for the differences in how the children turn out?" (Harris 2007, 61). However, apart from the mentioned kinds of care, she did not discover any fundamental importance of parents for the child, other than purely economic. Even if this is the conclusion of science, many people feel that parents are important. So what is the truth?

Whether parents succeed in influencing their children according to their own assumptions is one thing; whether their presence in the children's lives has any psychological effect on them is quite another. The parents' attitudes toward their children are one thing, and the children's attitudes—including the unconscious attitudes—toward their parents are another thing. The latter is of great importance, although Harris does not address it at all.

According to attachment theory, a child enters into adult relationships according to the patterns he developed in his early interaction with the mother. Harris questions such concepts, and is followed by Steven Pinker who says that "unlikely is the idea that a baby's attachment to its mother sets the pattern for its commerce with the world" (Harris 1998, xiii). On the other hand, Harris herself states, for example, that "it is going against nature to let a baby cry" referring to the fact that in hunter-gatherer bands babies were never left alone at night, as today, which is often recommended by advice-givers (Harris 1998, 343–44). Indeed, members of traditional societies did not think about "how to talk so kids will listen," but they never underestimated the prenatal period and the early bond with the mother. Harris writes:

> Babies in these societies are not read to; they are not even talked to very much. [. . .] Although these babies learn very little during their two years in their mothers' arms, that does not keep them from learning, when the time is ripe, all the things they need to know to become successful adults. (Harris 1998, 344)

So, can these "two years in the mother's arms" be important? Thanks to constellations, we know that the early bond with the mother and the perinatal events do matter. But we see this period and the processes related to it in a new way, absent in the old psychology. As for the perinatal period, we see that the disturbances that can occur here result, for example, in what I refer to as "incomplete birth." An incomplete birth means, in particular, that someone has not fully accepted his life, his being in the world, or does not fully feel he is alive. These are internal states of mind with great consequences for the individual's life.

Take the case of Claudia as an example. She came for her third constellation—the previous two improved many things in her life, but the feeling of constant sadness and lack of joy in life remained. When I stood as Claudia, I lay down on the floor quite quickly. I asked the client about her birth. It turned out that the birth had been difficult and the baby had had blood transfusions. Then it was Claudia who was lying as a newborn, and I stood as her "life."

It was difficult for her to accept it, she kept rejecting it. What was important here was the attitude of Claudia's mother, who was not sure if the child would survive and distanced herself from her probably for that reason. When it finally turned out that the daughter was alive, there was no visible turning point—something of the previous sense of "temporality" remained. Claudia looked at herself through the traumatized eyes of her mother. She did not let herself feel completely alive. The solution to the problem was in Claudia's hands. It was to deeply realize that: "It's over" and that "It's okay now, I'm here." The relationship with the mother was, however, crucial in this case, because Claudia had to stop feeling obliged to carry her mother's fear, and this was only possible when she accepted the mother as she was. Claudia had to understand and accept both her mother's fears and the fact that she never got a clear signal from her that she had already stopped being afraid and had begun to be happy about her birth.

Our parents are so essential for our success in life, health, our professional and personal success that almost every constellation leads to the issue of relationships with them. What is most important, however, is not that our parents, by this or that conduct, have shaped constructive or nonconstructive attitudes toward life in us. Parents are important because our attitude toward them is important. Which is often implicit and unconscious for ourselves. Our attitude toward them is related to how they treated us, but there is no simple correlation. Our attitudes are influenced by random events, our siblings, our unconscious perception, transgenerational factors, and finally, our own sensitivity.

Parents are important also for another reason. Constellations have discovered, for example, how strong disorder occurs as a result of concealment of paternity. Interestingly, its effects can be felt more strongly by later generations. Children, even grandchildren, and sometimes great-grandchildren remain internally unsettled due to the exclusion of their ancestors. I have encountered a case where the excluded was represented by leg problems manifesting in later generations. All of this also strongly influences those persons' fates, choices, and relationships. The powerful meaning of biological parents becomes apparent here, although—as we can see—not the meaning usually expected by psychology.

Methodological Limitations of Psychology

Does research indicate that the relationship with the mother may be of any kind and will not affect the child's life? By no means. Research only shows that there are no repeating relationships between identifiable personality types and behavioral patterns of people and what the researchers were able to identify as characteristics of their early relationship with the mother. This means that academic science has not found these relationships. Of course, this does not mean that they do not exist. The methodology of psychological research has many weaknesses. It very often involves simply remembering the facts of one's life. This is obviously encumbered by many distorting factors. The investigated persons do not remember or do not want to remember certain events, they do not want to admit certain traits or behaviors, and they understand questions in various ways. Parents describe their children, teenagers describe their parents, and adults describe their childhood in their own way, following their own motives. Harris herself points out that researchers tend to correlate statements with statements, not facts with facts. She gives an example of a study in which teenagers who *said* that their relationships with their parents worked out well and that their parents loved them *said* less often that they smoked cigarettes and had sex (Harris 1998, 322). Can we learn anything about facts from such studies?[10]

Researchers try to derive facts from statements, which is a task involving the risk of huge errors. On the other hand, when it comes to relationships and mental experiences, the very category of "fact" fails. External observation turns out to be insufficient to describe this multidimensional sphere, which is human relationships, emotions, and the inner world. What an observer considers to be violence or vulgarity, a woman who is in a relationship with her lover will judge as involvement, passion, or any other value. Or the other way round.

When working with constellations, I do not follow what the client tells me, for example, about his relationship with the mother. It is not that his words mean nothing, but what they mean and what is the deeper truth about the relationship remains an open question in the beginning. It is different in academic studies—the researcher must immediately "know" what the studied person's words mean in order to be able to put them in the right place in the table. That is why he touches only the surface from the very beginning of his research, and risks making a mistake.

Academic psychologists avidly study variables that are themselves complexes of mixed factors, often mutually suppressing one another. If we examine maternal behaviors based on mothers' statements about their ways of raising a child, we arrive at a collection of data that may say little about reality. The mother who says that "the child should always be kept an eye on" can understand this in many ways—as caring for him, criticizing him, supporting him, or living his life. She may repeat an opinion she has heard or something she thinks one should do even though she does not do it. The mother may try to create an idealized image of herself, she may not remember her true actions, or repress the truth. It may seem to her that she supports the child while she unknowingly burdens him. Her words alone will not build a true picture of her actions and impact on the child. This picture is built by the researcher.

Judith came for a constellation to work on her son's problems. He was her only living child, after him she had two miscarriages and one abortion for medical reasons, as she said. Judith declared—and there was no reason to doubt it—that she loved her son and was ready to support him.

In the constellation, there were representatives of Judith, her husband, son, and the unborn children. The son initially felt very bad, strongly empathizing with his mother, who was standing on the other side of the room, bending over, and expressing suffering (naturally, I am writing about the representatives). Finally, however, when the mother turned to her unborn children and her husband—expecting him to come over and help her in her suffering—the son felt relief. It turned out that the "abortion for medical reasons" worked like a normal abortion, causing the mother's internal pain and the partners to grow apart.

When at some point the mother approached her son, he felt worse again. He loved her, but needed her to be in a relationship with his father, while she felt rejected by her husband and turned to the son. But then she brought with her the whole burden of the unresolved attitude to the abortion and her husband. The son clearly felt this and weakened. What the representative felt during those few minutes was what had burdened the son's psyche for years.

And what would we arrive at through academic research? We would have a superficial description of the client's marriage, an abortion "for medical reasons" which is unlikely to affect the son's problems, and a loving mother who certainly does not intend to burden her child with anything.

Internal Attitude, Not Personality

During therapeutic work, the relationships between the child's psychic life and the figures of the parents are so evident that they cannot be denied. However, the exponents of academic psychology fell into a kind of intellectual nonchalance about these, as they thought, obvious relationships. There were many simplifications and too hasty "jumping" from parent figures to the functioning of children. Harris decided to take a look at this and the whole concept of the enormous influence of parents on children turned out to be more than questionable. This led to her radical thesis that parents do not matter psychologically. Here, however, she herself made an unjustified saltus without knowing any data other than academic research. Researchers speak of "personality traits" or "behavioral patterns" and these are generally quite rough constructions, as they must relate to larger groups and must be measurable. Therapists can see more diverse and subtle manifestations of the psyche. These are the dynamisms that affect our lives in a covert way. One of them is what I refer to as "internal attitude."

Working as constellation psychotherapists, we are hardly interested in our clients' personalities. Some of them are nice on the outside, whereas others are secretive, cheerful, or quiet. What really matters in their lives is beyond the usual "personality" traits.

Outwardly, two people may be quite different, and their personalities may not constitute any common category. And yet a rich businessman may have similarly conditioned problems with money as a person who cannot start any business. Those who seem to be very similar, for example, open, bright, proactive, travel-loving, and book-loving, may display completely different internal orientations. And while, as studies show, personality has little to do with parents, the "internal" attitude relates to them very clearly. However, it is difficult to determine it based on some external indicators. It is not a simple result of parental influences, but a result of one's childhood events, parents' inner attitude, intergenerational events and traumas, and the subject's own mental activity.

The importance of parents manifests itself in a different way than is usually presented. The parenting styles—the adopted tactics of dealing with children—are not of decisive importance for their future lives. Children brought up in one way or another may or may not have later problems, as this depends on a wider range of factors. What is important in the relationship with parents is also not what is typically mentioned. The most important thing is the child's attitude toward the parent, not the other way around. Naturally, the child's attitude is related to that of the parent, but there is no simple relationship here.

Harris writes, for instance, that boys raised without a father are not "less masculine" than those who grow up in nuclear families (Harris 2007, 256). This is probably a correct conclusion from the research. But does it really point to the insignificance of the father in the life of the son as a man? Let us see how many questionable points there are here. The first objection is the definition of "masculinity." What does it mean that someone is "masculine"? The researchers had to choose and assume some criteria. Perhaps those resulted from self-description, such as: "I consider myself masculine," or maybe: "I always carry the suitcases and read the map while traveling." Let us assume, however, that we know what masculinity is; then there is another question, whether the one presented by the subject is original "masculinity" or one that is supposed to compensate for the feeling of lack of masculinity? The latter—if it exists—will absorb additional energy, deprive of spontaneity, cause tension, and so on. So there will be no lack of "masculinity," but something completely different will fail, something that the researchers will not notice.

The fact that statistically there are no differences between men raised without or with a father does not implicate that the father does not matter. One can be without a father and respect him deeply, or one can be with a father and despise him or be afraid of him. And this alone affects one's attitude as a man. However, in survey research, this can be difficult to identify. As constellations show, people are generally not fully aware of their deep attitude toward their parents.

Harris also refers to the research which shows that children raised by widowed mothers fare better than children from other types of single-parent families (Harris 1998, 302). This has proved extremely difficult for the researchers to explain. From the point of view of family constellations, we could speculate that in such families, the children are more likely to internally accept the father than, for example, those raised by divorced mothers or the ones who were single from the beginning, where the father figure is more often excluded by the mother.

The Myth of the Influence of Upbringing

What Harris's stance and family constellations have in common is defending the parents—by showing the wrong understanding of their role. The unjustified belief in the supremacy of parental influence is responsible for blaming parents for their children's failures in Western societies. Harris, like Hellinger, opposes this widespread disrespect for parents and constant demands addressed to them. She writes:

> The nurture assumption is the product of a culture that has as its motto, We can overcome. With our dazzling electronic devices, our magical biochemical elixirs, we can overcome nature. Sure, children are born different, but that's no problem. Just put them through this marvelous machine here—step right up, ladies and gentlemen!—and add our special patented mixture of love, limits, time-outs, and educational toys. Voilà! (Harris 1998, 351)

> There is no evidence that the nurture assumption has done any real good. But it has done some real harm. It has put a terrible burden of guilt on parents unfortunate enough to have a child whose pass through the marvelous machine has for some reason failed to produce a happy, smart, well-adjusted, self-confident person. Not only must these parents suffer the pain of having a child who is difficult to live with or who fails in some other way to live up to the community's standards: they must also bear the community's opprobrium. [. . .] Parents are nervous about doing the wrong thing, fearful that a stray word or glance might ruin their child's chances forever. Not only have they become servants to their children—they have been declared unsatisfactory servants, because the standards set by the promulgators of the nurture assumption are so high that no one can meet them. (Harris 1998, 352)

Thanks to constellations, we know that there are more fundamental factors for human functioning than educational toys, praise, or even "showing" feelings to the child, although it is good and important. These factors are transgenerational influences, the parents' attitude toward their own parents and other family members, family secrets (e.g., related to the concealment of paternity or the existence of siblings), and the child's internal mental activity.

One of the basic guidelines of the constellation therapist's approach is respect for parents, even those who have "failed." Why do we have respect for them? Because we have respect for our clients. We must have respect for the client's parents because his psyche is irrevocably connected with them. How could we help him without respecting his parents? Of course, there are clients who do not have the slightest respect for their parents. However, we must not enter into an alliance with that part of the client that, influenced by the myth of upbringing, accuses the parents or, under the influence of the feeling of being abandoned, considers them unimportant. The real change and strength will come when we transcend these difficulties and move toward the bond that exists at a deeper level.

There are several ways here. The first one is to achieve what I call intergenerational consciousness—a person in the process of constellation begins to link facts that he has not linked before, that he did not think might be relevant, and also gains new knowledge about the relationships within the family. The mother was chilly and emotionally isolated? She did not do it out of spite or it is even hard to say that "she had such a character"—the constellation may show that she was emotionally attached to her older brother, who had died as an infant, or carried the trauma of her own mother, who had never met her father. Sometimes these are quite obvious things, but adult children, in their still infantile thinking, do not take them into account (for example, the fact that the parent lost his own parents in early childhood).

What we tend to see as the results of our parents' conduct usually has other and deeply hidden causes. I worked with Kristina, who had a terrible relationship with her mother. They did not speak to each other for two years, and when they did get together, her mother constantly manifested some sort of dissatisfaction. Kristina shared her thoughts that she would feel better if her mother died. Kristina said that she could not accept her mother, open up to her, because the things that had happened in the past did not justify her (for example, the fact that as a child she was afraid of rejection and because of that she stiffly looked up to her own mother). Kristina's view was that she was now an adult and was a mother herself, so it was her duty to manage.

Since Kristina's attitude was unchanged, I asked her to sit down and I stood as her myself—I wanted to know what else she could be hiding inside.

I immediately fell to the floor, assumed the characteristic fetal position, and began to emit muffled cries of pain. "There is still something here from the perinatal period," I said to the client. Kristina confirmed—she was born feet first and it was a very difficult birth. She said it was strange, but now she was calming down and felt fine (this was a standard reaction to the discovery and expression of repressed trauma). Her relationship with her mother also became clear—the bond had been broken in the earliest period, and then both the mother and the daughter faulted each other for being cold and distant, increasingly growing away from each other. Kristina recalled that she had never let her mother hug her, which the mother was resentful of. What was her attitude toward her mother now? She could no longer make any accusations.

Why is it that parents are so often brought to justice by their children? According to Harris:

> When you think about childhood you think about your parents. Blame it on the relationship department of your mind, which has usurped more than its rightful share of your thoughts and memories.
>
> As for what's wrong with you: don't blame it on your parents. (Harris 1998, 362)

One can agree with this. An important part of Harris's theory is the postulate that there are three systems in the brain (mind): responsible for relationships, for socialization in the group, and for social status. These systems work largely independently, reacting to different stimuli and evoking different types of motivation. In this concept—which is, of course, a certain idea and not a conclusion from research—there are intuitions that are parallel to what was discovered and conceptualized by Hellinger. In systemic constellations, we see the difference between what is personal or relational and what is conditioned by the intergenerational process. We are not aware of these processes, and most people do not know anything about their existence. It is not uncommon for parents to blame themselves for bad things happening to their child without knowing that the causes lie elsewhere. We simply see relationships, overt emotions, and what is happening here and now. Or what is clearly recorded in our memory. And these elements are generally not the core of the matter.

As in the case of Alexandra, whose seventeen-year-old son was apathetic for several years, and stopped getting up and going to school some time ago. Alexandra's husband blamed her for not showing him enough acceptance and love when he was a child. She was ready to agree with her husband's allegations—when her son was little she had a lot on her mind, and in her own childhood she herself had not felt her mother's full love.

When I stood as the son, I did not feel that I was addressing the mother and that I associated my condition with her. I rubbed my arms, thighs, stomach, buttocks,

I felt as if I did not know who I was and what I was for. I told Alexandra that there was something strange about the son's attitude toward his own body, and she confirmed that he was very focused on it—he went to the gym, whitened his teeth—but he was not happy with it and wanted to "be someone else."

The constellation showed that Alexandra's son was attached to some dead person. Only when this bond was shown and I, as the son, was lying on the floor, did I feel that I needed the mother to be there. At the same time, Alexandra approached me and began to caress me. Then, when I stood up, I wanted the mother to stand closer to the pillow representing the deceased (with whom she also felt connected) and give me some space.

When we work with constellations, we have no doubt that relationships with parents translate into our clients' lives. Even if one tries to negate these relationships, there is an obvious level at which parents influence their children and are of great importance to them. These are the accounts of the clients themselves, according to which it was the parents who contributed to their difficulties. These may be the result of the nurture assumption, but this "assumption" turns out to be so common that during our lives it is difficult to avoid seeing our parents as responsible for what happened to us. Therapeutic work generally verifies these simplified causal relationships—in which the father's alcoholism or mother's favor to the sister plays a decisive role—showing much deeper levels of our problems today. The fact is that many people experience their parents' behavior as extremely important for their lives. They bear the stories associated with them in their heads and dwell on them. They affect their emotions and behaviors. Parents prove to be important, and sorting out one's internal relationships with them and calming one's emotions results in many positive changes in life.

Harris's position was the opposite of that of Miller and Forward, who claimed that we are guided by the fourth commandment, not letting us admit how much our parents were at fault. Harris said that we are guided by the myth that makes our parents guilty even of what they could not really control. In my therapeutic practice, I have met people who idealized their parents, unable to look at the pain that was born in the relationship with them, as well as people who accused their parents of all the evil. Harris's ideas are more strongly justified, yet her final conclusions in which she minimizes the importance of biological parents are wrong.[11]

FAMILY IN A NEW LIGHT

Wonderful Families

Many people want to build a wonderful family. They really do their best to help their children develop properly. They spend time with them, solve conflicts, give advice, and are supportive and kind to them. They read guides and Internet forums, devote their time to school and after-school activities, talk, do not beat the child, but explain. They think that what they say and do for their children is all that shapes them. However, children take from the whole family system, of which they are only a part. They are shaped by unsolved and untold things that even their parents may not know about. "Ideal" parents sometimes forget about their own parents. They often want to be better parents than them, which involves judging and excluding them.

And what effect does it produce? Their children become arrogant and ungrateful, although the parents do so much for them. For the children look toward the whole family and toward their grandparents and the excluded. They want their parents to accept their parents. They automatically isolate themselves from the parent when he rejects his mother or father. And they open up when the parent accepts them with respect and love.

Accepting parents immediately improves relationships with children. This has been observed by many therapists. Martha Welch, the founder of the Holding Time method, wrote about one family:

> As small children both the grandmother and the mother had spent long periods in the care of aunts. Quite by chance the mother mentioned that she had never been held as a child and that, in fact, she had not be able to bring herself to hold or cuddle her son when he was a baby. The result was that he screamed and cried endlessly for most of the first eight months, then suddenly went into autistic withdrawal. Not long after telling me this, the mother brought a Mother's Day present to the grandmother. The grandmother was so surprised and thrilled at the unexpected gift that she grabbed the affection that she previously had not been able to express.
>
> The mother later told me that at that moment she had wanted her mother to let go immediately and at the same time never to let go. After this single dramatic moment of longed-for contact with the grandmother, the mother's ability to respond lovingly to her child increased. Within a few days, the child's behavior dramatically improved. He became more tractable and made much better eye contact with his mother and other people—a key sign of improvement in autistic children. (Welch 1989, 18–19)

Welch ascribes the child's reaction to the change in the mother's behavior, which undoubtedly took place. However, constellation therapists observe changes in children's behavior independent of their parents' behavior. Children change due to changes in the relationship between their parents and grandparents. They are influenced by the very change of the systemic situation and the parent's internal attitude. This often happens so quickly that the parent does not even have time to demonstrate his new behavior.

One can often hear: "I want my son to have it, because I didn't have it myself," "I don't want my child to experience what I experienced as a child," "My mother played so little with me, so I play a lot with my child." It is okay for the parent to give his child more than he received himself. As long as this desire does not conceal his reproach for his own parents. In this case, "giving what we did not receive" in a way shows the parents how "bad" they were compared to us. If we raise a child with the idea that we protect him from the deficits we have experienced, we actually confront him with our own deficit.

The current family is not always the first one. It happens that a woman, as a young girl, got pregnant and had an abortion, or a man has a child he has never seen. During constellations, the deep bond between these people and their first partners and children becomes visible. Often this bond is completely unconscious and is not taken into account. However, a constellation shows that this earlier relationship has the status of the first family. The one they currently form is their second family. The existence of the first family affects the present relationship as well as the children born from it. It may be that the man is not able to get fully involved, being driven by an unconscious sense of guilt, and the later children are identified with the parent's first partners, which makes their behaviors or difficulties hard to explain.

What Do Children Need?

It is a myth and an illusion that we can have the children we dream of. No matter how hard we try, there are forces that are stronger than what we can create through such or another upbringing. So is it possible to have any more advice for parents? Christian educators, Mariateresa Zattoni and Gilberto Gillini, wrote: "Every parent is worthy of being a parent if only for this reason: that they said 'Yes' to life" (Zattoni and Gillini 2002, 18). This is in line with the philosophy of systemic constellations, but at the same time completely different from the seemingly sensible, and in fact limited, view that these or other parents should not have children because they do not have adequate parenting skills. Thanks to constellations, we realize that our superficial judgments of families and parents mean nothing in the face of deeper processes of which we are unaware.

So what do children need? Family constellations show that children need completeness of the family most of all. What does this mean? Is it what we customarily refer to as a "complete family?" No, it is the completeness that can be achieved in any conditions, regardless of whether the parents are divorced or not, and even whether or not they both live. This completeness is

- knowledge about one's family, and
- the possibility to love all of its members.

A child is calm and develops when he knows his family and can have love for it, and when he can talk with his mother about the father and with his father about the mother. When he knows the biological mother and the real father and can turn to them in his heart. No matter if the parent lives or not. The child also needs to know and turn to the grandparents with love. He needs to know about his siblings, including those who are half-siblings and live separately. He grows and gains strength if he can talk to his parents about their parents and hear them saying the words of love toward the grandparents. When he speaks with love about the parents, grandparents, when he is interested in his cousins, uncles, and aunts, then he grows emotionally, and his personality develops.

Children must have the possibility of emotional and cognitive journeys through relationships within the family. And they must have a guarantee that they will never face the prohibition of thinking, speaking, and loving. If the child encounters a ban on thinking about someone or loving someone from the family system, his emotional balance will be disturbed. And when such a prohibition is targeted at the father or mother, in my opinion, it works just as a prohibition on thinking in general and may partially limit the child's intellectual development in terms of social competence.

One of the most important tasks of the parent is to respect the other parent and be glad that the child is attached to him. What does the child gain by this? In addition to the obvious thing—the possibility of contact with both parents—it brings him the feeling that he is loved in his entirety, also in the part that is related to the other parent. Otherwise, the child becomes insecure internally. He no longer believes in the love of the excluding parent. Sometimes, paradoxically, the child cleaves to him. But not because he starts to love him more. In fact, he is scared that the parent will reject him, that he will consider him to be disloyal. By excluding the other parent, the excluding one distances the child from himself.

Having the mother and father in mind and heart also has other advantages. It creates a safe space for the child. He can move from the mother to the father and from the father to the mother. He becomes freer and less dependent. Why is this important? Children want to belong and be loved very much. So much that they are ready to die to confirm their relationship with their family. That is why it is good when a certain distance is possible. It is provided to them by this space "between" the mother and father and the possibility to turn to the grandparents. A child brought up by one parent who does not mention the other and does not mention the grandparents, suffocates and wilts. The child needs both his parents also because the strength from the past generations flows to him through them.

Children Take on Themselves

The issue of "good" or "bad" upbringing is so difficult to assess because no matter what parents may burden their children with, it is children themselves who willingly find and take on difficulties. Children unconsciously share their ancestors' traumas, their losses, and their pain. They identify themselves with victims and perpetrators. They are subconsciously absorbed in the past.

Sometimes these things are so difficult that they start to behave in a disturbing way—they become aggressive or destroy their own lives. Other times they simply get physically ill. We were taught that we are autonomous individuals and that the past goes away. This proved to be untrue. Things that children unconsciously experience may concern even the fourth generation. Children look toward those of their relatives who witnessed some difficult events and were unable to cope with internal trauma all their lives. They mentally interfere in the past, trying to solve what has not been solved, or to take on themselves the pain of the witnesses, to honor the memory of the victims, and to bring about reconciliation with the perpetrators. During constellations, when they come to realize such attitudes, the clients are surprised how strong emotions and physical reactions are evoked in them by their grandfather's handicapped brother, about whom they never thought, or by the person who contributed to the death of their great-grandfather. Anger, fear, pain, and at other times deep sympathy and a sense of attachment to someone from the distant past emerge.

A child may be frightened that he will be abandoned by his parents, that he will lose them, that they will leave, or one day they will not pick him up from kindergarten. This seems to be his own set of fears and we will suppose that he has once experienced abandonment or that he is oversensitive. In fact, he may have taken on himself his mother's fear and act it out in the form of fear of being abandoned. Thus, although the situation of abandonment is terrifying in itself, the child is scared primarily because his mother is scared.

Children take on themselves the difficulties hoping that this will help the parents and extend their lives. However, they are sometimes angry with their parents, blaming them for all their failures. Why this inconsistency? Children are attached to their parents unconsciously, but they may consciously be angry with them and not want to have anything to do with them. If they adopt this attitude, they develop an even greater internal conflict. They feel guilty and unworthy of anything good in life. This is why during constellations we try to make people realize their bond and loyalty to their parents. Not to respect any moral or religious principles, but only to make their hidden loyalty revealed and stop affecting them without them knowing it. Then the internal conflict is resolved and the person regains energy and faith in life.

Parents may be hated because the child does not see the world beyond them and he associates each of their behaviors with himself. When the parent is angry, it means to the child that the child is guilty; when the parent is sad, it must have something to do with the child; when the parent laughs, the child must have made him happy. This perception is not unusual. Even as adults, we rarely consider a person's condition to be related to a broader context than the current relationship. We usually do not say to someone who is angry with us: "I have the impression that it's not me you're angry with" or "I can see that something went wrong for you at work." Instead, we look for causes in ourselves and in the current situation. Associating everything with ourselves becomes our curse. Many people are convinced in their adult life that their parents did not love, accept them, or even hated them, precisely because of this childlike view.

Andrew felt all his life that his mother "did not love him." He mentioned the situation when she came to his grandmother, where he was staying, and immediately started "attacking" him. He said that she was "motivelessly aggressive" toward him. Andrew felt that there was always a child in him, that he lived a double life. In a constellation, the mother figurine really emanated anger. But this anger was not targeted. Adding an additional figurine showed the mother as a person connected with something in an unclear way. In this relationship, there were, as it were, suppressed emotions or memories that she could not even think of. It was probably a painful event (from the mother's biographical past or from an even earlier period). As soon as the mother moved away from her son (who had chosen a child figurine to represent him), he felt great relief, which he enthusiastically communicated to me. When the mother's attachment to something from the past was displayed, Andrew felt unburdened. Now he saw that what was coming from his mother was not directed at him.

However, the question arose: "Why? Why did you burden me with this for so many years?" Looking at the mother figurine, entering her information field, I did not see that the mother had any answer. But she could say, "I am sorry." In my opinion, in Andrew's question: "Why?" there was another question hidden: "Should I leave it that way? What will I be left with then?" For we are shaped not only by good things but also by bad things. We do not want to lose not only the good things but also the bad things. We build our identity and sense of belonging from the latter too. Therefore, leaving what burdens us is not always an easy step. It requires overcoming the fear of loneliness and agreeing to build a new identity.

The child has the right to leave what is not his with the parents. How to distinguish it? The parents' matters as a couple are not the child's concern, and yet he is so interested in this! It is obvious that the child is very interested in the parents' relationship and wants it to continue in love. When the parents divorce or stop loving each other, the child suffers. Is there any way out here? The parents can stay together for the sake of their child. They can also part if they want to. Because there comes a time when the child himself must realize that trying to repair the parents' relationship needs to be stopped. The child really has the key to this relationship, but it is inside his heart. There, his parents' relationship lasts forever, no matter what happens.

Siblings—The Bond Above Jealousy

Many people have a grudge against their parents because, in their opinion, their brother or sister was favored and loved more. They present it as the worst, the most determining factor in their lives. When they are to say something about their life problems, they usually say in the second or third sentence that they were not loved by their parent. They almost always talk about the mother, and the unloved child is often the daughter.

The feeling of being unloved, someone on the fringes, worse than one's siblings, is deeply rooted in one's psyche. It causes that the child turns away from his mother and becomes a walking accusation. He also turns away from happiness, because the worse it gets for him, the more accurate the accusation. Nursing the injury and the need for balance become more important than health and success. The psyche becomes caught in resentment against the parent and in envy for the sister or brother that they received something that we were allegedly refused. In the child's fantasy, it assumes a picture of a treasure. It is difficult for him to derive from life, because he feels that what is most valuable has been taken away from him anyway.

Harper claimed that her mother had favored her younger sister in her childhood. Later the mother took care of her sister's children, and Harper's children were only taken care of by her mother-in-law. All the time Harper held a grudge that her mother lived with her sister's family and cooked for them. She said once to the mother: "Pick me instead of Lucy," meaning that the mother would let her live with her, to which the mother replied: "What do you want from me?" In a constellation, Harper was very resistant to accepting her mother. The reason was the interrupted movement toward her. During the constellation, the client, lying on a blanket, learned to open her hands and take from the mother, which was difficult for her. I set up a representative of her sister. Then I asked the sister and mother to stand in front of Harper, who was still lying on the floor, and said: "It's ordinary here." This sentence referred to her fantasy about something special that her sister had been given and that was completely invisible in the constellation. Blinded by jealousy, Harper was not able to take what is—true love. Jealousy builds a persistent fantasy of a lost treasure, which later does not allow to enjoy what one has.

It is not rare that parents actually treat siblings differently. They spoil one child, and they require work from the other one. Often the daughter becomes the father's darling and the son becomes the mother's darling. Why does this happen? It often tells us about something that the parents themselves have derived from their own family systems—about the disorders that make their children have to represent someone, to perform some "extra functions" in addition to being a child.

Neglecting one of the children may be quite real, but it may have nothing to do with "lack of love." The reason for this may be the care of another child, who was very ill and needed more attention. The healthy child grows up, so to speak, in his shadow. Interestingly, many people do not see the objective fate here, focusing on the parent's "injustice." These are a child's feelings—greedy and wanting exclusivity from the mother. Then, persisting in the adult person, they can be the source of the need to balance the alleged wrongs.

What is the solution? To accept one's fate as it was, along with the strength that flows from it. It is necessary to see what was objective and beyond the parent's decision, such as the sibling's sickness or the parent's family background. The solution is to go beyond the external aspect of the experience to love and bond. To leave behind thinking about single events and words. The solution is to look from the perspective of the family, instead of looking only at the mother. And when necessary, to start moving toward the mother, instead of waiting for her to move. It is also necessary to open up more to the bond with the siblings, not to block love for the sister or brother, to get out of the blind need for "justice," for which we are ready to sacrifice ourselves.

Joanna was plagued by recurring migraine attacks. She was born almost exactly one year after her sister had died at the age of six months. She maintained that she became a "substitute" for her deceased sister. Her name was even supposed to prove it: the client's name was Joanna and her sister's name was Anna. I set up Joanna herself and a representative of her migraine. Quite quickly it became clear that the migraine was her late sister. I also set up a representative of the mother. The basic dynamics concerned Joanna's childhood feelings toward her sister and mother. Joanna wanted the sister to disappear, as she wanted to have all her mother's love for herself. She was unable to understand what her mother was saying to her through her representative's mouth: "You both have a hundred percent of my love." She thought she would have to share and she experienced her sister's close presence as unbearable.

In this constellation, the client contacted her infantile jealousy, anger toward her sister, and possessiveness toward her mother. In the framework of another psychotherapy, we would perhaps believe her claim that she was a "substitute" for her deceased sister, because her parents chose that role for her. Here, however, it was clear that it was more difficult for her to acknowledge the existence of the older sister and the fact that she had received her "part" of the mother's love than to be a "substitute." The idea that the mother gave all her love to her younger child, Joanna, was not a trauma at all, but a wish. What did the migraine represent in her body? The bond with her sister, suppressed by anger and jealousy.

When we have siblings, and we do not know about it—because it is a half-blood sibling or a sibling who has died without being brought to light, also an unborn one—it is always a source of of inner anxiety. A bond that cannot be realized is an element that disturbs mental life. An additional factor is that we cannot take our rightful place and unconsciously usurp our brother's or sister's place. The awareness of seniority, the order of births, and therefore of the hierarchy between the siblings are important. Perhaps the most important thing is to know who was first and not to usurp that place.

The Way to One's Own Life

Our Parents and Us

We are connected with both our parents and other members of the family. However, everyone is responsible for themselves, has their own fate and the right to live independently, which Hellinger put into words: "Me for myself, you for yourself." By identifying and recognizing ties, we do not become our parents' slaves, but we liberate ourselves from needless loyalties and can focus on our own lives.

Many people find it difficult to leave their parents and go into their own life. In some, it is visible on the outside; in others, it happens on an internal level. Some have not moved out; others live separately, but in many ways are attached to and emotionally dependent on their parents. Some believe that they were not loved enough, that their parents did not give them enough attention or hurt them. So why do they continue to stay with their parents? They are bound to their parents by a mixture of resentment and loyalty. It is like a glue that blocks their inner freedom. Resentment isolates from the parent, and excessive loyalty is a reaction to this separation.

There are children who are overly involved with their parents as a couple. They also find it difficult to live their own lives. They keep their finger on the pulse of the parental relationship, advise them or try to fix their relationship. What happens between the parents is more important to them than what they could build themselves. Such a child imagines that he has to heal the parental relationship, that he cannot leave them if they are in conflict. He may also think that everything that concerns him, all his problems, are due to the failed parental relationship. He does not understand that by meddling in the things that should remain with his parents, he harms himself. He cannot take what he has received because he thinks that it is only when he has repaired his parents' relationship that he can live peacefully. Naturally, the parents' relationship is important for every child, which is why it is so difficult for him when they part. Children can unconsciously experience the relationship of their parents, organizing their lives accordingly. Then, some elements represent the father and some the mother. An example would be the case of a person who lived her life traveling between two cities, one of which represented her father and the other represented her mother to her; or the case of another person who could not choose or combine two work activities that likewise represented her father and mother.

What makes one stick to one's parents is not necessarily related to them. Conrad came to me because his relationships failed regularly. He felt that he took too much on himself, that even when he did not like something, he did not say a word to his partner, and tried to somehow bypass the problem. All his life he was entangled in his parents' marriage, and in their affairs. His parents were constantly "fighting with each other," he said. When I sat with him in the office and he presented his problem—and I saw his parents and relationships in my mind—I could clearly feel that he was strongly attached to his parents and their problems. It was as if he was devoid of his own energy. I said to him: "It's—I don't know how else to put it—as if your life remained with your parents, as if you left it at home. Conrad froze and told me that my words about "life" resonated very much in him; he felt something in his chest and a surge of emotions. How could he develop? He should leave his parents' marriage with them, leave the suffering and hypochondriac mother with the father, and the alcoholic father with the mother. He should go beyond the child in himself, who—like many children—believes he is the savior of his family, someone who can and should help. Feel and regain his own energy, fight his own "battle" and not continue to feed on the life of the parents. But how can this be done? Only by keeping the inner bond with the parents. Only then will a sense of guilt and a misconceived duty not take him back to the old way.

Guided by this very intuition, I said, "I will stand as 'something that took your life,' or maybe 'someone who took his own life.'" I turned my back on Conrad, the thought "I'll leave and you won't see me again" came to my mind, but I did not share it and remained silent. Conrad was strongly attracted to this person, he bowed spontaneously, or he "got bent" this way, and started weeping. I suggested the following words to be uttered to this person: "You wanted to disappear, but I can see you." Conrad started crying even more intensely. Eventually, he calmed down, could withdraw, and stand upright. He smiled meaningfully while saying goodbye to me: "Something has changed, yes, something has changed."

There are people who speak highly of their parents, and their father and mother are "wonderful people" to them. However, they do not have the strength that should come from having loved parents. Quite the contrary, they feel weak. When they talk about the love and care that their mothers gave them, they fall apart and fight back the tears. As if their mothers' love did not give them strength, but caused their weakness. These people feel painfully obligated that they have to pay back the debt and that living their own life would be detrimental to their parents. They may get confused: "Is it the parent who needs me? Or is it me who needs the parent?" Sometimes it seems that it is the mother who needs the child, and only a constellation reveals how strong the child's need to stay with the mother is. Such persons need to return to their parents and take him deeper into their hearts so that they can finally acknowledge that they have every right to go their own way. Constellations leave no doubt that one of the orders of love is children's right to leave their parents and go in their own direction. When we say about the bond and leaving, is there a contradiction? No. The more the parent is in our heart, the greater the right we give ourselves to not interfere in his life. The parent and I become separate people—so strongly connected yet so autonomous.

Some fathers and mothers are extremely controlling. They expect the child to follow the path they have chosen. There are mothers who cannot imagine that their adult son or daughter will leave them and start to live independently. They raise or even mold the child in such a way that he is incapable of emotional separation. Arousing guilt in the child and the need to compensate the mother can contribute to such molding. The mother may say how much she devoted herself to the child, how many things she gave up. She may make the child a companion of her misery and share her pains and disappointments with him. It happens, however, that the mother finally lets the child know that he can already live his own life, and even that she has had enough of his dependence. Then a sense of rejection arises in the child. He has always felt overwhelmed by the mother and dreamed of freedom, and when there is a chance to become independent, he clings back to the mother. The mother finally allows her adult child to stay with her again and thus strengthens his dependence. After some time, she may again suggest to him that he should go his own way and the whole pattern repeats itself.

Why is the mother sometimes controlling, intrusive, living the life of her adult child and does not allow him to emotionally separate? It may not be about this child at all. The mother may be attached to someone earlier. It may be her lost first child, an early deceased sibling, or a loss that has affected someone from an earlier generation. The mother cannot imagine being separated from her child, but in fact, it is not about her son or daughter, but about a completely different person. When in a constellation, the mother's representative reaches the person she is attached to, then the mother can finally withdraw her projections and truly see her own child.

The child can say "No!" to his mother's demands. "No, I won't do it, even if you're unhappy." The idea that a child can make his mother happy by limiting his life is an illusion. It is also not true that by doing the opposite, the child will break the bond with his mother, that it is tantamount to cutting himself off from her. On the contrary, the more he accepts his mother as a mother, the easier it will be for him to say "No."

The father is a break from the mother for the child and a barrier against what is destructive in her. If there is no father, the child has little chance to protect himself from the overwhelming impact of the mother. However, it is fathers who are most often excluded because they "are alcoholics," "use violence," "are absent," or "aggressive." Even if they provide for the family, they are condemned for having "only worked." The father-tyrant, alcoholic, or even a hothead, becomes an explanation for all the family's problems. However, a constellation may show that the causes lie elsewhere. Interestingly, they often lie on the part of the mother, not the father. It sometimes turns out that this quiet and suffering woman brings much more difficulties into the life of her children than her partner. The connection between the mother and her child is so strong that if there is an inner "You for me" ("Die for me") in the mother, the child will not resist. In such a situation, finding one's way to the father can be of great importance. Fathers, as well as grandfathers, are more often the ones who keep us alive. More children turn away from life for their mothers than for fathers.

We all know the saying, "It is not an art to conceive a child, it is an art to raise him." However, family constellations reveal a different level on which the biological parent remains the most important one, regardless of his behavior toward the child. The child is related to the parent not only through genes but the parent is also a part of the child's life and a transmitter of what flows from the family lineage. All parents have been, as Hellinger says, "taken into service," into service of life, no matter how it all went later on. Accepting the father who never existed in the individual's life and "only" begat him is a very important developmental factor. Someone who previously felt insecure or incomplete deep inside themselves, can now feel that, like any other person, they too have a mother and a father. This results in a large increase in the sense of strength and often also enables us to build better relationships with our own children.

A child may be the fruit of rape. Such an event can have multigenerational consequences, which arise because the rapist is very strongly excluded. The terrifying secret continues from generation to generation. The child from rape cannot take his father into the heart. He does not accept his origin, and thus his life and himself. When he has his own child, this gap in the family tree has an impact on the child and then on the next generations. The result is that subsequent children in the family do not accept their parents. They rebel. As was the case with Molly, who could not accept her mother during a constellation (she came to work on her difficulties in entering into relationships with men and skin problems on her hands). Even setting up the multigenerational sequence of women did not calm her. The group of representatives had the impression that a man from a distant past mattered here, and then they had a feeling that there was also a child who was probably born from rape. When this man appeared in the constellation, Molly felt relieved. Now she could accept her mother and her family without the feeling of untruth and unresolved mystery. Her inner problems and rebellion were in fact speaking up for her great-great-grandfather.

Saying "Yes" to Life

Psychoanalyst Carlo Strenger mentioned two competing visions of man in psychoanalysis, which he described as "classic" and "romantic" (Strenger 1989).[12] "Classicism" finds that in child's development, pain, disappointments, and suffering cannot be completely avoided. Accidental and sometimes painful situations leave indelible marks. The way out is to accept and understand what shaped our character and fate, because it is impossible to change it.

Among the "Classics" there is Melanie Klein, whose perspective on this topic has many common points with the optics of systemic constellations. Klein states, for example, that the child must "find his way between his hate which is increased by frustrations, and his love and wish for reparation which bring in their train the suffering of remorse. The way the child adapts himself to these problems in his mind forms the foundation for all his later social relationships, his adult capacity for love and cultural development. He can be immensely helped in childhood by the love and understanding of those around him, but these deep problems can neither be solved for him nor abolished" (Klein 1975, 316).

The "Romantics"—represented by Heinz Kohut and Donald Winnicott—make demands on the external environment, including the parents, and not the child. They argue that our development could be fully harmonious and no accidental and painful events should shape our *self*. The Romantics expect parents to be good enough, empathetic, and attentive to their children, so that the latter can fully develop their potential. In therapy, they try to provide a "corrective experience," where the analyst becomes a good parent to the patient.

The "Romantics'" expectations are justified, and it is best if the parents are good. However, there are situations when we have to abandon such expectations. The parents of children born during wars, famine, and social unrest could not meet them. Nor did those who took particularly much upon themselves as children and had serious mental problems in later life. Were they bad parents? Did their children lose what was so easily received by children living in peaceful times and raised by peaceful parents?

The "Classics" do not so hastily reject fate. Is it not part of what every person is? Can a person be considered independently of his fate? Of his parents, for example? In his work on Leonardo da Vinci's childhood, Freud wrote:

> But may one not take objection to the findings of an enquiry which ascribes to accidental circumstances of his parental constellation so decisive an influence on a person's fate—which, for example, makes Leonardo's fate depend on his illegitimate birth and on the barrenness of his first stepmother Donna Albiera? [. . .] We naturally feel hurt that a just God and a kindly providence do not protect us better from such influences during the most defenceless period of our lives. (Freud 1989, 99–100)

How can one overcome one's fate that is "not optimal"? By rejecting it, if it is possible at all, or by accepting it? Focusing on the "losses" we have suffered may lead to the world of claims and fantasies. It seems that our mind is constructed in such a way that we can go really far in fantasizing. For example, blame one's mother: "I would be better off if you had gotten involved with another man, and not with my father." This is surprising, but such words are said, and those who say them do not see any contradiction in them. The mother was supposed to choose another man before they were conceived! This is how Freud describes a similar attitude:

> We all think we have reason to reproach Nature and our destiny for congenital and infantile disadvantages; we all demand reparation for early wounds to our narcissism, our self-love. Why did not Nature give us the golden curls of Balder or the strength of Siegfried or the lofty brow of genius or the noble profile of aristocracy? Why were we born in a middle-class home instead of in a royal palace? (Freud 1997, 155)

Where do these ideas lead us? Do they do us good? And if not, what is the solution? Hellinger writes about it:

> It is thus part of the orders of love that the child takes his life as his parents give it, as a whole, that he accepts his parents as they are, that he does not wish for anything else, that he is not afraid of anything, and that he does not guard against anything. Taking in this way is an act of humility. It means accepting the life and fate that my parents gave me. The limitations set for me, the

> opportunities given to me. Entanglement in the fate of this family, and even in its guilt, in the difficult and easy issues in this family, whatever they may be. (Hellinger 2006, 120)

The act of accepting, our "Yes," as Hellinger put it, has great transforming power. The acceptance Hellinger speaks about does not mean going into the problems of the past or carrying burdens. Such acceptance makes it possible to regain strength, capableness, and autonomy. It is rebellion that causes us to be tied to the past, blocked, and held in negative emotions. Any freeing oneself from burdens in order to finally live one's own life needs to be preceded by a fundamental acceptance of our fate and those through whom life has come to us.

VARIANT IDEAS FOR THE CHILD

Adoption

Someone who adopts a child brings many people into their home. Are they aware of this? Are they able to deal with it without harming the child, their own family, and themselves? Every child is attached to his biological parents, siblings, and other family members. The fact that the child knows nothing about his real parents and does not consciously miss them does not matter. Adoptive parents may sometimes feel the wall that exists between them and the adopted child, which makes them frustrated and sad. The child is sometimes mean, aggressive, does not obey, or is self-aggressive. One girl tore her hair out when her adoptive mother stroke her; she scratched her skin when the mother kissed her. In such cases, it seems that the parents do their best and the child is not able to love.

Adoptive parents may think that the cure will be to separate the past with a thick line, as they believe that the problems of their adopted child are due to the difficulties they experienced earlier in life, in their family of origin. Naturally, he may have experienced neglect and injuries, and may have been beaten or maltreated. But providing a safe and loving environment is not enough. His bond with his real parents demands to be respected. If this does not happen, the child will rebel, fall ill, or will not use all his potential.

Excluding the adopted child's biological family seems to be frequent. Possessive love comes easier than love that respects differences and autonomy. Loving one's own daughter or son comes easier than loving a child from another family that one decided to raise. In the latter case, one has to sacrifice a lot, show humility and acceptance. I have to love someone I cannot expect to be like me. Someone who is attached to strangers more than to me. I have to accept his parents and siblings into my heart. Am I ready for that? Accepting the hidden bond between the child and his family is a challenge. Adoptive parents may deny it and try to make the adopted child "their own." However, this will fail to bear fruit. Instead, they should acknowledge that there is a part of his family in the child that they will not have access to. This can bring peace.

The adopted child needs to be like any other. That is, to be someone who has biological parents. Otherwise, he will be internally torn or suffer in other ways. When the adoptive parents do not respect the child's birth parents, they do not respect the child himself. They weaken him. The same may happen when the parent who adopts a child from his partner's first relationship excludes the child's biological parent. For instance, when the stepfather does not honor the adopted daughter's father, but instead calls himself her "real father." In a constellation, we can see how much chaos such behavior brings to the family.

If the child, attached to his biological parents and siblings, does not know that they exist, he cannot realize this bond, which becomes a disruptive factor in his life. An invisible rope holds him and prevents him from fulfilling himself. The child lives in a gigantic secret that shapes his own and his descendants' fates. Bringing the biological parents into the child's life is not easy. The point is not to "drag" the child to his parents; besides, sometimes, the adoptive parents do not know his birth parents. The problem is that they often consider themselves better and disdain the biological parents. This attitude may be shared by the child himself, unaware of the fact that he is much more connected to the fate of his biological family than to that of his adoptive family.

The caregivers should have in their minds a picture of the real parents. If they do not know anything about them—a picture of the couple who are parents of their child. If they care about their child, they respect the couple regardless of what they have done. They avoid judging, calling the family "pathological," referring to the father as a "drunkard," and the mother as a "degenerate." They see the birth parents as inalienable roots and a fragment of the vast family of the person they chose to care for. When the adoptive parents respect the child's family in this way and are able to recognize its existence in the child, then they are a true support for him.

When the adoptive parents remember about the child's real family, they protect the child from their own unconscious expectations of the child. Every child, when born, enters a family that existed before. With all its past, shaped by ties and events. He also enters the mental world of his parents, the sphere of their fears, desires, ideas, and limitations. In the case of adoption, the parents' expectations can be particularly strong and binding the child. These may involve a need to "save" someone, fear of having a child of one's own, a desire to feel superior, and so on. The couple may want the adopted child to replace their deceased child, they may want "someone to love" or someone who will make their family "complete" if they are childless. Of course, parents' unconscious fantasies also play a role when their biological child is born—but in the case of adoption, the child is more defenseless because he is deprived of the strength coming from his own family.

But it does not always have to be like this. Ivy had an adopted sister, and during the constellation, one could see that even though Ivy's mother and father set the adopted girl a task: to carry the pain of the death of their own child, the girl was not particularly burdened, as she felt strong support from her family. However, the fact that the parents, particularly the mother, were not able to cope with the loss had a great impact on their biological children, who unconsciously tried to take the burden off the mother.

I have observed that adopted people are often torn. They love their adoptive parents and are grateful to them. However, they cannot pay them back and feel guilty about it. A client, Sarah, asked: "Why do I have such a messed up life?" Her mother died when Sarah was five years old. Sarah was raised by her stepmother, who "became a mother" to her. It turned out to be difficult for her to accept the birth mother, and thus also her life. When I represented the mother, Sarah said, "But I've always treated her like a mother." I clearly felt that this sentence confirmed that Sarah did not really accept her mother. At one point, she asked about her adoptive mother: "Who is she then?" Her confusion was evident. She was torn between loyalty to her adoptive mother and the nascent awareness of her bond with the biological mother. I told her to imagine her mother, grandmother, great-grandmother, and so on standing behind her back. I asked if she felt the strength. And I answered myself: "You feel it, but you still defend yourself against it." Sarah said that this was exactly the case.

Adopted people continue to be torn apart because they were not given the opportunity to thank their biological parents for their lives. The whole world told them that "it is not an art to conceive a child, it is an art to raise him." That is why they believe that they have nothing to thank their birth parents for. What happens to their body and life then? They turn away from it and consider it worthless. The failure to accept their own family and the inability to pay back their adoptive parents—tears them from within. What is the solution? First accepting the biological parents and gratitude for life, then saying "Thank you" to the adoptive parents. The latter is sometimes difficult because the child thinks he owes them more than that.

I once represented a man who had been raised by his biological mother and adoptive father. At the beginning, I proposed to the adoptive father to tell his son that he was "father number two." However, I saw that this did not work and understood that there is no such thing as "father number two." I looked at this man for a long time as the son, until I finally realized that there was one thing that was right: "the man who raised me." I felt that this was "something fantastic"—I could not express it any other way. A strange man raised me! It was a great gift. I felt that the word "father" would be inappropriate here, especially as I was getting closer, as a representative, to the real father. When I looked at the adoptive father as a father, I felt attached to him, but at the same time, I was powerless. On the other hand, looking at him as the "man who raised me" was initially almost staggering and I needed to get used to it. Also, the adoptive father, although he always referred to himself as "father" and was even over-responsible toward his adult son, felt relieved when he stopped being his father (he stood in the constellation in person).

Abortion

Consequences of Abortion

Constellations show that abortion affects the child's mother, father, their relationship, and their living children. Our hidden conscience reacts to abortion as it does to the killing of a family member. Some children die early, the main reason for which is the abortions in the family. Children "follow" their deceased siblings, which is particularly strong when parents do not accept responsibility and blame. Hellinger says that when it comes to abortion, the parents tell the child, as it were, "I have a right to live, you don't." This is, in his opinion, an extreme sense of superiority. Conscience does not tolerate such hubris and those who have excluded are attracted to the excluded. They want to get sick and die. And if they push away their responsibility, then the pain is taken by the next. I remember a sick boy and his mother staying in the pediatric oncology ward, where I had a short internship. While drawing the family tree, the mother admitted that she had had two abortions before her son. Now she was a converted Christian, watching over her son by his bed with a big cross on her chest. It seemed, however, that her unborn children still had not found their place in the system, and her son wanted to restore "justice" and the bond with his siblings through his illness.

Melody experienced anxiety for years, and she slept with the lights on and sometimes woke up with terrible sleep paralysis.[13] She tried to be very rational and "keep her feet on the ground," but she was afraid that one day she would "see a ghost" and "go crazy." The constellation showed that she probably had siblings who had been aborted. Her fears disappeared, and at the next meeting she said that she "changed her mind about abortion." She also asked her mother about that matter, and she admitted that soon after she was born she had an abortion.[14]

The impact of abortion can also have a more complicated dynamics and can have consequences in completely unexpected areas. Juliette was married and had a teenage daughter. She lived abroad and her problem was her dependency on her parents who lived in the country. She bought a house in Poland, even though she did not intend to live there—that was what her father wanted. She said "they" or "my parents," but described only the situation with the father. When she was a child, her father was usually away because he worked abroad, and she lived with her mother and brother in her mother's parents' house. As the session progressed, Juliette's real suffering became apparent. She spoke with tears in her eyes, she said that she could not see a solution—if she kept agreeing to her father's expectations, she would not be able to live an independent life, and if she cut herself off, it would not work either, because she could not cope with a sense of guilt. When I asked her about her relationship with the mother, Juliette was taken aback: "With my mother . . . What about my mother . . . I don't know what to say." She mentioned that she had very difficult experiences with her female bosses many times, which even ended in her quitting the job. Now it is enough for the boss to enter the room where Juliette is, and she starts to be extremely stressed, almost paralyzed, "her whole body reacts."

In the constellation with figurines, one could see a blockade and lack of movement from the beginning. I observed the same blockage in the client sitting opposite me. She said that she felt increasing tension. Her figurine was standing behind the mother, at a certain distance. I turned the mother's face toward the client's figurine and asked what was happening between them. The client found it uncomfortable. No specific movement appeared, something was missing. I asked Juliette if something had happened in her life that she did not tell me about and that could be relevant. Then the client said, "I had an abortion when I was 17, mother talked me into it." I placed a boy figurine between her and her mother. I asked her to set up the father of the child, and then also the daughter the client had with her husband. I suggested the words of resolution: "You are my child. You are a child who was not born." I also said that this child was solely her responsibility—despite her seventeen years of age, her mother's pressure, and the difficult situation. Juliette herself positioned the children by her, in the right order. She felt good now.

Accepting the fact that the child's fate was her responsibility, not the mother's, and accepting it into the family was a way to resolve Juliette's conflict with the mother. It was also a step toward "living her own life." Holding the mother responsible for the fate of the unborn child reinforced Juliette's dependence on her. Paradoxically, it also led to the client's inability to cope with the underlying guilt that weakened her. In contrast, accepting the unborn child, and thus her adulthood, made Juliette's position in relation to her mother as well as superiors clearer.

Psychiatrist Philip Ney noted that the accounts of children admitted to psychiatric wards involved an imaginary companion and discovered that it was a deceased brother or sister. When he talked to the children, he realized that they had suspicions and sometimes even certainty about their aborted siblings. That knowledge—according to Ney—caused a deep crisis in those children (Foà 2015, 108). When a woman decided to tell her nine-year-old son about her abortion, which she had done many years before he was born, he replied that he also knew about it, as he always had nightmares about knives, and that the mother wanted to kill him in those dreams. He also stated that he had an imaginary brother who wanted to kill him (Foà 2015, 108). Of course, based on what we know from constellations, a dead child does not want to kill his brother. It is him, driven by the bond and the need to balance, who imagines that he deserves to die.

A failed abortion or a risk of it also has a psychological impact. Ney addressed the "post-abortion survivor syndrome" (Foà 2015, 93–94). It concerns children whose parents planned to terminate their pregnancy, whose siblings have been aborted, or who have been told words such as: "I should have aborted you," also those who know that they could have been aborted because they are handicapped or were born out of wedlock, children who were not aborted because their parents were late in deciding on the procedure, or those who survived the abortion procedure. All these children have experienced a kind of trauma, and there is a fundamental uncertainty in their psyche. Grof writes:

> For many individuals, memories of fetal traumatization seem to be among important factors underlying general emotional instability and various specific forms of psychopathology. Similarly, the question of having been wanted or unwanted by one's mother appears again and again as an issue of critical importance. (Grof 1988, 75)

Cole came to me because of problems with his ex-wife, with whom he could not reach an agreement. However, at the end of the initial conversation, he mentioned the mother and the fact that he was probably an unwanted child, perhaps the mother considered an abortion. He felt he was losing his vitality, and since he was a psychologist and a person capable of introspection, he said that it was as if he had problems since fetal life. This did not sound like a fantasy to me; on the contrary, I felt that there was something important here. I put a piece of paper on the floor that said "mother" and I asked Cole to touch me and say, "You are me, as a fetus in the womb."

I lay down on my side opposite the card representing the mother and trembled slightly. I quickly felt that there was also someone/something near me and I put a piece of paper there. I felt that there was a threat from that side, but I did not say anything about my feelings to the client. Seconds later he himself said, "There's a pressure point there, a threat as if someone wants to extort something." I felt something similar and I thought that this was a person who opted for an abortion. Cole felt that he wanted to get closer to me—he put his hands on me, which meant that he connected with his "fetal part," did not separate from those feelings any longer, did not run away from his primal fear. He said that he felt strongly connected with me.

When representing the client—through "displaced introspection," that is, probing his condition in myself—I realized what the core of the problem was: Cole felt the danger in his mother's womb, which caused him to isolate himself, shrink, not take fully the life that flowed to him. However, the danger was not caused by his mother's attitude; the fear had some other source (represented in this constellation by another sheet of paper). Continuing to represent the unborn Cole, I felt that I was calming down and opening up to the mother, to her womb. This is how I felt it. After a while, Cole himself described his feelings that were identical to mine. In place of fear and isolation, there was a sense of openness and richness that flowed to him from his mother and family, along with peace.

And how does an abortion affect the couple? At a deep level it ends the relationship, breaks the subtle thread that tied two people together. For our evolutionarily shaped psyche, the couple's greatest achievement is a child. If the child is killed, the relationship ceases to matter. After the act of abortion, the partners grow apart, even though they will remain parents of the conceived child forever. So they are connected on a certain level, and on another level, there is a wall between them. Perhaps by destroying their relationship they try to atone for their guilt? Maybe they feel an unexpressed anger toward each other? Is it still possible for such a couple to stay together? Yes, if they accept the lost child into their hearts, admitting to themselves that they have lost him and recognizing themselves as his parents. In other words, they must accept him into their family and live together with him. Internally.

The Fetus Is a Member of the Family

Mothers and fathers feel their aborted children's presence. One woman reported:

> I feel that he is close to me. I was on the street and suddenly I felt he was here. [. . .] I have a feeling that the air around me is moving. As if it were my child's soul. (Chazan and Simon 2009, 151)

Another one said:

> I was standing in the subway when at one point it seemed to me that I saw my unborn child playing hide and seek. (Foà 2015, 106)

All these could be considered symptoms of psychosis or mere illusions, but they are completely different phenomena. Although not all women consciously experience the negative psychological effects of having an abortion, it seems that such phenomena as grief, depression, guilt, emotional numbness or obsessive reminiscences, and tiring associations are frequent and culturally universal (Chazan and Simon 2009, 133 et seq.). The absence of any feelings about having an abortion is sometimes only external. Representatives of women, who claimed that they had coped with their abortion and that it was not a problem for them, felt great pain. This was particularly strong when a woman had several abortions. A person who represented women who had had several abortions said it was a dramatic feeling. In such situations, the feeling of pain reaches also the real mothers, which has a healing effect on everyone in the family.

Many people build their attitude toward abortion based on biological data: a fetus does not have a developed nervous system, there are many idiopathic miscarriages in nature, the length of a zygote is 1 mm, and so on. Attempts are made to determine the maximum age for abortion by assuming that a child of one or another age is not yet—if such terms can be used—"an organism sentient enough" or "something important enough" to deserve protection. This is how Hellinger comments on such attempts:

> When you try to pin down exactly when life begins, what effect does that have in the soul? If I look at it broadly, it seems to me that this kind of exact definition sets you in the place of God, or in the place of greater forces, whatever it might be. (Neuhauser 2001, 203–204)

An example of the "biological" approach to abortion is the reasoning of Richard Dawkins, who states:

> Early embryos that have no nervous system most certainly do not suffer, And if late-aborted embryos with nervous systems suffer—though all suffering is deplorable—it is not because they are *human* that they suffer. There is no general reason to suppose that human embryos at any age suffer more than cow or sheep embryos at the same developmental stage. (Dawkins 2008, 336)

Dawkins declares that he is not concerned with whether the embryo is a human being—he is only interested in when the organism becomes capable of suffering. Following—as he puts it—consequentialism, he concludes that the embryo does not suffer, while it is very probable that the mother and her family will suffer if the embryo is not aborted. Perhaps the point is that a kind of pool of suffering is greater if the pregnancy is not terminated.[15] Even if one were to agree that this kind of thinking about ethics is correct, the facts are different—the pool of suffering always increases. Hellinger wrote:

> My observation is that an abortion usually has much greater consequences than consenting to have the child. [. . .] The burden of having an abortion is much greater than that of having the child. (Hellinger 2018, 190)

For killing a family member, someone always has to pay. It will be the mother or father, one of their children, sometimes grandchildren, in various forms and various proportions. Such is the ruthless ethics of the family conscience.

Dawkins states that an embryo, at the early stages of development, has the sentience "of a tadpole" (Dawkins 2008, 335–36). I will not speak of sentience at the earliest stages of embryonic development, but fetal sentience exists, and the experiences during this period can have a serious effect on later life. Grof wrote: "Having witnessed over the years countless episodes of embryonal and fetal experiences in other people and having experienced several prenatal episodes myself, both in psychedelic sessions and in nondrug contexts, I find it impossible to discard them simply as figments of imagination" (Grof 1988, 76). According to Grof's experience, people are able to remember events from their fetal life during drug sessions. They remember states close to miscarriage, attempted abortion, and the mother's emotions.

Those who advocate abortion usually think that if a child who is likely to be disabled is aborted, it will spare suffering for both him and his parents, who would otherwise have to watch his pain. Does such a child really "vanish?" Hellinger states:

> Can something that exists disappear? Where else could it disappear if not into further existence? How strange, then, is our idea that we could get rid of something, especially the idea that we could get rid of a person. For example, through an abortion; and vice versa, the idea that we could create something new. Everything that we think we create already existed, including the new life. (Hellinger 2014a, 131)

Family constellations leave no doubt that the aborted child still exists—he will appear during a constellation session, even if not mentioned by the client.

The unborn child already has his own biography. He originated from the life, desires, and conditionings of the parents, and developed in the mother's womb, physically connected with her body, and spiritually connected with the history of the family. The changes in his life—over days, weeks, or months—happened at a speed unknown to an adult. And above all, he has come into being. This moment of transition from nonbeing to existence is fundamental, and yet so underestimated, even in relation to our own lives (hence the statement of those who do not respect their mothers: "She only gave birth to me").

Apart from the fact that the child has come into existence and already has a biography, he is, so to speak, more than what he currently seems to be. This is because many of his characteristics have already been determined by his genome. In a sense, then, he is already this person and no other. But that is not all. The idea that it is possible to "terminate a pregnancy" without killing any child is based on the concept of time that in physics is no longer valid. Advocates of abortion seem to follow the Newtonian or thermodynamic definition of time that consider time to be linear, so the past is strictly "separated" from the future. Time passes and what has not yet come does not exist, just as what is past no longer exists. Well, there are many data in science that show that this vision of time is not sufficient. Quantum mechanics seriously considers retrocausality, that is, the impact of the future on the present, and for physicists, it is nothing unimaginable to consider retrograde time. A living organism or consciousness may be—and the existence of prenatal memory indicates that it is—rooted in a space other than Euclidean space and in a time other than Newtonian time. In such a case the embryo would be a "group of cells" only from the perspective of the thermodynamic arrow of time, while on a more holistic level it would exist also in a "fuller" form. It seems that the Christian writer Tertullian, who lived at the turn of the third and fourth centuries, said something similar: "He is a man, who is to be a man."

Dehumanization

Many tend to underestimate prenatal existence. Those who live for a short time, those who cannot speak, those who are small in size, seem unimportant. Rana Awdish, a doctor who almost died due to pregnancy complications, shares her feelings after losing her child:

> I would be driven frequently for blood work and imaging studies, and once for the baby's burial. I hadn't thought there would be a burial. I'm not sure exactly what I had thought would happen to her body. In the hospital when I was told they would keep her body for us in the morgue until I managed to get home, I thought it was an odd place for the remains. I had imagined that the very premature baby, being only twenty-seven weeks, would perhaps be sent to the pathology lab to be examined in the same way they would examine the placenta, sliced and sectioned so the pathologist could issue a report that covered every microscopic abnormality [. . .]. And after she was examined, I didn't know what would happen next. I thought of surgical terminations of pregnancy I had seen performed in the operating room as a medical student. Those remains went to pathology, not cemetery. I recall the term "medical waste" entering my mind before I reprimanded myself. (Awdish 2017, 94–95)

The author of these words was under the illusion that the difference between a twenty-year-old woman and a several-month-old child is so radical that the latter is just "waste." At a spiritual—though empirically penetrable through a constellation—level, this difference is much smaller, if it exists at all.

We succumb to similar illusions all the time. Our approach to unborn children involves a tendency to diminish the importance of other people, to search for "less important ones." This is an omnipresent psychological phenomenon. It escalates to its highest level during wars, when the enemies are called "bandits" or "vermin," depicted on posters as caricatured and generally downgraded. Adrian Owen—a psychologist who detected consciousness in people commonly considered to be in a vegetative state—wonders how "our sense of consciousness and humanity influences the ease with which we kill" and states that this sense is "closely related to the physical form and the behavior of what is being killed and its similarity, or not, to human form and behavior" (Owen 2017, 173). It is easier to shoot someone who is far away, because he becomes just a point; it is easier to deny humanity to someone who is handicapped, ugly, deformed, or even simply dirty. SS men in concentration camps did not show mercy because hungry prisoners falling on potato skins did not resemble people dear to them. Arthur Greiser, the governor of the Wartheland (a part of Poland incorporated into the Reich during World War II), stated that during the inspection of Łódź (a city with a huge Jewish community) he had the opportunity to see "figures who can scarcely be credited with the designation 'person'" (Epstein 2010, 167). In Sweden, between 1935 and 1975, there was a sterilization law, introduced on the basis of "race hygiene," which deprived more than sixty thousand people labeled "feebleminded," "imbecile," "asocial," or with "gypsy traits" or "vagrancy blood" of the right to reproduce (Zaremba Bielawski 2011, 35). Sometimes it was enough to show "signs of epilepsy" to be sterilized (Zaremba Bielawski 2011, 30).

As can be seen, we can always find those who deserve to live less. Owen writes that "if patients don't behave like humans and no longer even look human, then it's much easier to believe that they don't think like a human either" (Owen 2017, 175). And from this, it is only one step away from denying them the right to be called humans at all. It is a great taboo of psychiatry that psychiatrists often do not see schizophrenics as fully human. A different kind of thinking of a schizophrenic makes the psychiatrist confused; he loses any power of understanding and persuasion. The only way out is to depersonalize the patient, to administer strong medication, and to withdraw from interpersonal contact with him.

We should remember how easy it is to stop seeing a human in another person. It is enough that they are unborn, mentally ill, mute, and sometimes simply strangers or old. We often consider such people to be "incomplete" and their lives to be less important. In the case of unborn children who show certain defects during prenatal examinations, our tendency to dehumanize can be particularly evident. The point of abortion is not to "force" the mother to see "something that will not live anyway." However, even if one knows that the child will live with, for example, Down or Turner syndrome, most such pregnancies are terminated and the bodies of these children are "utilized." The lack of respect for the child's existence, the lack of a real or even symbolic burial, will not be unnoticed by the consciences of the next who will strongly desire to connect with him.

When one justifies abortion, one also speaks of "quality of life." If the person to be born is destined to live a low quality life, it is better for him not to be born at all. This is astonishing, but many people really believe that they can judge this. However, it turned out that 72 percent of those with the so-called locked-in syndrome (completely paralyzed) declared that they were happy and their level of happiness increased in proportion to the duration of their illness (Owen 2017, 186). Would any healthy person foresee this result?

Systemic constellations provide a vision of man similar to that of Christian anthropology—as the person who has his dignity. We see that unborn children or handicapped people have their own individuality and inner life. They are persons, although they may not be recognized as such by biological knowledge and social standards. Religion advocates recognition of the mystery and peculiar depth of the human being, while science claims to be able to tell where man "begins and ends." Religion maintains a non-mercantilist approach to man, trying to admonish those who put themselves as the measure of the humanity of others. Similarly, thanks systemic constellations, we stay away from establishing "degrees" of humanity, if only for the reason that, in the course of constellations, we see that handicapped people or those regarded as of little value often play an important role in the family system. They form, together with others, an inseparably interwoven whole. We see that the human person is and remains present even where the dominant culture denies his existence. A sick or disabled person has a place that belongs to him and his own inner life that is no less valuable than that of a healthy person.

Abortion is and probably will remain part of the human world. Family constellations help to overcome the fears of the siblings of the aborted children and of the children who could have been aborted as well as the parents' feelings of guilt related to the abortion they had. We know that parents are always directed by a wider, also transgenerational, context. Their decisions are not fully free. We also know that each terminated pregnancy generates pain; even if it is suppressed in the parents, it is present in the next generations. However, those who have received life can accept this gift with gratitude and leave all fears behind. Those who are not born—the aborted children—can also find peace. In constellations, we see that they do not blame their parents, even if they still fear them. All they expect is that they are seen and that their belonging is acknowledged. When their parents take them into their hearts, then everyone breathes a sigh of relief. As if in a wider movement and a greater whole, everything is in the right place. Even the act of abortion. Looking at this wider context is important because when we speak of abortion, we are in the sphere of conscience, which means

> that we look at the perpetrators and the victims, at the good and the bad. So the parents who aborted the child are the "bad ones," they are murderers and the children are their victims. If we think this way, then we do not give the perpetrators a place in our soul. We say, "You are guilty" or "I am guilty." Then we feel a need to atone for this, for example, to fall ill or even die. We feel sorry for the aborted children. We say, "These poor children, they were not meant to be born." In this field of good and evil, misery repeats itself. (Hellinger and Nehrebecki 2012, 309)

New Parenting Phenomena

In our era, we witness a revolution in the understanding of gender, procreation, parenthood, and raising children. Never in history did all these elements together undergo such a profound transformation. Until now, children could be orphans, half-orphans, the fruit of rape or love, the result of the so-called misalliance, posthumous children, and illegitimate children, and they could be raised in families, communities, or institutions. They could either suffer or be happy for all these reasons, but these variations never exceeded the limits set by biology.

Nowadays, children can be brought up by single-sex couples; and the situation when a child is brought up from the beginning by one parent (practically by the mother) is increasingly regarded as normal. Children are born as a result of fertilization with sperm from an anonymous donor; through in vitro fertilization; the egg cells of one woman are taken, fertilized in vitro, and then implanted in another woman who becomes a surrogate mother for the time of pregnancy (surrogacy). Egg cells are produced from somatic cells, which will make it possible for a woman who went through menopause long ago to have a genetically related child. Another woman's mitochondrial DNA is implanted into egg cells.

Medically assisted procreation methods make it possible to manipulate the parental figures. Until now, the parent could be separated from the child (which is unfortunately a common divorce practice), but now he can be ignored in a more fundamental way, as is the case with insemination with semen from an anonymous donor. And with the latest bioengineering techniques it is possible to intervene at an even deeper level. In the case of surrogate pregnancy, the baby has in fact two mothers—the egg donor and the one who was pregnant and gave birth. The mother in a way "splits." There may be a situation in which there is a donor of an egg cell and a sperm donor, a pregnancy surrogate and two caregivers who are formally named parents. This gives five people in the parental role related to the child.

A famous football player, whose son was born by a surrogate mother, carefully selected to ensure that the child would resemble him as much as possible, said: "Some children never get to not know their parents, neither mother nor father. Having a father is enough." By the way, the football player continued to live with his mother as an adult, and his father did not participate in his upbringing. In the past, we would have wondered what was happening in his psyche that made him think this way. Now we think that he simply follows social trends.

All these procedures limit the child's freedom and increase the parent's impact. A woman choosing semen for artificial insemination determines the physical characteristics of the offspring to suit her preferences. She does not have to take into account anything else but herself, her desires and fantasies. Hellinger once said that fathers are lost crowds that are despised today. He said that many women elevate themselves above their children's fathers. For these women, the child's father is nobody important. They usually fault him for many things, which is perhaps often justified, but, what is characteristic, they do not suffer at all if their child is deprived of him. What happens to children deprived of fathers in this way? Hellinger states that they become incapable of living.

Indeed, we can often observe that people who are disconnected from their fathers have a breakdown or weakness at some point. This is particularly evident in sons who, raised only by their mothers, start to be aggressive, disorganized, and often enter into conflict with the law. At the same time, one must keep in mind that it is not only due to a "lack of relationship" with the father, but primarily due to the fact that the father has been excluded from the son's heart.

A child born from a donor's sperm is related to his biological father, his family, and his other children. How often is this taken into account? Common practice in society is rather to deny these influences. Not taking into account the biological father and his family is even part of the donation process. Women who participate in it believe that the donor's genetic characteristics, physical health, and intelligence will guarantee the successful development of their child. However, it may be otherwise. Because they do not know or even do not want to know anything about what flows from his family. They want to believe that they have "their" child, while in fact they take his ancestors into their home as well. Unfortunately, without any invitation or respect. This is an avenue to make the child or his offspring suffer.

As I have already mentioned, the mental life of a parent is an important factor influencing the child's psyche. The child absorbes the parent's sadness, confusion, unfulfilled desires, self-destruction, and unsettled matters. What protects him partially from this? Being between the two parents. The "in-between" area gives him space and guards him against the excessive influence of each parent. The child alternately escapes from one parent to the other, keeping his mental health this way. A child who is the effect of a desire of just one person and stays with one person lacks this space. The influence of the parent's psyche is stronger in his case. Therefore, it may be more difficult for him to reach his individuality and achieve mental independence. The developmental space of which I speak can appear even when the parent is physically missing—provided that the other parent respects him in the child and is grateful to him for the fact that the child exists thanks to him.

In vitro may also involve abortion, since several embryos are implanted to increase the chance that at least one of them will survive. When all fetuses develop successfully, abortion is used to reduce the number of children that can be born. Also, surplus zygotes are frozen or eliminated. The question arises about the impact of these actions on the child that will be born. Will he be connected with the zygote as with siblings? What will be the transgenerational effects of killing the embryos in the IVF procedure?

According to the so-called dogma of molecular biology, DNA encodes the structure of proteins, but proteins and the whole organism do not affect DNA. It is a one-way transmission of information. It seems that this paradigm is a basis for the functioning of pregnancy surrogacy. The DNA donor is important, and the woman carrying the fetus is of little importance. However, the biological dogma has been seriously modified. It turned out that the external environment, including intrauterine, plays a huge role in gene expression. The closer science examines genetic mechanisms, the more complex and less transparent they become. In other words, a different baby will develop in the womb of a different mother (despite identical genetic material).

During pregnancy, the fetus is embedded in the uterus and is kept relatively isolated from the rest of the mother's body. The barrier is the placenta that lets only selected substances pass through. However, it turns out that some cells also pass through the placenta. The child receives them from the mother and the mother from the child. This exchange causes the child's body to be genetically nonhomogeneous and every pregnancy changes the genetic pool of the mother. The cells which enter the child's body are not only the mother's own cells but also those which she received during previous pregnancies from her children. In addition, also those she received from her mother when she was a fetus herself. The mother's mother, in turn, could be the carrier of the cells of her siblings and her mother. In this way, the cells of closer and further relatives are mixed from generation to generation. The discovery of this phenomenon, called microchimerism (the mother and the child become, as it were, chimeras—individuals composed of "parts" of different origins), indicates the biological relationship between the mother and the fetus, regardless of the origin of the zygote.

During family constellations, one can encounter a surprising phenomenon. People who have been in the incubator for a long time after birth develop a kind of bond with it, as if it were their first "caring object." Not only as a physical object, but as a manifestation of the help that the child received from medicine. In any case, this unconscious bond connects them to another primal "object" other than the mother. In the cases I encountered, it involved distancing from the mother. It resulted not only from the internal attitude of the child himself but also from the mother's attitude. I noticed that in such a situation, the mothers were unable to accept the fact that their child had a "second mother," the incubator. Of course, with the surrogate mother, a similar primal bond develops. Will this child have a chance to respect this bond within himself?

NOTES

1. Alice Miller showed elements of mental instability, and it was not difficult to make her feel persecuted and see her interlocutor as a perpetrator. She found her mother to be "destructive" and her "building up her own power at the expense of her children" to be "criminal" (Miller 2018, 6). Miller felt she was a victim of her Jewish origin, her husband, her son. One could say that she was always a victim, and that is why she was able to empathize with victims' experiences. Her defensive attitude toward others, using "lawyerly" vocabulary referring to criminal actions (of parents), holding accountable, accusing, etc., and stressing the need to remember "what has been done to us" and to hate our "persecutors" are indicative of the writer's paranoid mindset. Martin Miller, too, stated that, fearing that the true story of her life would come out, his mother became increasingly paranoid.

2. Alice Miller had cancer too.

3. Martin Miller was taken care of by his mother's acquaintance for two weeks right after he was born, then he was taken care of by his aunt for six months. At the age of six he and his younger sister were placed in an orphanage, where he spent two years and his sister spent a year. At that time his parents were writing their doctoral theses.

4. Does the term "unwanted existence" not resemble the Nazi *Lebensunwertes Leben* ("life unworthy of living")? Was it not the disappearance of "evil" that all eugenicists and those who organized the T4 action (the name of the program carried out in the Third Reich in 1939–1944, whose goal was to eliminate the handicapped and mentally ill) aimed at? Do not most of those who kill expect to destroy some "evil?"

5. She went through her entire life with this false identity. Her maiden name was not Rostowska, it is not true that all of her relatives died, many other elements of her biography are also not true, but she never corrected these lies, nor did she reveal her past to her environment. Quite the contrary, she was terribly afraid that it could go public.

6. "Most traditional individual therapists regard the family of origin of their clients as the enemy, as noxious, and as undermining their therapeutic efforts. This attitude is epitomized by the book *Toxic Parents*" (Framo 1992, 8).

7. Forward reaches her conclusions in an instant and is fully convinced of them. The therapist is intrusive in many points. Instead of listening to her patients, she tells them that their feelings are "myths" they should get rid of. She describes convincing the patients of her own opinion as eliminating "denial." Forward's therapy may be founded on her own problems and simplifications (the author of *Toxic Parents* herself was allegedly molested by her father, she also claims that she had a bad relationship with her mother), as was the case with Alice Miller.

8. All the patients' names and identifying details have been changed in the book.

9. According to Harris, this direct influence of genes comes with an indirect influence that consists in a given response of the environment to certain innate traits. For example, parents of calm and pretty children will probably more often smile at them and show them to their friends, which will create an "environment" different from that of children who are ugly or cry a lot. However, both these "environments" are ultimately shaped by genes.

10. Based on this study, perhaps we can, but we will not learn what the researchers assumed. What is more important for our functioning is *our* attitude to our parents, not their behavior toward us. So in this case, it is the *statements* of the adolescents that may be more important than attempts to objectively assess family relationships.

11. Harris believes that it was not until Freud that it was recognized that parents are to blame for what goes wrong with their child. Freud, however, did not discuss raising broadly, and in addition he meant mostly educators, not parents. If he spoke of inadequate raising, which too often leads to neuroses and other mental illnesses, he meant raising as a general social practice. He wondered whether, by acting appropriately, a certain compromise could be reached between infantile sexuality and demands of social life. However, he was far from a vision of some perfect raising that would not harm the child's psyche in any way. For he believed, and this is the essence of psychoanalysis, that there is no cure for the existing conflict between the drive-life and social requirements. If one were to search for differentiation of raising practices in his works, one would find such a thing in the

description of the case of "Little Hans." But it is not what we would expect. Freud writes about Hans: "But since he was brought up without being intimidated, and with as much consideration and as little coercion as possible, his anxiety dared to show itself more boldly. With him there was no place for such motives as a bad conscience or a fear of punishment, which with other children must no doubt contribute to making the anxiety less" (Freud 1964, 178). This is not a common knowledge about upbringing, but I do not need to point out that one should not deduce from this that Freud recommended "intimidating" the child. Regarding his vision of modifying parenting, we could use the following quote: "Parents who have themselves experienced an analysis and owe much to it, including an insight into the faults of their own upbringing, will treat their children with better understanding and will spare them much of what they themselves were not spared" (Freud 1990, 185–86). Although "faults" are mentioned here, this should again be understood primarily as universal mistakes that are common to the whole society or social class. What parents can do is, through analysis, to get to know themselves better and thus to unburden their children. We must remember, however, that in this way they would only be able to push away only a part of the pathogenic factors from their children. They would not eliminate the immanent conflict between drives and reality.

12. In making his distinction, Strenger referred to the British poet and literary critic Thomas Ernest Hulme, who wrote: "Put shortly, these are the two views, then. One, that man is intrinsically good, spoiled by circumstances; and the other, that he is intrinsically limited but disciplined by order and tradition to something fairly decent. To the one party man's nature is like a well, to the other like a bucket. The view which regards man as a well, a reservoir full of possibilities, I call the romantic; the one which regards him as a very finite and fixed creature, I call the classical" (Hulme 2003, 70). It should be mentioned, however, that this distinction is only partially consistent with what we discuss.

13. Sleep paralysis—a state that occurs when falling asleep or waking, in which no movement is possible while the person is conscious. It is usually accompanied by unpleasant sensations such as anxiety and sometimes hallucinations (waking dreams).

14. Melody visited me after two years and shared a few more details. When she was a child, she often felt nostalgic, then she would lie down and say to herself "Where are you, where are you, I miss you." She did not understand these words herself; she assumed that she meant her future partner. She once told her mother that she did not open up to people because she felt as if she had some secret that she could not let them know about. The mother became upset at these words and said, "What are you talking about? You're acting like you killed someone!" Melody said she "never knew herself," studied a demanding faculty but never worked in her profession, as if not knowing what she wanted. After the constellation described above, she had a dream: she saw a dove flying, which was the Holy Spirit ("I don't actually know what the Holy Spirit is") and a levitating naked infant who made, as it were, the sign of the cross over her.

15. In his book *The God Delusion*, Dawkins, who refers to the integrity of the argument, repeats in the subsections on abortion, for example, that abortion involves aborting an "embryo" or even a "little cluster of cells" (Dawkins 2008, 336). If so, he means the period before organogenesis, which is before four weeks of pregnancy. This is when many women only find out that they are pregnant, and abortions are often performed much later. And no matter how one approaches the matter, it is then more like "killing a child" than "eliminating a cluster of cells."

Chapter 6

A New Picture of Human Motives

THE QUESTION OF CONSCIENCE

The question of conscience and ethics is one of the most difficult issues addressed by psychology and philosophical anthropology. Why do people act this way and not differently? Are their motives egoistic? What is the origin of altruism? What is the origin of morality?

From a philosophical and psychological perspective, conscience was described, for example, by Arthur Schopenhauer, Ludwig Feuerbach, and Friedrich Nietzsche, who indicated that it is complex, that it develops in the process of education, that it is the voice of social norms and authorities, and that its judgments are not errorless. Nietzsche even stated that a good conscience is "a physiological state which at times looks so much like good digestion" (Nietzsche 1998).

Freud, who first recognized conscience (superego) as the source of crucial psychological processes that shape mental disorders such as melancholia and obsessional neurosis, pointed out in particular that its operation often remains unconscious. He stated, inter alia, that some people "by their behaviour during treatment and in life [. . .] give an impression of being morally inhibited to an excessive degree, of being under the domination of an especially sensitive conscience, although they are not conscious of any of this ultramorality" (Freud 2001b, 168–69). This is manifested in what he described as an unconscious need for punishment, a kind of clinging to one's own failures and provoking humiliation.

Is the superego directed toward the good? Klein stated that it is the "excessive severity and overpowering cruelty" of the superego, not its absence, that can be responsible for criminal behaviors, because the fear of the internal persecutor in the form of the superego causes hostile behavior (Klein 1975, 251). So one can see that the operation of conscience understood this way is quite ambiguous—at times it seems too flexible, at other times too rigid. At times it is the cause of self-punishment, and at other times of wrongs done to others. It certainly does not seem perfect, and yet conscience has often been called "the voice of God" in man's soul. Hellinger said that when he started observing what happens when people say they follow the voice of their conscience, he was struck by the fact that "many people who refer to conscience say or do something that humiliates and harms others" (Hellinger 2006, 13). He wrote:

> So I saw that conscience serves not only good but also evil. That is why the respect shown to conscience in our culture seemed questionable to me. [. . .] Over time, I have come to realize that conscience is something ordinary, something of a drive. Like other drives, it constitutes and strengthens human relationships, within certain limits, and beyond those limits, it fails. (Hellinger 2006, 13)

According to Hellinger, what we call conscience is a psychological mechanism, rather a drive than a metaphysical compass. The fundamental function of conscience is to prevent our exclusion from the family, the group, and the community.

CONSCIENCE AND BELONGING

Conscience is a multidimensional phenomenon, in which several basic mechanisms operate. One can say that there are levels or circles of conscience. The level we are aware of is the "conscience" that we usually refer to when we use the term. This conscience primarily cares about our belonging to the family and to the group, and for this reason it leads us to respect the unwritten rules that exist within it. Loyalty to the rules is felt as innocence, a feeling of guilt appears when conscience signals that we go beyond the rules of the group or community. It is a warning against exclusion. For it is only when we follow our conscience that we feel that we have a right to belong and gain a sense of security.

Freud himself stated that at an early stage of man's development "the sense of guilt is clearly only a fear of loss of love, 'social' anxiety" (Freud 1989c, 85). This process was similarly seen by Jung, who wrote that conscience "is a psychic reaction which one can call moral because it always appears when the conscious mind leaves the path of custom" (Jung 1978, 453).

The fact that conscience is related to the need for belonging is not surprising. This need is one of the strongest, and exclusion has always been one of the most severe penalties. That is why we even speak of social "death" of people who live in infamy. Naomi I. Eisenberger and her colleagues examined the neural correlates of social exclusion using brain imaging (Eisenberger, Lieberman, and Williams 2003). The brains of the subjects in the experiment were scanned during a game that involved virtual balls being passed by allegedly three individuals. Each of the subjects was excluded because the other two persons (in fact simulated by a computer) started passing the ball only between themselves. It turned out that the situation of exclusion activates the same brain areas that are responsible for feeling physical pain.[1]

Hellinger writes about conscience:

> With a clear conscience we feel good, with a guilty conscience we feel bad. We get a guilty conscience when we think, feel, and do something that is not in line with the expectations and demands of the people and groups we want to belong to and often must belong to. These are important for our well-being and survival. We experience this secured belonging as beneficial and good. We do not have to worry about being suddenly alone and defenseless. So our conscience is watching over our connection with these people and groups. It immediately notices when we put this belonging at risk and move away from the others. Then it reacts with a feeling of fear. This is why the importance of personal conscience cannot be overestimated. This is also reflected in its high status in society and culture. (Hellinger and Heilmann 2018, 141)

The primary role of this conscience—which Hellinger describes as "personal"—is to secure our place in the community. Conscience thus also serves the sense of being part of the community. The other side of this sense is rejecting those who do not belong to the community. The sense of greater national unity, *Volksgemeinschaft*, was said to be the result of Germans' wartime hardships (Fritz 1997). It also helped to keep people from paying attention to the suffering of other nations. Soldiers who feel they are a community are capable of heroic deeds. A soldier who feels abandoned dies of fear. The same soldier who cries over his companion's plight, kills another soldier, the enemy, with no feelings. A man just like him. Someone who protects his family, kills another man's children. During wars, the limitations of human conscience are clearly visible.

Hellinger says that conscience "holds us to our group like a sheepdog holds the sheep together in a herd" (Hellinger, Weber, and Beaumont 1989). And when we change our environment, our conscience also changes to protect us. So we have a different conscience in front of our mother and a different conscience in front of our father, a different conscience in the family and a different conscience at work, in church and at the football stadium. But it always concerns "bond and love and the fear of separation from the group and of losing membership" (Hellinger 2006, 77). These statements are similar to the thought of Freud, who believed that each individual has "a share in numerous group minds—those of his race, of his class, of his creed" and has only little autonomy (Freud 1975, 61). Collectivities generate pressure, which shapes individuals' conscience and behavior. Even social gatherings "obey some unformulated and sometimes consciously unrecognized rules, which keep them coherent over some period of time" (László 1972, 44).

The fact that our conscience can be flexible, changeable, and context-dependent was demonstrated by Stanley Milgram in his famous experiment, in which people agreed to subject other people to the shocks of increasingly stronger currents (although in reality these shocks were fake). Milgram described their obedience to the experimenter and their ruthlessness to the person "subjected to the shocks" as entering an "agentic state." He explained that in this state, an individual does what he does "because conscience, which regulates impulsive aggressive action, is per force diminished at the point of entering a hierarchical structure" (Milgram 2009, 161). In the agentic state, morality "does not disappear—it acquires a radically different focus: the subordinate person feels shame or pride depending on how adequately he has performed the actions called for by authority" (Milgram 2009, 177).

As we can see, morality does not have to be related to the good of another person; it can also be based on other values. In the case of the Milgram experiment, the individuals examined subordinated their consciences to a social phenomenon called "science." They became as if members of a "scientific community" and stopped considering those who, like the "person subjected to shocks," are not part of it. Many people did not feel well and felt that they were doing something wrong. Milgram stated, "Many subjects make tentative movements toward disobedience but then seem restrained, as if by a bond" (Milgram 2009, 180). Was the thing that restrained them the fear of being stigmatized by the experimenter and excluded from the "community?" Conscience specifies what is allowed and what we are not allowed to see in a given group. The "scientific community" could not do anything wrong, even though the "person subjected to shocks" shouted that he had heart problems. The group we belong to is always good and has no dark sides.

Of course, conscience is not simply "selfish." It goes beyond ourselves toward others to ensure our belonging. It undoubtedly has a lot to do with compassion and empathy, which may seem conflicting in view of the above facts.

Schopenhauer even considered compassion to be the "real basis of all *voluntary* justice and *genuine* loving-kindness" (Schopenhauer 1995, 144). He believed that it consists in experiencing someone's harm as my own, which "requires that I am in some way *identified with him*, in other words, that this entire *difference* between me and everyone else, which is the very basis of my egoism, is eliminated, to a certain extent at least" (Schopenhauer 1995, 143–44).

So conscience derives from the sense of unity of all people, but its—so to speak—most external layer, the circle closest to consciousness, and thus the one that shapes our choices and judgments, always refers to some limited group: nation, friends, family. History shows many examples that people's consciences remained unresponsive to the suffering of others when they did not belong to their nation or race. Even by acting wickedly, people were able to keep a "clear conscience" because their victims belonged to a foreign group. Rudolf Höss, commandant of Auschwitz, probably actually thought he was doing something useful and necessary. His conscience did not speak up when thousands of people of other nationalities were killed. Islamic terrorists also do something "good" when killing innocent and unarmed people. Their conscience connects them with their own group, and the act of suicide makes their delusional merit even greater. Although they die, they feel that they belong, as their fantasies go beyond death, into a vision of continued existence (Janus 2019, 202 et seq.). All these people do not lack conscience, but their conscience is narrow. This is in line with the observations of psychologists and ethologists. It has been found that empathy is activated primarily in relation to people of the same race and similar to us (Bloom 2016).

ETHICAL MOTIVATION

The first, narrowest circle of personal conscience is not all. Systemic constellations have clearly shown how strongly our lives are determined by the mechanisms that we can link to ethics, conscience, or a sense of justice. Man turns out to be not only more "egoistic" than we assumed, but he is also more "moral." This was already noticed by Freud, who wrote:

> If anyone were inclined to put forward the paradoxical proposition that the normal man is not only far more immoral than he believes but also far more moral than he knows, psycho-analysis, on whose findings the first half of the assertion rests, would have no objection to raise against the second half.
>
> This proposition is only apparently a paradox; it simply states that human nature has a far greater extent, both for good and for evil, than it thinks

> it has—i.e. than its ego is aware of through conscious perception. (Freud 1989b, 53)

We unconsciously want to suffer and be punished when we have done something wrong to someone, especially a family member. We feel obligated to carry the burdens of our parents or more distant ancestors and repeat their fate. We find it difficult to accept that we deserve to live when someone else is dead, such as our twin who died in the womb. We carry within us the conflicts of past generations, such as our grandmother's anger toward the grandfather, because subconsciously we want justice to be done. And in addition to this, which is the wider circle of our conscience, we desire reconciliation between perpetrators and victims.

We can see how some of the mechanisms of hidden conscience work by looking at the example of abortion. Hellinger writes that after an abortion:

> The mother wants to go back to her child, the father to his child, and the siblings, if there were or are any, wait for this sibling to appear among them.
>
> How does this desire to come to her aborted child manifest itself in the mother? She wants to find a way to him by dying too. This secret desire accompanies her throughout her life.
>
> What is the consequence? [. . .] she secretly communicates to one of her living children, "Die too, die instead of me."
>
> How does this child react, even though he knows nothing about the background? He acts in accordance with his mother's wish. He says to her, "I for you, I in your place." (Hellinger 2014b, 193)

What can happen later? The same child who wanted to die for his mother, if he survived, says "the same sentence, 'You for me.' Either to his own child, or to his life partner" (Hellinger 2014b, 194). In this intricate way, they seem to combine the instinct of self-preservation with the need for justice and love. However, I would like to stress that, according to my observations, the "altruistic" aspects are stronger and more fundamental. It is these that lead above all to difficulties in life or health. However, even though they stem from the bond, empathy, and the need for justice, they do not bear good fruit, becoming a cause of destructive atonement and a vehicle for negative transgenerational transmissions.

Conscience cares about fundamental justice, reflected in balancing what is taken and given, profits and losses, of one's own and others. The balancing mechanism works in such a way that if we get something from someone, we feel compelled to give something. The need for compensation makes us feel guilty when we are indebted or obliged. When we give back, we feel innocent and even entitled to claims. If someone hurts us, we expect harm to be done to him. And when we hurt someone, we expect ourselves to be hurt. This level of conscience has a significant unconscious part—we are often not aware that we expect punishment and failure due to our own actions (or imagined guilt). For, all this works automatically, regardless of the ethics and views we declare.

These debt and obligation dynamics are very similar to the so-called reciprocity principle—well known to social psychology—which "is one of the strongest and most common principles governing social interactions" (Wojciszke 2017, 286).[2] The balancing mechanism separates, judges, and demands equality, compensation, and revenge from an early age. This is confirmed by research on children (Bloom 2013).

Nietzsche observed that the balancing principle that functions in conscience relates to the purchase and sale category:

> Whence has this age-old, deeply-rooted, perhaps now no longer eradicable idea taken its power—the idea of an equivalence between injury and pain? I have already given it away: in the contractual relationship between *creditor* and *debtor*, which is as old as the existence of "legal subjects" and in turn points back to the basic forms of purchase, sale, exchange, trade, and commerce. (Nietzsche 1998, 40)

> The feeling of guilt, of personal obligation [. . .] had its origin, as we have seen, in the oldest and most primitive relationship among persons there is, in the relationship between buyer and seller, creditor and debtor [. . .]. Making prices, gauging values, thinking out equivalents, exchanging—this preoccupied man's very first thinking to such an extent that it is in a certain sense thinking *itself* [. . .] it was out of the most rudimentary form of personal legal rights that the budding feeling of exchange, contract, guilt, right, obligation, compensation first *transferred* itself onto the coarsest and earliest communal complexes. (Nietzsche 1998, 45)

The concept of debt and obligation to pay would therefore be deeply rooted in us; so deeply that it directs the foundations of our morality. "Guilt," according to Nietzsche, originated in the processes of purchase and exchange—indeed, the German word *die Schuld* means both "debt" and "guilt." He also believes that thinking that everything has a price and can be paid for is the oldest moral canon.

Hellinger writes about balancing in the form of atonement:

> So we can see that the need for balance works against life and against love, because then we see ourselves, and not the other person. Let me say more. Such atonement is blind and hostile. This atonement is completely against reason. (Hellinger and Nehrebecki 2012, 70)

This is a paradox of conscience: although it commands us to transcend our own narrow interest, it may lead to new forms of egoism and blindness. At the same time causing harm to ourselves.

These hidden processes can be seen during a constellation, for example, when the mother, unable to forgive herself for the death of one of her children, considers herself "unworthy" or "no good" for her living child. Her conscience punishes her, dictates that she should remain in the pain of the past, so the woman distances herself from both her life and the living child. Consideration for the demands of her conscience does not allow her to move toward what is right now.

Persistent remorse, constant blaming oneself, and no forward movement contain a certain hidden attitude—a refusal to accept full responsibility for what happened. Being stuck in the past, guilt, and the need to atone, we do not have to be fully confronted with the event and our deeds, and above all, we do not face the victim. In constellations this is clearly visible—someone cannot transcend the sense of guilt toward the victim, but at the same time does not want to see him, he is not interested in the victim as a person, he avoids looking at him.

When we atone for fault, we aim for the well-being of our conscience. We want our conscience to be "clear" again. This desire may obscure our seeing the other person and any constructive way out of the difficult situation. For moving forward requires that we accept that our conscience is "troubled." Many people find it difficult to accept this and some prefer to die rather than live with a bad conscience, even if their death would hurt even more people. This is how strong the balancing mechanism is. The desire to have a "clear conscience" can lead to deeds that are worse than those that have caused it to be troubled. Someone, for example, feels guilty about cheating on his wife, so he decides to have his lover terminate her pregnancy. In this way, his narrow conscience is against life.

While an "unclear" conscience causes suffering, a "clear" conscience makes it possible to nurse one's own pride, which is the road to hubris and egoism. And one's conscience becomes "clear" not only due to good deeds and refraining from causing harm. Our consciences also become "clear" as a result of the wrong that others do to us. Hence, for example, the "moral" superiority of some children over their parents, who in their opinion have failed. These people do not want to look at the past in a different way and see the context of their situation, because they would have to abandon the pride of the victims. There are also those who never expect compensation from the perpetrators, for example, some wives who have been wronged by their husbands. They do not seek compensation for the wrongs so that there is no balance. They want to keep their role as a victim and, through their "clear conscience," tower over the perpetrator.

FAMILY CONSCIENCE

Boszormenyi-Nagy spoke of an internalized tribunal, guarding the balance of give and take, even across several generations. This conscience is based on the unconscious bond with the family members and watches over the belonging of everyone, even at the expense of our happiness.

The fact that conscience is not something entirely individual was intuited by anthropologist Francis M. Cornford, who wrote:

> The collective consciousness is, thus, superindividual. It resides, of course, in the individuals composing the group—there is nowhere else for it to exist—but it resides in all of them together, and not completely in any of them. It is both in myself and yet not myself. It occupies a certain part of my mind, and yet it stretches beyond and outside me to the limits of my group. And since I am only a small part of my group, there is much more of it outside me than inside. (Cornford 2004, 80–81)

From this it follows that conscience "like a traitor within the gates, acknowledges from within the obligation to obey that other and much larger part of the collective consciousness which lies outside" (Cornford 2004, 81).

Driven by the dictates of the family conscience, descendants take on the guilt of their ancestors or suffer from the disorder and trauma they experienced. Sometimes they try, as it were, to repair the past or compensate for past injustice with their own suffering. These astonishing processes are completely unconscious to the subject. It is only during a constellation that the subject finds the true causes of his failures or depression. This circle of our conscience does not care about our own belonging, but is directed toward other members of the family, especially those who are excluded. It commands us to unconsciously remember them, which is manifested in taking over their emotions and following their fate. For the first guideline of this conscience is the principle that we can put in the words: "Everyone in the family has an equal right to belong." No matter how long they lived, what their merits were, or what they did wrong.

We often put our personal conscience, closer to our consciousness, before the requirements of the family conscience that we do not know. We see the family in its narrow sense, but do not see the wide system of the family. We remain, for example, loyal to our parents, but we are not aware that the family conscience demands that we respect our father's first wife. We love our living siblings, but we do not know that we are unconsciously attached to the unknown deceased siblings, and that this loyalty shapes our lives much more strongly.

Hellinger cites the example of a wealthy business owner who was on a slippery slope. His mother sent her first husband, the father of the businessman's step-brother, away, considering him a "loser." The constellation showed that the young businessman, under the influence of the family conscience, sought to become a loser himself, and in this way represent his mother's first husband who was excluded. In the constellation, the older brother's father was given his rightful place, and the businessman was able to recognize that the marriage of his parents was connected with the loss suffered by his brother and his father. In spite of all this, he accepted his success and considered himself equal to the others. He also decided to find his brother's missing father and make them meet (Hellinger and Heilmann 2018, 153).

The family conscience is embedded in the knowing field. Its operation is possible only because the individual has unconscious knowledge about the members of the family and the most important emotional events that affected them (abandonments in childhood, losses of children, murders, deep guilt, great fear, etc.). This is not, of course, knowledge of the details of their lives, but knowledge of the existence of these people, and empathy with what was particularly difficult and painful for them. So it can be said that the family conscience is par excellence a transpersonal part of our mind.

Another circle of conscience is the one that sees to the hierarchy in the family. When we disrupt the hierarchy, when we put ourselves in the place of others (driven by nothing other than our bond with them and our conscience), we may, on a superficial level, feel superior, significant. But internally, the circle of conscience that sees to the maintenance of hierarchy demands reparation for our usurpation.

The order of birth matters and has certain consequences. The affairs of the older ones should be left with them, although very often things go differently and the younger ones take them on themselves. For instance, when children meddle in their parents' affairs. They do so consciously when they educate their parents, suggest divorce, or are concerned about fidelity or infidelity in their marriage, or subconsciously when they co-experience the parents' guilt or want to stop them from going into death (the latter is an extremely strong factor that shapes the child's fate and is sometimes difficult to stop). In both cases, they put themselves in the place of the older ones, which is a violation of the hierarchy and is not without an internal response.

SPIRITUAL CONSCIENCE

Because the family conscience takes the innocent and unconscious "into service," forcing the descendants to carry the plight of their ancestors or to compensate for their guilt, Hellinger said that this conscience is archaic and unjust. But family constellations, which made it possible to discover these unconscious processes, showed something more. The same constellation that identifies the subject's entanglement, his blind following of the imperatives of this conscience, leads to a solution, suggesting to the therapist, representatives, and client what is right. As if there is a force that leads to good solutions for all. A special feature of this movement, which led Hellinger to distinguish the next level of conscience, the spiritual conscience, is that it regularly leads to reconciliation between perpetrators and victims and causes their descendants to unconsciously want such reconciliation. In constellations, this is manifested through the fact that representatives of perpetrators and victims are always eventually attracted to each other and together they find peace. In turn, clients discover their identifications with perpetrators of crimes, for example. Although the clients wanted revenge or condemned the perpetrators on a conscious level, they now realize that they are part of their family system and want to give them a place. These processes obviously go beyond our narrow personal conscience.

Such observations caused Hellinger's work and views to evolve. He originally claimed that although the family conscience takes care of everyone's belonging, there is one exception—murderers, especially if they killed someone from the family. The conscience allegedly demanded that they should be excluded. These views—perhaps shaped by common morals—changed when Hellinger noticed the spontaneous movement of representatives toward reconciliation between murderers and their victims. He then began to speak of the spiritual conscience, stressing that it turns toward peace and does not judge anyone. Based on this experience, the term "movements of the Spirit" was coined (German: *Bewegungen des Geistes*) to define a therapeutic technique in which the therapist withdraws to the maximum extent possible, giving room to these teleological processes that go beyond our judgments and expectations.

The personal conscience can lead to very archaic reactions, because, as Hellinger says, if someone "does something very bad to us, we experience violent feelings. What feelings? We want him to die. Then justice will be done. There is something murderous in the idea and demand for justice" (Hellinger and Nehrebecki 2012, 73).

The question of "justice" was similarly illuminated by René Girard, who wrote that all "who are enveloped by the scapegoat mechanism, and completely convinced by it, live in a world that always conforms to the demands of Justice. If, momentarily, this world ceases to be just, sooner or later the scapegoating process will intervene to re-establish its perfection" (Girard 1987a, 122). "Perfect justice" is the goal of the primordial mechanisms of conscience. Everything must be carefully balanced, all debts paid. It involves vengeance, for example. To stop it, it is not enough to convince people "that violence is detestable—for it is precisely because they detest violence that men make a duty of vengeance" (Girard 1977, 15).

The idea that murderous impulses come easily to us is backed by the research of David M. Buss, which shows that fantasizing about killing people who have somehow fallen afoul of us is common (Buss 2005).

Hellinger asks: "How can we protect ourselves from the destructive effects of our conscience?" and answers: "By getting rid of the conviction that when we act in the name of a clear conscience, we cause something good" (Hellinger 2014c, 34). For, what do people with a clear conscience do? They always exalt themselves above others. And those who want to keep it clear? By atoning, they destroy themselves and often do not care about others. In order to get out of this situation, it is necessary to accept the fate that we have been given. Also to accept a "bad conscience." This has nothing to do with denying the act that caused our guilt. On the contrary, it is only in this way that we really bear its consequences.

Constellations show us more fully the determinants of behaviors, including the bad ones. We can see that someone follows a "plan," the roots of which are beyond him, lying in the period before his birth. During a constellation, we see, for example, that the brother who sexually abused the female client in childhood is unconsciously connected with the trauma of his grandmother, who was probably raped. We see his shame, insecurity and guilt, perhaps never clearly articulated. The client's love is also brought to light, her representative is clinging to her brother without fear, and then the client herself admits that only the events related to her brother gave her the closeness she needed. Could we judge all this? We see love at the heart of all movements and events.

NOTES

1. The same areas are activated also by a sense of injustice and the loss of an important person—this confirms the fundamental meaning of balancing and bond.

2. The principle of exchange in relationships proposed by Hellinger, which consists in giving more good in return for good and less evil in return for evil, is in line with the tit-for-tat strategy described by evolutionary psychologists, a successful strategy forpromoting cooperation (Buss 2016, 259). Three principles of this strategy have been identified: (1) never be the first to defect, (2) retaliate when the other has defected, and (3) be able to forgive.

Chapter 7

New Paths in Anthropology and Religious Studies

THE TRUE FOUNDATION OF THE BELIEF IN SPIRITS AND THE MEANING OF ANCESTORS

The Influence of the Dead on the Living

In all ancient cultures, people believed that their loved ones did not cease to exist after death and that their influence on the living continued. As we read anthropological studies, we can easily see that great value was always placed on mourning rites and, if I may put it this way, on the management of relationships between the living and the dead. Some peoples focused on protecting the living from these "spirits" that were feared; other peoples focused on winning their grace as benefactors, though usually the two elements were mixed together.

Native peoples, many of the traditional religions of the East, but also native Americans or pagan Slavs and Germans, saw to it that the dead take their intended place, do not trouble the living, but become their support. To some extent, this approach has continued in our Christian Western culture, although it seems that by entrusting the dead to God we have taken the burden of taking care of them off ourselves. Respect for the dead has remained even in the secular world, for we have not yet abandoned all funeral rites, even if we no longer really know what their purpose is supposed to be.

Why were funerary rituals never neglected and why did people try—as many anthropologists emphasize—to separate the world of humans from the world of spirits? Why was it believed that these worlds remain mutually connected? Why was it so widely believed that one had to be particularly vigilant so that their interaction would not harm the living? Was paying so much attention to these matters in all cultures and for millennia a sign of a gigantic waste of mental and physical energy? Is the widespread belief in souls being active after death rooted in fear of death, being an expression of dreams and projections?

Systemic constellations provide solid premises for the thesis that the ideas and rituals of traditional cultures were based on real psychological phenomena different from those considered before by science. They were not known to any of the anthropologists who described aboriginal cultures, so the researchers understood the natives' rituals as resulting from errors in thinking or having only symbolic or social meaning.

The phenomena referred to are much more aptly described by the natives themselves. The living do indeed commune with the dead, the dead may be in various conditions, and contacts with them may produce good or harmful effects. To see this and to be sure of it, we need not renounce rationality or leave the realm of facts. Quite the contrary, we need to confront them.

Some anthropologists, such as Alfred Radcliffe-Brown, came very close to finding out the real reasons why traditional peoples placed so much importance on mourning rituals. He said:

> The dead man was bound by ties of solidarity to those still living. Now that he is dead those ties have not ceased to exist, but continue until the society has recovered from the effects of the death, for they are based on deep-seated and elaborately organised sentiments. I believe that the mourning customs of the Andamanese are to be explained on this basis, as being the means by which the social sentiments of the survivors are slowly reorganised and adapted to the new condition produced by the death. The severance of the dead man from the society is not a sudden but a gradual process, during which his relatives and friends, being still attached to him by social ties, are in an abnormal condition which may be defined as a partial separation from the world of living men and women and a partial aggregation to the world of the dead (i.e. the spirit world). (Radcliffe-Brown 2013, 288)

The author notes that the essence of the mourning ritual is the emotions of the living and the ties that connected the survivors to the deceased. These ties do not cease to exist when the loved one dies, but they demand to be remodeled. They need to be addressed during the mourning ceremonies that last a long time. The Andamanese studied by Radcliffe-Brown say that "if the burial and mourning customs are not properly observed the relatives of the dead person will fall sick and perhaps die" (Radcliffe-Brown 2013, 298).

Radcliffe-Brown finds that the basis of the above beliefs

> is that the near relatives of the deceased, being bound to him by close social ties, are influenced by everything that happens to him, and share in his good or evil

fortune. So that when by sickness and resulting death he is removed from the community, they are as it were drawn after him. (Radcliffe-Brown 2013, 298)

This "drawing after" is not a fantasy; it involves phenomena known to the constellation therapist—the ties between the living relatives and the deceased, and the unconscious movement of the living toward death. Without being aware of these factors, Radcliffe-Brown calls these ties "social" and says that this "society" must reorganize itself after its member dies. He is probably right, but the impact that the Andamanese try to cope with through rituals goes deeper. It is a powerful psychological force.

What effect do "ghosts" have on the living? Anthropologist E. E. Evans-Pritchard concludes that, according to the beliefs of the African Nuer people, when the ghosts "return to the living [. . .], it is only to cause trouble, to fetch the living to join them in the place of the dead or to punish them for faults and shortcomings" (Evans-Pritchard 1956, 161). He also writes that "the living do not want the dead to take any interest in their lives. The dead had best look after their own affairs and let the living look after theirs" (Evans-Pritchard 1956, 161).

In light of what systemic constellations show, the fear of neglect toward the dead is justified. "The dead," continuing to be an active part of the family system, influence the psyche and fate of the individual. The early deceased older sibling influences the next children; the kind of relationship with the deceased mother is an important factor shaping the life of the daughter; unknown traumas of the grandparents are present in the psyche of the grandson. These processes affect people, regardless of the society in which they have been raised. For this reason, members of modern societies also have something to fear from their ancestors. This is particularly true when their lot was so hard that their suffering was unconsciously taken over by the next generations—when they were excluded or treated very unjustly by the family, or when, thanks to their loss, we could be born, as is the case with the former wife or husband of our father or mother.[1]

Evans-Pritchard speaks of the relationship between the notion of "behind" and of the "ghosts" that can be seen in the phrase "to go behind" used by the Nuer, which means "to go to the ghosts," that is, "to die" (Evans-Pritchard 1956, 161). This phrase is not a mere euphemism, as the author defines it, but refers to a real psychological process that we repeatedly observe during constellation work. The person entangled in the ancestor's hard lot is driven by just this sort of movement (which he realizes during the constellation). It is a hidden desire to connect with the one who departed earlier. This inner movement is essentially against his own life and sometimes turns into moving toward death. There is no better phrase here than to say that someone "follows the dead." And this is precisely the phrase we use in constellations.

The African Bahima believe that illness can be caused by a deceased king, witchcraft, natural causes, and ghosts (muzimu), "which take possession of people for various causes, and have to be exorcised" (Lévy-Bruhl 1966, 245). Does the last assertion make any sense? In constellations, we see that, as Hellinger puts it, the organ that is in dissonance with our body is in resonance with some other person. Illness often represents someone, and it is like his embassy in our own body. It arises when, because of our unawareness or attitude, we cannot give that person a place in our hearts. When the bond cannot be consciously experienced, unconscious identification occurs, which has its bodily dimension in the form of illness.

Although in the beliefs of native peoples we can distinguish certain universal elements—such as that spirits exist and act, and something must be done about it—there are differences in understanding the nature of their influence. Often anthropologists themselves were not able to adequately portray what the natives really think on these matters. It is generally said that they consider spirits to be dangerous, even hostile, wishing to intentionally harm the living. Sometimes, however, the picture is more subtle. Radcliffe-Brown cites a legend of a tribe from the Andaman Islands in which the spirit of a dead man comes to see his brother and causes his death. The story, however, does not imply that the brother died because of the spirit's evil disposition:

> On the contrary it was his attachment to his relative that caused him to return to visit him, and death followed as a result of this contact of the living man with the spirit. [. . .] Thus it appears that the Andamanese conceive that the spirits do not cause death and sickness through evil intention, but through their mere proximity. (Radcliffe-Brown 2013, 299)

This picture is closer to the knowledge we derive from constellations. The problems with "spirits" are caused by the ties that exist between the members of the family. This primal love is responsible for most of the difficulties that the constellation therapist deals with. It causes the living to internally turn toward those who have passed away, even if they have never met them in person. This results in turning away from life to a greater or lesser degree, causes sicknesses, and sometimes is even a substantial "trigger" for death. This mechanism has nothing to do with the hostile disposition of the dead. Even if it was someone aggressive or brutal during his life, what attracts the living person to the "spirit" is always unconscious love. The truth, the Andamanese say, is that it is the "proximity" of the "spirit" that can be the cause of sickness or death. However, it is not the "spirit" that produces this proximity. Constellations have discovered that it is the activity of the living toward the "spirits" that causes problems, not the other way round. It is not the "spirits" that draw us to them, but we ourselves, on an unconscious level, long to connect with them.

Freud, too, wondered about the reasons why traditional cultures attributed evil intentions to their dead. He compared their mentality to the emotional lives of neurotics. He wrote:

> When a wife loses her husband, or a daughter her mother, it not infrequently happens that the survivor is afflicted with tormenting scruples, called "obsessive reproaches" which raises the question whether she herself has not been guilty through carelessness or neglect of the death of the beloved person. [. . .] Psychoanalytic investigation of such cases has made us acquainted with the secret mainsprings of this affliction. We have ascertained that these obsessive reproaches are in a certain sense justified and therefore are immune to refutation or objections. (Freud 1946, 80)

The justification Freud refers to is an unconscious death wish against a beloved person. Such unconscious hostility, hidden under the mask of love, exists, according to Freud, in every strong emotional relationship. The reaction to this hostility, which is contrary to the conscious attitude, is guilt and self-reproach. In neurotics, it is particularly strong, and among aboriginal peoples it is experienced in the form of projection—it is not the survivor that had bad intentions, but it is the spirit that wants to do him harm.

Family constellations have shown that beneath the layers of conscious positive attitude and unconscious hostility, there is a third layer—that of bond and love. After a mother dies, her daughter feels guilty because she turned away from this deeply hidden bond. Because of her experiences with the mother, such a daughter has not fully accepted the mother as a mother. At a certain level, she rejected her. However, as a "good daughter" and a "good person," or perhaps because she was completely unaware of her negative attitude toward her mother, she had a "good relationship" with her or simply cared for her "because it was the right thing to do." After her mother died, the daughter's poor condition was in fact a reaction of her conscience. But it was not driven by the social prohibition of aggression or the religious imperative of honoring parents or by purely individual motives. What activated the most persistent aspect of it was the regard for the irreducible bond with the mother.

The Influence of the Living on the Dead

Members of traditional cultures believe that it is possible to influence the dead, their "dispositions" and "actions." For example, the Dagara believe that "it is the duty of the living to heal their ancestors. If these ancestors are not healed, their sick energy will haunt the souls and psyches of those who are responsible for helping them" (Somé 1995, 10). While the influence of the dead on the living that I wrote about above can be fairly easily imagined—even within a slightly expanded scientific worldview—for example, as an effect of the "memory" contained in the field of the family on the mind of the individual, the reverse influence, of the living on the dead, may seem quite extraordinary.

Family constellations show, however, that "healing the ancestors" is not a fantasy or an anthropological curiosity. Ancestors may be "sick" because they never made it to their parents, or because there is an ongoing movement toward death in them, toward their deceased siblings, or for other reasons. The suffering they carried in their lifetime—being more or less aware of its source—continues in the family system, and through the knowing field becomes part of the mind and life of someone younger. Constellations display these internal dramas and enable the ancestors' movement toward resolution. This in turn unburdens the descendant's mind. Is this not the "healing" of the ancestors, through remembering and respecting them?

The aforementioned practitioner of ancestral medicine, Daniel Foor, states:

> We also bring honor and joy to our ancestors when we heal intergenerational challenges, support healthy families, and live as good and ethical people on Earth. Remember that death in our world is the start of a rite of passage for the recently deceased. This journey is completed only when they fully join the ranks of ancestors. The living can play an important role in this transformation. When we assist the recently dead and those who are not yet well in spirit to complete their transition, we support the ancestors' health. (Foor 2017, 29–30)

All of this could be considered a set of peculiar beliefs, were it not for the fact that therapeutic practice emphatically corroborates the "effect" of the dead on the living and vice versa. German therapist Heinz Stark wrote:

> One of the many surprises encountered when setting up constellations with the dead is that one is confronted with the very many conditions that the dead are in. There are many different ways of being dead, ranging from soul's restless wanderings or tormented feelings of being unredeemed, to a peaceful passing, just to name a few. These states of being can change drastically in the course of the Constellation Work. (Stark 2005, 37)

Stark states that these phenomena cannot be explained by the "memory" contained in the morphic field because, as he puts it, "they are not something historical that is still vibrating, but instead something current that relates to a state of being" (Stark 2005, 37). At the same time, however, he states that, in fact, no one knows what the field we encounter in systemic constellations actually is. And precisely for this reason, we can stick to the field concept. It is a fact that in constellations we can see mental states of people we know nothing about, whether they are alive or dead. It is also a fact that through the constellation process, we can make the representatives of the dead feel better. And this only happens when the orders discovered by Hellinger are respected, whether the representatives have any knowledge of them or not. It is also a fact that as the condition of the dead in the constellation improves, the functioning of the client improves.

In the Japanese Buddhism-related practice of *mizuko kuyō* (literally "water-child"), which is a form of ritual coping with the loss of a child (through accident, miscarriage, or abortion), the idea is to give the deceased children a sense of well-being and calm them so that they can become a source of benevolent effect on the living family members (Harrison 2008, 128). Elizabeth G. Harrison writes that the essence of *mizuko kuyō* is that it provides

> a formal, public, ritualized way to acknowledge the existence of a child—both its potential existence in this world as a result of its conception and its continuing existence somewhere else after death, to (re)establish a relationship with it, and to care for it wherever it may be. In this construction, although the child might be absent from this world, it nevertheless remains a child to its parents and a sibling to its living brothers and sisters. (Harrison 2008, 135)

Mizuko kuyō makes it possible for women "to mother their *mizuko* that is conceptually similar to the way they care for their living children" (Harrison 2008, 136). To participate in this ritual is to acknowledge that "there was (by virtue of its conception), would have been (in that a child conceived is the seed of a child born), and still is a child, even though that child is not now present in the mundane sense of the word" (Harrison 2008, 136).

What we deal with in the case of *mizuko kuyō*—and we know this thanks to family constellations—is much more than a "belief-based" religious practice. The calming and benevolent effect reported by participants in this practice is not necessarily based on the suggestion or wishful thinking. The deceased children "really" exist, and acknowledging their importance as equal to that of the living children, as in this practice, can bring not only comfort to the parents but even save their living children from death or from failures in life. For the latter follow their deceased siblings internally, and the movement is especially strong when the dead siblings are forgotten by the family. Therefore, recognizing the deceased children as still living is not a bizarre act of faith, but an adequate response to the psychological processes that have a significant impact on the living.

Ancestral Support

According to James George Frazer, ancestor worship is most likely a common form of primitive religiosity, and Claude Lévi-Strauss states that there is probably no society that does not revere its dead (Frazer 1996; Lévi-Strauss 1961, 216). This does not mean that ancestors are paid "religious reverence" everywhere. Respect for ancestors or awareness of one's ties to them takes many different forms.

Ancestors may be something that is a threat to us, but they are also a source of irreplaceable strength for us. An expert and practitioner of modern shamanism, Daan van Kampenhout, based on traditional beliefs, speaks of the aspect of flame and heat brought by ancestors (Kampenhout 2006, 75). The "flame" shapes us; it is brought by those who raise us in childhood. The "heat" gives us strength and is brought by the distant ancestors who most often did not have a direct impact on our development. If we do not cut ourselves off from our parents and other ancestors, we can take life that flows through them, which brings us strength and health.

In Madagascar, the energy of life, *aina*, was and still is believed to exist. *Aina* is one for all, and on its basis, a spiritual community of *fihavanana* is formed and connects the living with the spirits of the ancestors. The integration and communication within the family, which includes both the living and the ancestors, enables one to participate in the flow of this energy and find one's own place in the world (Marcinkowska 2016, 90). A concept similar to *aina* is *hasina*, the power that the ancestors emanate after death (Szyjewski 2005, 273).

The above ideas capture very well what we can experience in family constellations. When those who are full of resentment and cut off from their parents work through their difficulties and are finally able to get closer to them, then they can also open up to their distant ancestors. The universal sensation is then a strong feeling of "energy flow." This can be felt most fully when we stand in the so-called the generational string—the client, followed by a representative of his father, then a representative of his father's father, great-grandfather, great-great-grandfather (the same applies to women—mother, grandmother, etc.). What occurs during such a session is a completely specific phenomenon, which cannot be reduced to other phenomena, including those that may occur during bioenergetic therapy and similar practices. The "energy" appears only as a result of previous work on the client's attitude toward his parents and distant ancestors, and after "healing the ancestors," in the form of uncovering their traumas, losses, or interrupted bonds.

It has been difficult for anthropologists to understand the fact that the natives, on the one hand, manifest fear of spirits of the dead, which makes them seek to "cut themselves off" from the dead, and, on the other hand, cultivate their relationship with them so that "a participation between the living group and its dead [. . .] is most intensely realized" (Lévy-Bruhl 1966, 304). Lucien Lévy-Bruhl writes that we can neither clearly define "the personality of these dead, nor form any satisfactory idea of the way in which the living group participates in their existence, and in which it is 'participated' by them" (Lévy-Bruhl 1966, 304). It is equally difficult, according to this author, to understand such ideas as that one can be "entirely dead" (Lévy-Bruhl 1966, 304).

In the face of the experiences offered to members of Western culture by family constellations, these exotic assertions cease to be unusual or illogical. We see that the dead in the family system are, on the one hand, "energies" that can entangle us in their suffering, but on the other, life-givers and the source of our psychophysical strength. Constellations are a process through which we transcend the first kind of influence and open up to the latter. Some of the dead, or rather their fate, are a source of subconscious concerns and anxieties. They are scary areas in the family's unconscious memory. They can be described as "restless," or "not entirely dead." However, addressing their fate in a constellation, consciously confronting what has hitherto been unconscious, changes this situation. They too may eventually become strength that supports us. This is the meaning of what members of traditional cultures had in mind when they said that someone dead joined, or did not join, their ancestors.

Our ancestors are our parents, grandparents (and sometimes some unrelated people). However, being an ancestor is a little different than being a remembered relative. It is this gratitude that makes our deceased loved ones "ancestors" in the full sense of the word. If our resentments, memories of wrongs, or everyday events are in the foreground, our loved one has not yet achieved the status of an ancestor for us. Foor stated:

> In my experience of supporting others in making repairs with recent ancestors, I have encountered situations in which the spirit of the deceased seemed to be bright, loving, and available for connection, while the living—often adult children of the deceased—were not able to move beyond memories of their parent during life. (Foor 2017, 27)

Similar experiences are frequent during constellations—the "spirit" of the mother or father is open to the client, but the movement toward the "spirit" is blocked by the client's negative memories. This disposition of "spirits," different from the one the client is familiar with, is nothing but a manifestation of the existence of a deeper level of relationship in the family where bonding and love predominate.

Evans-Pritchard finds that the Nuer "do not so much think of the ghost of their forebears as being those members of their lineage who are in the home of the dead, but rather as names numbered, as it were, in the archives of the lineage. They think of the dead continuing in this way in the living" (Evans-Pritchard 1956, 162–63). For the Nuer, the lineage is a collective of the living and the dead. Among the Nuer, there is no "cult of the dead" in the sense of reverence paid to images, remains, burial sites, or other symbols that denote a particular person. "A man's memorial is not in some monument but in his sons" (Evans-Pritchard 1956, 162). As Evans-Pritchard writes, "Theirs is a this-worldly religion, a religion of abundant life and the fullness of days" (Evans-Pritchard 1956, 154). Is it any different in constellations? We do not "worship" our ancestors, but welcome them with love into our hearts, leaving their affairs with them. And we do this perhaps primarily to make our own lives successful.

Realness of Ghosts

Constellations acknowledge the realness of the influence of "ghosts," while leaving aside the question of postmortem existence. Until now, such a solution seemed impossible. The reasoning was that since it is impossible to agree on the—scientifically unfounded and even incompatible with the paradigm of science—postmortem existence of the self, any statements regarding the influence of the dead on the living should be regarded as errors in judgment of reality.[2]

These rationalist views were moderated by psychoanalysis and Jungian psychology that saw the effects of "ghosts" as manifestations of the unconscious. Jung argued that "ghosts" are a result of the autonomous activity of psychic complexes hidden in the unconscious (Jung 1990, 167). Although they are part of our psyche, to our consciousness they appear in the form of uncontrolled projections. That is why one can "meet" a ghost in the form of a hallucination. From this point of view, spirits of the dead gain a certain degree of autonomy and "real" influence on the individual, although they remain creations of his psyche.

Family constellations take us even further toward acknowledging the "reality" of influences from the dead. While we do not enter the realm of metaphysics, we are already close enough to what members of traditional cultures feel and claim to have a chance to truly understand them. The dead who are "healed," "appeased," or "honored" in the course of constellations are part of the client's family memory. The dead understood in this way can still be distinguished from the dead found in religious ideas and spiritualistic theories—the dead who are aware of their existence and live an afterlife. The dead who appear to us during systemic constellations are the dead who exist "for us." We do not know anything about their existence "for themselves."

We feel, however, that we must not approach them without respect, as if they were merely a voice recorded on tape. They exist in a much more significant way. The person who faces his deceased parent or sibling in a constellation does not—as he feels—participate in a symbolic psychodrama, nor does he "read" a dead record about his ancestor. He participates in an emotional encounter with him that takes place internally rather than externally. This encounter is interactive, and in the course of it, words addressed to the client often come to the mind of the representative of the deceased. These are always simple words like: "You are my daughter," "Live," "Go to your life," "I can see you now." These words are not the therapist's projections, and they really express something on the part of the mother, father, or another person.

When I represent, for example, someone's deceased mother and her suffering of being abandoned by her own mother, of which her son had no idea, comes to me in a dramatic form, then I "do something" for that woman, as if I allow her to release repressed pain. That pain was in her childhood, and she is no longer alive. So what actually happens? The "mother" that the son carries in his psyche becomes more transparent to him, and he can come closer to her, which improves his mood. However, this is not all. The "mother that appears in the constellation" must not be reduced to the client's "internal mother." After all, neither I nor her son had any idea of her inner pain. What is more, this feeling may no longer have been available to her in her adult life, because it had been repressed. And yet it appeared, as if it still vibrated "in her."

THE MECHANISM OF MAGIC AND RITUAL

Magic—the Greatest Illusion of Mankind?

One of the most important elements in the lives of members of traditional cultures was magic. Magic includes rituals related to hunting, farming, healing, war, human relations, and the burial of the dead. Yet none of the famous anthropologists—such as Tylor, Frazer, Mauss, or Malinowski—recognized magic as a process that could produce material effects. It was obvious to these scholars that magic does not work even to the approximate extent as assumed by those who practice it. Here is the comment of Marcel Mauss (who additionally refers to the standpoint of W. Lehmann):

> We have now arrived at the conclusion that there are affective states, generators of illusions, to be found at the root of magic, and that these states are not

> individual, but derive from a mixture of sentiments appertaining to both individuals and society as a whole. Here we find ourselves in close agreement with a theory advanced by W. Lehmann. Arguing from the point of view of individual psychology, he explains, as we all know, that magic derives from errors of perception, illusions and hallucinations, as well as acute, emotive and subconscious states of expectation, prepossession and excitability: all range from psychological automatism to hypnosis.
>
> We also agree with this writer that the expectations and illusions which are produced are the primary phenomena of magic. (Mauss 2001, 159–60)

Bronisław Malinowski's stance is the same in essentials. In his opinion, magical activity consists in replacing practical actions with symbolic ones, which happens in moments of helplessness in the face of the natural world. Malinowski, referring—after Frazer—to magic as "pseudo-science," writes:

> The spurious character of this pseudo-science is not hard to detect. Science, even as represented by the primitive knowledge of savage man, is based on the normal universal experience of everyday life [. . .] Magic is based on specific experience of emotional states in which man observes not nature but himself, in which the truth is revealed not by reason but by the play of emotions upon the human organism. [. . .] The theories of knowledge are dictated by logic, those of magic by the association of ideas under the influence of desire. (Malinowski 1954, 87)

Even my respect for the great anthropologists cannot stop me from expressing a negative opinion about this kind of "explanation." These are constructs created from what is at hand, in fact, not only of an anthropologist but of every member of Western society. "Errors of perception," "hallucinations," "subconscious states," "excitability," "prepossession," "hypnosis"—a whole range of terms that are supposed to explain something, although they themselves demand an explanation, denoting the phenomena that are among the least understood. There is a symptomatic convergence between the standpoint of anthropologists and the opinions of opponents of the systemic constellation method. One of the critics claims that systemic constellations are "seances probably based on psychodrama and perhaps collective hypnosis." He also claims that they "are so popular because people participating in them want to see and experience certain things very much" and that "everyone who takes part in this madness becomes infected with euphoria and enthusiasm, characteristic of most new and trendy therapies" (Doliński in: Szulc 2009, 13). We have here an identical collection of terms that are supposed to "explain," or discredit, the phenomenon incomprehensible to this psychologist.

According to Malinowski, magic does not have an effect on its object but affects the magician's psyche. Unable to cope with a problem, we calm down through magic, relieving our tension in words and gestures, after which "the desired end seems nearer satisfaction" and "we regain our balance, once more at harmony with life" (Malinowski 1954, 81). The effect of magic, then, is a kind of relaxing abreaction. Ultimately, it is nothing more than "a system of collective suggestion, which at that critical season tells the Central Australian that all will be well, on condition that man obeys the behests of tradition and enters into communion with the supernatural essence of his world" (Malinowski 1962, 323–24).

Is it possible to trivialize the issue of magic any more? "Everything will be all right" as long as you perform pointless rituals and believe in a nonexistent power. In the same way, opponents of systemic constellations try to portray their therapeutic effects—a group of "blinded" enthusiasts begin to feel better because they believe they should feel better. These explanations, however, are false. Practitioners and clients of constellations know that the effects of sessions go beyond any suggestion or momentary appeasement (Konkolÿ-Thege et al. 2021). And the effects do not arise as a result of beliefs, traditions, or perceptions shared by the therapist and client. Despite cultural, linguistic, worldview, and educational differences, there is a common ground of feeling and understanding, and a real impact that transcends the commonly known phenomena.

Mauss gives examples of "magical judgments" found among traditional cultures: "The magician conjures up his astral body; clouds are produced by smoking such-and-such a herb; a spirit is moved by the ritual" (Mauss 2001, 150) and states that:

> Objective reality has never imposed any proposition—of the kind we formulated above—on the human mind. Obviously you need the eyes of faith to see an astral body, the smoke that brings rain, and (most particularly in this case) an invisible spirit which obeys ritual. (Mauss 2001, 151)

Things are not so simple, however. Even if the world is divided into the realm of experience on one side and the realm of fantasy and belief on the other, the line between the two is somewhere else. I will not comment on the subject of smoke and astral bodies because I have no experience in this respect. However, the question of the effect of a rite on the deceased does not lie solely in the realm of faith. There is a clear, sometimes decisive for our lives, "effect of the dead" and there is also some kind of our "effect on the dead." I wrote about this above. Even with the most cautious approach, there is no doubt that we deal with facts here. The same processes were recognized by the "savages," who conceptualized them in their own way, and constructed their rituals on that basis. These rituals need not be perfect, and they may contain many imaginary or redundant elements, and may even at times be completely wrong. However, to judge what comes from identifying the mechanisms of the psyche in magic of the natives, and what comes from imagination and wishful thinking, anthropologists would first have to have the correct vision of man. Since they do not know the important psychic characteristics of Western man, how can they judge representatives of quite different cultures?

Gnothi Seauton

The way a researcher understands the world, especially when it comes to the realm of the psyche and emotions, depends on the experiences available to him. All people probably know pain, fear, desire, and they are also inclined to assume the existence of suggestion based on their own observations. However, they generally do not have telekinetic experiences, and do not have premonition dreams or visions. Such phenomena, if they occur manifestly, concern a small portion of the population, so telepathy or precognition do not serve as explanatory processes for other psychic or cultural phenomena. The writer Elias Canetti gives the example of an old Bushman who has a wound in his body:

> When the son thinks of his father he thinks of his old wound, but it is more than just thinking. Not only does he visualise it exactly, but he feels it at the corresponding place on his own body. As soon as he feels it he knows that his father, whom he has not seen for some time, is approaching. (Canetti 1984, 337–38)

Canetti believes that the Bushmen practice the skills, which we have lost, in their daily lives. He states that

> their descriptions of the way in which these presentiments announce themselves are among the most valuable material we have on the nature of transformation; there is nothing comparable to them, for, whatever myths and fairy stories can teach us about the subject, they are all open to the objection that they are something "invented," whereas here we learn what an actual Bushman in real life feels when he thinks of an ostrich or a springbok in the distance, what then happens to him, what it really means to him to think of a creature other than himself. (Canetti 1984, 339–40)

As a practitioner of constellations, I think I can understand the above quotes a little better than the average anthropologist. Feeling what someone else feels, personating another person, is not an abstraction or an incredible thing to me, but part of my everyday work. I also know that every person is much more strongly attached to their father than mainstream psychological theories would have us believe. Therefore, I am not particularly surprised that the Bushman feels his father's wound. However, I am not unique in this respect. The same abilities will be available to any average person if he attends a constellation workshop.

Frazer writes that "one of the great merits of homeopathic magic is that it enables the cure to be performed on the person of the doctor instead of on that of his victim, who is thus relieved of all trouble and inconvenience, while he sees his medicine man writhe in anguish before him" (Frazer 1996, 19). He then describes one such medicine man treating persistent vomiting, which was believed to be the result of the patient's stomach being "unhooked": "He at once throws himself into the most horrible contortions, for the purpose of unhooking his own stomach. Having succeeded in the effort, he next hooks it up again in another series of contortions and grimaces, while the patient experiences a corresponding relief" (Frazer 1996, 19–20).

A similar procedure was practiced by the Dyaks of Borneo, where in the case of a difficult labor a wizard "pretended"—as Frazer put it—"to be the expectant mother" himself, moving a big stone about on his abdomen, imitating the birth of the real infant (Frazer 1996, 17).

The British anthropologist did not refrain from irony and, describing the medicine man's efforts, referred to the patient as his "victim." Yet he was wrong to think that the doctor's experiencing the patient's pain could only be a trick or a sign of stupidity. Almost every week I conduct individual (non-group) sessions in which I experience my clients' "pains." Although these are rather psychological pains (perinatal traumas, the feeling of early separation from parents, inherited fears, or a feeling of confusion), it happens that I recognize "in myself" some physical symptoms that really plague the client. In such moments, I repeatedly writhe, curl up as if in pain, or clutch my "aching" head while kneeling on the floor.

To someone who has not participated in constellations, the description of this kind of activity must seem bizarre and absurd. He will assume a priori that this is a rather silly role-playing, whose possible effect can only be based on a suggestion. Things are different, however. During the session, I do not enact the events told to me by the client, but I discover them myself. Standing as his representative, I start to feel what his psyche hides. It is very simple, but it goes very deep.

Whether the medicine man actually experienced the patient's condition and, if so, how clearly, we do not know. What we do know, however, is that these methods did not necessarily develop from "imaginations" but may have been based on real processes of transferring feelings from one person to another (or rather, from one person's personal and family field to another person). How effective these methods were, we do not know. For some practices, the actual processes may have been more fully utilized, while for others, the ritual proved empty and ineffective.

Ritual as Prevention and Therapy

Rituals have primarily a psychological and psychotherapeutic meaning. They can be a kind of prophylaxis, like many of the so-called rites of passage (French: *rites de passage*), used in moments of major life changes, or a way of treating both physical and mental ailments. This does not necessarily apply to all rites of passage in their current form, but in general, their origins are basically psychological. Anthropologist Victor Turner writes that rituals are "a set of evocative devices for rousing, channeling, and domesticating powerful emotions, such as hate, fear, affection, and grief" (Turner 2008, 42–43).

Most ancient societies used rituals related to birth. Birth was never limited to a purely biological act; it always demanded a symbolic completion. It was referred to as "introducing the child into the world" (by the Yao of East Africa) or "launching the child into the world" (by the Dyaks of Bakarang, North Borneo) (Gennep 1960, 50 et seq.). Arnold van Gennep, who developed the concept of rites of passage, draws attention to these practices (Gennep 1960, 50 et seq.). Some of them can be called, following the author, rituals of "assimilation into the kin group"; in other rites, as I would put it, "assimilation into life" comes to the fore. For example, in the rite practiced in Vedic India, which is accompanied by the following recitation: "Take possession of this charm of immortality . . . I bring you breath and life; do not go toward the dark shadows; remain safe; go before you toward the light of the living" (Gennep 1960, 54). Many of these rituals involve a symbolic washing with water that symbolizes life, as in Christian baptism, which is also sometimes referred to as a "new birth."

In the light of psychotherapeutic knowledge, attempts to ritually complete one's birth make deep sense. As I showed in the book *Systemic Constellations: Theory, Practice, and Applications*, one's birth can psychologically be a process, as it were, incomplete, not quite successful. Many people "are not fully here," "are not completely alive," "do not quite believe that everything has ended well," "do not fully accept their lives." These are very real, though hidden, processes whose impact on the individual's life is extremely powerful. If someone in the perinatal period has not fully accepted his life—for example, because of identification with his parents' fear for his life—he carries an inner blockage that will impede his fulfillment in almost every sphere of life.

According to ethnographer Alfred Burdon Ellis, when on the Slave Coast (the Bight of Benin in West Africa), "one of the twins happens to die, the mother '. . . to give the spirit of the deceased child something to enter without disturbing the survivor, carries about, with the latter, a little wooden figure [. . .] roughly fashioned in human shape, and of the sex of the dead child'" (Lévy-Bruhl 1966, 35).

Did the "savages" think the figure was alive and coped with feelings of loss or anxiety in this primitive way? We do not know this. But there are mental processes in the light of which practices, as described above, are completely rational. We can then assume that it is them—and not mental incapacity—that were the basis for the development of practices of this kind.

The suffering and psychological problems of many people are caused by the fact that they lost a twin in their fetal life. These people experience states of irrational guilt, sometimes they oscillate between submissiveness and excessive emotions, anger and narcissistic withdrawal. They are often depressed and feel that their lives have no meaning. Of course, these people know nothing of the loss that took place at the beginning of their lives; only a systemic constellation suggests that such a thing may have happened in their case.

The practices of the African peoples described above involve a child who died after it was born, but even in this case, the twin bond remains strong. The mother, realizing this—or merely performing a traditional ritual—preserves the memory of the deceased child and gives him a place next to the living one. This is very important, because when listening to the experiences of people who have lost a twin, one can observe that they speak of emotional shifts from a "winner" identity to a "victim" identity, as they unconsciously imagine the fate of their brother or sister. The process of getting out of this psychologically difficult state is not easy, but it must include recognition of the existence of the other twin as a separate being. The solution can be expressed as follows: "There are two of us. I am alive, my brother/sister was not born/is not alive, but he/she is with me."

Turner refers to a ritual of the Ndembu people of northwestern Zambia that is a healing ritual. It is intended to cure the procreative problems of women who have experienced multiple miscarriages or stillbirths. The Ndembu believe that "either for his own default or as representative of a group of kin, a person is believed to have been 'caught,' as Ndembu say, by a shade [ancestor's spirit]" (Turner 2008, 11). Such a fate menaces "a woman who is either quarrelsome herself or a member of a group riven with quarrels, and who has simultaneously 'forgotten her [deceased mother or mother's mother or some other senior deceased matrilineal kinswoman's] shade in her life [. . .]'" (Turner 2008, 12). In addition, the Ndembu claim that a woman's procreative problems relate to the woman's identification with masculinity, with the shade of one of her past ancestors, called *Mvweng'i*.[3]

For a therapist, there is nothing unusual about the above beliefs. Experience shows that female procreative disorders, such as infertility or a tendency to miscarry, are largely psychosomatic. These problems are usually, if not always, caused by disturbances in the female family line, often manifested through the negative and grudging attitude of the subsequent daughters toward their mothers. In such cases, the woman internally "detaches" herself from her ancestresses or from her mother, whether the latter is still alive or not. When such a woman becomes pregnant or gives birth to a child, she "activates" in her own psyche her, often hidden, rejecting attitude toward her mother. Thus she becomes a kind of resentful child, and her ability to assume the role of a mother becomes impaired. In rejecting her mother, she rejects the role model that she considers bad, but quickly faces the fact that she cannot construct any other "mother" without it. Thus, she is unable to fully become a mother to her own child.

The problems we discuss here can also relate to the grandmother or another woman in the family who, for instance, had a dramatic delivery or, in extreme cases, died during the delivery. In this case, unconscious identification with her can cause anxiety and a variety of blockages, including a subconscious aversion to becoming pregnant and having children. It is somewhat puzzling for Turner that it is the female patient herself who is identified with the shadow, while it is the shadow that is said to cause her affliction (Turner 2008, 18). This is understandable in the light of constellations because entanglement, as that is what we are discussing here, is precisely a kind of identification that at some level can be so deep that there is an implicit identification.[4]

The Ndembu say that procreative problems menace a woman who is a member of a family group riven with quarrels, which can be explained by the fact that mother-daughter problems tend to be transmitted between generations, and that they affect many people.

The issue of identification with masculinity as an additional cause of procreative problems is also understandable. Rejection of the mother is partly a rejection of femininity and is related to identification with male figures, generally the father. He may become an ideal and role model for the daughter, who tries to be like him, forgetting that the most appropriate model for her is her mother.

Given that the spirits of matrilineal ancestors are the cause of problems, the purpose of the *Isoma* rite is, according to the Ndembu's claims, to "cause [. . .] to remember" these female matrilineal spirits. Another purpose of the ritual is *ku-solola*, which means "to make appear, or reveal," for "it is the 'hidden' [. . .] that is 'dangerous' or 'noxious'" (Turner 2008, 25). Turner writes that naming "an inauspicious condition is halfway to removing that condition" (Turner 2008, 25). The above statements are fully consistent with how therapy with the aid of family constellations is carried out. Its essential aim is, in Hellinger's words, to show what is. This aspect of therapy is fundamental and indeed is about halfway to therapeutic success. The invisible ties of love and loyalty and the effect of the client's identification with one of his ancestors on him must be revealed, and when this happens their influence is automatically reduced (although the client's internal work may still be needed for full success). These ties, when left unconscious, are indeed "dangerous" and "noxious," and lead to failures and suicides.

It seems that during the *Isoma* ritual healing is achieved on two planes—the same I wrote about in my book *Systemic Constellations: Theory, Practice, and Applications*, on the systemic plane, related to the ancestors, and on the individual plane, related to the patient's inner attitude (Janus 2021, 89 et seq.). According to the Ndembu, as a result of the ritual the woman must "measure up" again to the role of a fertile woman. After undergoing the *Isoma* ritual—as Turner wrote—she has "a sharpened awareness of where her and her children's ultimate loyalties lie" (Turner 2008, 13). The idea is probably that she identifies more strongly with the matrilineage, with its fertility and strength, and gives up excessive male identification. All this translates into her psychophysical state, increasing her procreative capacity.

Maurice Leenhardt described another tradition related to women, found among the Melanesian Canaques. When "a mother dies before giving birth to the child she is carrying" a "legend takes over her existence so that she can complete her function. Touching accounts are given of the mother's attentions to her child" (Leenhardt 1979, 33). When the child is bigger, the mother sends him back to the world of the living, at the same time saying that she stays where she is. "As soon as her maternal function is complete, the mother withdraws into the darkness; she is truly defunct" (Leenhardt 1979, 34). Are such actions merely sentimental additions to the brutal reality that will go unchanged anyway? Not necessarily. We know from family constellations that one of the events with the strongest transgenerational impact (if not the strongest) is a death of a woman in the postpartum period or in childbirth (the same may be true of a death in advanced pregnancy). In such a situation, women of several successive generations experience a variety of procreation-related fears and blockages, and men experience guilt, inhibitions, and other symptoms. From this perspective, allowing the deceased woman to continue her life in a somewhat mythical way, by remembering and engaging the psychic energy of community members, can help to mitigate or eliminate negative transgenerational transmission.

Let us return to burial rites, which are so vital for members of native societies. Malinowski distinguished two basic psychological tendencies that accompany the phenomenon of death: the centrifugal tendency, manifested by disgust for everything associated with the deceased and the urge to break all ties with him, and the tendency to preserve the memory of the deceased and the bond that connected the survivors with him (Brozi 1983, 152). Religion, through the ceremonial of death, "ties the survivors to the body and rivets them to the place of death," it "counteracts the centrifugal forces of fear, dismay, demoralization, and provides the most powerful means of reintegration of the group's shaken solidarity" (Malinowski 1954, 53).

This has not only social but also individual function. During family constellations, we can observe how the "centrifugal forces" in the form of disgust or fear of a corpse get in the way of proper mourning when a loved one, for example, the mother, is lost in childhood. This can happen in particular when the unprepared child has come into direct contact with the mother's corpse. In such cases, there is a problem with accepting the mother into the heart, with the internal bond with her. Here, a constellation makes it possible to experience the "mother as a mother," one may also say, as an ancestor and as a "spirit," and to abandon the picture of the corpse. This contributes to the recovery of mental balance. Confronting one's feelings about the deceased, expressing pain at the loss of the deceased, and at the same time acknowledging—as traditional cultures do—the continued existence of the deceased after death (in the form of his influence on the living) prove fundamental in the grieving process and necessary to fully cope with it.

Traditional cultures placed a strong emphasis on expressing feelings about the dead and losing them. Perhaps, at times, it was even exaggerated when loud weeping and lamentation were expected. A teacher of African traditions, Malidoma Patrice Somé, writes that "a spirit who is not passionately grieved feels anger and disappointment, as if their right to be completely dead has been stolen from them" (Somé 1995, 57). In his view, grief should be maximally expressed, which the ritual helps with, and if suppressed feelings are not freed, another person may die. The Nuer, on the other hand, recall the deeds of the deceased during mourning ceremonies, and every relative listening to the ceremony is expected to express his grievances against the deceased (if he does not do so, he is expected to remain silent forever) (Evans-Pritchard 1956, 150).

If someone holds a grudge against his own father, mother, or one of his grandparents, his grudge after that person's death does not vanish. It persists in him and affects his life in a negative way. When a mother turns away from thinking about her deceased child out of unbearable pain, she excludes her child from the family circle. Without fully confronting the loss, she stops "inwardly looking" at the child and sometimes behaves as if she denies the child's existence. Then her living child or his child may "follow him into death"—that is, become ill due to a psychosomatic reaction, and sometimes become the victim of an accident or suicide.

THE RITES OF EXCHANGE, THE EFFECTS OF GIVING AND RECEIVING

The "Energy" of Things?

Members of traditional cultures believed that not only man but everything around him had souls. Since the objects they used were also not just "inanimate objects" for them, they considered matters of exchange to be extremely important.

Anthropologists explained in many ways the complicated customs of exchanging goods that they observed in indigenous peoples (e.g., *potlatch*, *kula*). Many of the patterns they discovered explain, to some extent, the observed behavior. However, the approach of the "savages" to these issues may result from their sensitivity to the processes that Western anthropologists were not aware of. It is primarily what we refer to in constellations as the balancing mechanism or the psychological effects of balance or imbalance in the process of giving and taking.

In traditional cultures, rituals of exchange were an essential part of life, and their members paid much attention to the giving and taking of gifts. A gift could not be rejected, and there was an obligation to repay for gifts with gifts. Referring to the laws and customs of exchange—in which the aim is to "produce a friendly feeling between the two persons concerned" (Brown in: Mauss 1967, 18), Mauss writes:

> Souls are mixed with things; things with souls. Lives are mingled together, and this is how, among persons and things so intermingled, each emerges from their own sphere and mixes together. This is precisely what contract and exchange are. (Mauss 2002, 25–26)

This statement by the famous anthropologist—which he probably treated as expressing the primordial mentality rather than objective reality—perfectly reflects what we encounter in constellations. There is a kind of "mingling" of objects and persons. Persons are subject to certain laws, unconscious to them and not controlled by them, and this we usually understand as a kind of "objectification." Objects, on the other hand, cannot be manipulated entirely freely—because they are integrated into a wider system, they resist and appear to "demand" this or that attitude from us, as if they had their own "souls." In a constellation, we represent the client, his "money," his "debt," the "clients of the company," the "partner" or the "premises" within one system. The material or abstract objects animated by the representatives, like the persons represented, link together into a dynamic system.

Mauss cites a Maori informant who speaks of the *hau*, the spirit of things (Mauss 1967, 8 et seq.). It implies that there is a certain spiritual power in personal belongings, property, and creations. This is particularly evident in exchange. When, for example, someone receives an object from another person and then gives it to someone else and receives something in return, he should give it to the first person. This is due to the relationship between the *hau* of the first object and the second object. As one can see, this is a kind of "transaction memory." If we do not manage it properly, we risk unpleasant consequences, including health consequences.

When we acquire or establish a business, buy or build a house, come into an inheritance or incur another debt, we do not start anything from scratch. We always function within something that already has a history and a dynamic. The goods that we get, convinced of our own profit, may bring something negative into our lives, but it is not because of the "bad energy" in them. By receiving them, buying them, or coming into possession of them illegally, we modify the configuration of systemic and mental "tensions and forces" in which we function. For we function also in the sphere of unconscious expectations and projections, unconscious perception, unconscious conscience, and hidden intergenerational loyalties. The hidden activity of this whole sphere makes the object appear as a being equipped with a "soul" or "energy."

If we buy something stolen, for example, we know that our gain is based on someone else's harm. This demands a balance and triggers an unconscious compensation mechanism within us or those attached to us. Similarly, when we gain a lot from another person's tragedy, for instance, when we buy a house at a deeply discounted price from a young widow who cannot afford it herself. Or when we receive an inheritance that someone else was entitled to. Then a situation arises as if it were the money or things that have a negative impact on us. In fact, our conscience comes into play here, demanding that certain orders be acknowledged. It does not care about material matters, counting every penny like a bookkeeper, but significant injustice, harm, or taking someone else's place are "recorded" in it and call for a balance.

In constellations, inanimate or even abstract objects seem to be somehow directed by invisible orders. The ease or difficulty of selling a house, the success of running a café in a given building, and the ability or inability to take over a family business are not only dependent on personal skills or ordinary external conditions. Systemic processes also come into play here. These are neither subjective factors nor mere material factors, but a separate class of processes.

When we set up our company, the money we earn, or the house we want, it turns out that they are part of a dynamic system. The most important elements of this system, apart from the money or house, will be us, maybe our mother or father, maybe also some other person or matter. This system will not be chaotic; we will see inner coherence and mutual connections in it. Its dynamics will not be something mechanical, but will turn out to be governed by laws with something "human" about them. In describing them, we will refer to the terms of justice, respect for memory, gratitude, and loyalty. If these relationships are displayed, and we become aware of the important issues and agree with the introduced orders of love, then the representative of money, home, or work will feel a specific openness and we will want to move toward him. We are not dealing here with a directed psychodrama, immersed in a sea of projections and wishful thinking. During the constellation, the information that we did not talk about before will be revealed, and everything will arrange into clear patterns without any planned action on the part of the participants. Often it will also turn out that the problem we came with will be unexpectedly resolved.

Of course, inanimate objects do not function systemically alone, and there are always people involved (owners, employees, cooperators, customers). But what happens in such systems we cannot reduce to the functioning of individuals and human minds. It appears that everything that is part of the human world is incorporated into an order with certain rules. My house, put up for sale, remains a physical object, but it is also a carrier of information, a letter in the book of my life that combines into sentences with many other letters of other people and speaks to them on an unconscious level. These unconscious messages are not merely passed on "from person to person," but are anchored in a certain field that "remembers." Thus, in cases of transactions, companies, ventures, and exchanges, we have at least two hidden realities involved: our unconscious conscience that may believe that we are entitled to something or not, and a supra-personal system of relations.

Between the Dead and the Living

Lévy-Bruhl writes that in the Congo, one dresses the dead "with all his ornaments, and everything he possesses that is valuable, for all this must perish with him" (Lévy-Bruhl 1966, 292). In New Guinea, a deceased man's bows, arrows, and other objects are "broken to pieces on his grave and left there to witness to the fact of his incapability to use them more" (Lévy-Bruhl 1966, 295). There is a similar practice with regard to a woman's utensils and belongings. The clothes, weapons, and utensils of the deceased are buried with him, his boat is turned over on the grave or thrown on the water, and objects that cannot be buried in his grave are sacrificed (burned, thrown into the water, or hung on trees). With the Ba-Ronga, when someone dies, all his belongings are thrown into his deserted hut, dishes and drinking vessels are smashed on the grave and "nobody dare touch them again" (Lévy-Bruhl 1966, 296). The Hos of Bengal and the members of a hill tribe from Assam destroy and burn the dead man's belongings and the money he had with him because they do not want to "derive any immediate benefit from the death of a member of their family" (Lévy-Bruhl 1966, 296).

In the old days, there was also a "custom of burning or pulling down the house in which the death has occurred [. . .] to avoid any risk that the dead man, exercising jealous supervision over the survivors, may be tempted to return and seek his possessions" (Lévy-Bruhl 1966, 292). In ancient Egypt, old Europe, and Asia, equipment, weapons, and valuables belonging to the dead were laid in graves. Sometimes their wives and slaves were also buried.

These practices were associated with beliefs about the world of souls and the afterlife. They were seen as manifestations of fear of the dead who might "claim what is rightfully theirs" or as an expression of concern for them—the equipment placed in their graves was supposed to serve the deceased in the underworld (not in a physical but in a spiritual form—the "spirit" of an axe or a boat could be useful to the "spirit" of its owner).

Lévy-Bruhl explains the above customs with "mystic participation" (French: *participation mystique*)—the objects used by a man participate in his person, as if they were part of himself or were a continuance of his individuality. As he writes, a person's objects cannot be deprived of this mystical relation to him and become someone else's objects. Because this bond between the soul of the dead and his possessions does not disappear after he dies, as Lévy-Bruhl writes, it opposes "to any use being made of the things" and determines the practices that "put them, as it were, at the disposal of the dead" (Lévy-Bruhl 1966, 297).

The concept of mystic participation well describes the essence of the beliefs and traditions of the natives. However, its author believed that he only described a primal and strange kind of thinking (prelogical thinking), not the observation-based conclusions of people seeing relationships that he and other members of his culture did not see.

Why were the belongings of the dead destroyed or stored in his grave? It was for fear of disturbing the invisible balance between the dead and the survivors. For such a disturbance could pose a threat to the health and well-being of the living. The objects of the deceased remain in mystical connection with him in that, on an unconscious level, their possession—whether legitimate, illegitimate, debatable, or otherwise—brings a certain factor into the relationship between the living and the deceased. The desire to receive them may involve greed or even a death wish for the holder. This obviously does not bring harmony into the relationship with him. Nor does it serve the internal relationship that continues after his death. If it were a parent, this inner relationship is of great consequence to the life of the son or daughter. This is why—as Lévy-Bruhl writes—"primitive mentality regards the mystic features of things and their occult properties as by far the most important" than practical gains (Lévy-Bruhl 1966, 294).

To make this clearer, I will give an extreme example. Imagine a son, desperately wanting his father's money, whom he disdains or hates. After the father dies, the son receives the money. Will it serve him well? Will his life be successful? Will he be a man who achieves something? In all likelihood, no. The internal rejection of the father weakens the son and activates the mechanism of compensation in him, which may manifest itself as a need for punishment or identification with negative aspects of the father's personality. If this is compounded by an unconscious need for compensation for money taken without respect or gratitude, the son's defeat is clinched. Traditional cultures intuitively knew that sometimes gaining something material can seriously disrupt the inner world, which will ultimately outweigh any benefits. Leaving the belongings of the deceased with him facilitates a proper relationship with him, which may be more critical to a person's well-being than a few arrows or even a gold bracelet.

SACRIFICIAL RITUALS AND THE CONTROL OF CONSCIENCE

Sacrifice and the Hidden Dimension of Conscience

The Roman author Sextus Pompeius Festus defined ritual in the second century as an "approved practice in the administration of sacrifice" (Ratzinger 2000, 159), and in the nineteenth century William Robertson Smith recognized that the Latin word *sacrificium* covers the whole of ritual activities (Barnard and Spencer 2002, 497). From Oceania, India, and China, through the Middle East, Greece, and Rome to Africa, sacrifice was at the center of every religion and cult. In Christianity, too, the sacrifice of Jesus is the most essential element. What in fact is sacrifice? What is the point of these bizarre rites of slaughtering an ox, burning a ram, pouring wine, or eating the "flesh and blood" of Christ? And the Bible speaks of human sacrifices too, especially of one's own children.

René Girard, the author of the groundbreaking *Violence and the Sacred*, sees the genesis of human civilization in the religious sacrificial mechanism. For cultures and human communities to emerge and persist, they must cope with the interpersonal violence growing within them, which the author describes as "mimetic"—resulting from imitation and rivalry. What makes it possible to channel and limit aggression is the scapegoat mechanism—neither more nor less than choosing innocent individuals who are accused of any wrongdoing and then killed. This collective murder relieves tensions and reintegrates the community. Instead of going for one another's throats in the war of all against all, people, with a sense of unanimity, attack one randomly chosen person. From such events, whose calming effect is a surprising discovery for the community, sacrificial rituals and myths were born. The very object of unanimous violence became both "cursed" and "sacred"—he was rejected and at the same time glorified for the fact that his death brought peace to the community. Through a more or less symbolic reenactment of the original act of unanimous violence, all religions have sought to suppress violence, the threat of which has accompanied every human community. As Girard stated, religion "protects man from his own violence by taking it out of his hands, transforming it into a transcendent and ever-present danger to be kept in check by the appropriate rites appropriately observed and by a modest and prudent demeanor" (Girard 1977, 134).[5]

Walter Burkert, too, concentrates on violence in his analysis of the origins of culture. In his book *Homo Necans*, he presents the theory according to which sacrifice derives from ritualized hunting (Burkert 1983). This author also noted that interspecies aggression, associated with sexuality and rivalry, had to be channeled and was given vent through projection onto the prey in the act of hunting. This heightened the role of the act of hunting itself, which was already important as a source of food, and the prey, which began to be anthropomorphized. These processes demanded that the hunt be ritualized so that it could carry such a large set of emotions and meanings. From this ritualization, religious sacrifice was born.

I agree that sacrificial rituals are essential to the continuance, and perhaps the very emergence, of human societies. I believe, however, that they are not based only on simple affects reduced by Burkert to "biological" and by Girard to "mimetic" aggression.[6] I consider the roots of sacrifice to be more complex. My basic thesis is that ritualized sacrifice is meant to frame and stop the escalation of balancing dynamics that threaten the individual, the family, and the community. Religion not only and not primarily "takes man's violence out of his hands," religion takes man's need for balance out of his hands and takes control of his conscience.

Systemic constellations seem to support the thesis that manifest human aggression—although commonly regarded as primordial "energy"—may not be so primordial in nature. According to Freud, aggression arises from the death drive, which is redirected toward others, but perhaps what he called "the drive"—observing his patients' self-destructive behavior—is in fact the result of the operation of conscience. For, a huge part of aggressive behavior stems from primordial morality, the unconscious pursuit of justice. It may be rooted in the events of the family past, inaccessible to the subject and unknown to him. But because his conscience demands justice, an attempt is made to bring about justice using a surrogate object. A person or a group of persons becomes the enemy, the guilty party, and the whole process of rationalization is involved in proving them evil. In its most nuclear form, this person can be a spouse. In the mass one, it can be Jews, kulaks, homosexuals, or Christians. In the latter case, individuals somehow combine their personal resentments in an illusory sense of unanimity. Aggression and violence have erupted because persons have been sought who could be blamed and held responsible. Persons on whom one could exact a just revenge, defeat them, banish them, or exterminate them. Underlying this violence has always been the rudimentary movement of conscience.

Even the greatest criminals, such as serial killers, act out of early experiences, transgenerational perceptions, and conscience, rather than out of the "pure" drive toward destruction. Their sexual fixations, too, most likely have ancestral roots and become so strong not only because of the strength of their drive but because of the strength of their attachments to the dramatic past (rapes, murders, child deaths, etc.). Their rage is most likely motivated by the transference of feelings, whose original object are people and situations from their family past, to the people and situations they encounter now (of course, this does not fully explain *why* they became what they became, but it could explain much of their behavior).

However, alloaggression is only one of the manifestations of conscience, the more conspicuous one; an equally important one is self-directed aggression, self-sabotage, unconscious penance. If our ancestors suffered, were abandoned, got separated from their loved ones, or were excluded, our hidden conscience seeks balance. Therefore, we do not let ourselves live a happy life; we may wish for diseases or accidents.

Girard claimed that stopping bloody revenge, reciprocal retaliation, is essential for the survival of the community. One must agree with this. However, reciprocity and balancing mechanisms do not work only at this overt, behavioral level. They operate just as strongly, if not more strongly, at the internal level. The balancing mechanism, arising from entanglement in the guilt or trauma of one's ancestors, is a primordial morality that expresses itself: (a) in the need to make amends through one's own harm for alleged or real wrongs done to others, and (b) in "reparative interference" in the lives of one's ancestors, when the descendants feel obliged to share the fate of those who lost much, to devote their lives to those from whom they received them (parents), to avenge the wronged and forgotten.

The course of systemic constellations and their effects leave no doubt how strong these processes are. Loyalty to the family and the family conscience are stronger than the fear of death. Similarly, the mechanism of atonement has no regard for the good of the individual. These processes could not and did not go unnoticed, and were at least in part managed by sacrificial ritual.

Sacrifice as the Equivalent of Balance

Evans-Pritchard states that among the Nuer "most sacrifices are made to prevent some danger hanging over people, for example on account of some sin, to appease an angry spirit [. . .] they [sacrifices] involve ideas of propitiation, expiation, and related intentions" (Evans-Pritchard 1956, 198). "The suppliant asks God to take the offering and spare him" (Evans-Pritchard 1956, 197).

The anthropologist writes that although studies of African peoples often recognize that sacrifices are associated with weather, soil fertility, sowing, and hunting, the Nuer generally do not perform rituals for these purposes, and their sacrifices "are concerned with moral and spiritual, not natural, crises" (Evans-Pritchard 1956, 200).

The author gives the example of a Nuer who destroyed his herd of cattle for sacrifice. His relatives criticized him, claiming that he destroyed the herd out of his love of meat. However, he defended himself by saying that he sacrificed the herd only for his family's sake. He even killed his favorite ox. The man offered the cattle to the spirits of the deceased family members, because they were "frequently troubling his children and wife and her brother with sickness" (Evans-Pritchard 1956, 222). It was "the ransom of their lives with cattle" (Evans-Pritchard 1956, 222).

This type of behavior was invariably understood by interpreters as an anthropomorphization of natural forces (in this case, the biology of illness), which the natives saw as the result of the activity of spirits or God. Family constellations offer a different perspective on these issues. First, illnesses, regardless of their biological aspect, are surprisingly integrated into the life history of the individual and the family. We do not know exactly how this happens and we do not know all the relationships that are involved, but constellations leave no doubt that illnesses are much more "psychosomatic" than is commonly believed. During constellations, representatives who do not know the client experience all sorts of sensations that turn out to represent illnesses in the family. These disorders seem, albeit in variable forms, to be transmitted from generation to generation. The client's representative feels nausea and abdominal sensations, for example, and the client says that he does have a digestive disorder. But that is not all. Several other representatives of the client's family members have similar feelings. It is as if the family is under the influence of some kind of "gastric energy." The client confirms that many of his family members suffer from gastric disorders, and some of them have been operated on. One might think that it is all genetics, but it turns out that some distant ancestor—according to the representative's feelings—was wounded in the abdomen rather than ill. The client recalls that he once heard about a homicide in the family.

The very fact that the representatives can "detect" significant illnesses of the living and the dead, unknown to them, suggests that there is some "energy" associated with illness. Thus, illness is not something purely physical, in the narrowest sense of the term. This view harmonizes with the concept of illness found in traditional cultures—illness here is "not limited" to the body, but is "spiritual"—it somehow relates to the attitude and actions of the individual, as well as to the attitude and actions of his environment, including those who have already died.

Illnesses, as they are shown by family constellations, are connected with systemic disorders and with a reaction of conscience that causes the individual to unconsciously try to fix these disorders, even at the cost of his own life. These mechanisms, repeatedly confirmed in work with thousands of clients, cause the "primitive" ideas to cope with the disease through symbolic-psychological actions to make sense. The Nuer, like other peoples, sought to find out the cause of the illness or misfortune, which could be a sin, the action of a spirit, or the anger of the dead. Often only then did they make a sacrifice.

Because Western civilization has taken a completely different direction, exploring biological causes of illnesses and reducing most of life's unexpected events to chance, the thinking of representatives of traditional cultures in this regard has been regarded as unfounded. However, participants in systemic constellation workshops have the opportunity to experience a different reality. During constellations, it becomes clear that what doctors consider to be purely somatic is deeply psychosomatic, and many life events turn out to be connected within a broader causal system. Even if we do not notice or understand everything here, it becomes clear that the "somatic-random" model is not adequate.

Evans-Pritchard says that "in a sacrifice for sickness what is said is not so much may the sick man be healed as that his sickness is of no account and that he will be healed in the moment of sacrifice" (Evans-Pritchard 1956, 211). Since the Nuer assume that sickness is related to "sin," the sacrifice, in wiping out the sin, "wipes out also the material form in which it is manifested and known" (Evans-Pritchard 1956, 211). I see parallels here to the constellation work with somatic diseases. Sickness is indeed sometimes a sign of some sort of "sin," though it does not necessarily result from the actions of the sick person. It generally involves transgressions of the orders of love by ancestors (such as excluding someone from the family system).

The Nuer's sacrificial rite thus goes beyond what we customarily understand as religious, toward something akin to psychotherapy. During an offering, the Nuer do not simply ask God or Spirit for this or that, do not just make ritualized gestures, and do not just utter conventional words. The ritual has a self-reflective and self-expressive part. As Evans-Pritchard writes, the invocations before the animal is sacrificed contain "all sorts of affirmations, exhortations, reflections about life, anecdotes, and opinions," and in addition, "the speaker must reveal any grievance he may have in his heart" (Evans-Pritchard 1956, 209). The Nuer stress that even in speaking of "the most trivial details in a history of events which have led up to a situation in which sacrifice is necessary every statement made in the presence of God must be true" (Evans-Pritchard 1956, 211). "What counts in sacrifice," Evans-Pritchard writes, "is not the outward, physical, state of the sacrifice, but his moral state, the sincerity of his intention" (Evans-Pritchard 1956, 317).

Evil as "Matter"

Among the Semites, there was the scapegoat ritual, in which one of two goats was chosen and herded into the desert, with the sins of the whole community symbolically placed on its back prior to the expulsion (the other goat was offered in a blood sacrifice). A very similar custom was practiced by the Caffires of South Africa, who brought a goat to a sick person, confessed the sins of the entire kraal over it, and then herded it into the wilderness. The sickness was supposed to be lost together with the animal (Frazer 1996, 648–49). Similar rituals, based on the belief that guilt or sickness and suffering could be transferred—from human to animal and sometimes from human to human—functioned in many other cultures.

Frazer stated that the belief that it is possible to transfer suffering and guilt to another being who will carry the burden for us "arises from a very obvious confusion between the physical and the mental, between the material and immaterial. Because it is possible to shift a load of wood, stones, or whatnot, from our own back to the back of another, the savage fancies that it is equally possible to shift the burden of his pains and sorrows to another" (Frazer 1996, 646–47).

However, this conviction, whether right or wrong, has a more solid foundation. During family constellations, the basic signal of an emerging solution and sign that it is time to end the session is the client's feeling that he has become "lighter" or that "some weight is off his shoulders." These feelings occur for the majority of clients, being surprising to them, as they do not occur in obvious situations. When we pass a long-deferred exam, we can also feel lighter. Here, however, a sense of unburdening comes at unexpected moments, when the issues of ancestors are resolved, and not when we realize that a problem has disappeared. We carried this burden completely unknowingly—not because we "tortured ourselves" with some thought. On the other hand, looking at the matter from the side of the representative or therapist, we see that when they enter the field of the client, they feel the burden independently of any reflection and attitude—there is a feeling of "heaviness," a sudden sensation of weakness, and sometimes pain or "stiff legs."

The concept that sickness has a similar status to a physical object and that it can be rid of in a similar way to things is therefore not based on fantasies, but is grounded in facts. The phenomena occurring during constellations show the strength of the pressures to which the individual is subjected from the field of his family system, although in everyday life, he does not feel them due to a kind of habituation (only a stranger, a representative, can uncover them to him). Sickness thus turns out to be, to some extent, something external to the sick. Asthma or headaches or other health problems may not be, and generally are not, conditioned solely by the state of the organism, but have an "external" source in systemic disorders that affect the individual's mind and, through this path, also his body.

The observation of quasi-physical phenomena concerning man could have led to a whole host of different beliefs and practices involving casting out of evil, driving demons out of the village, and transferring illness to objects or people. An example would be the Hos of Togoland in West Africa, who, while running, shout: "Out to-day! Out to-day! That which kills anybody, out to-day! Ye evil spirits, out to-day! and all that causes our heads to ache, out to-day! Anlo and Adaklu are the places whither all ill shall betake itself!" (Frazer 1996, 667). These few sentences show that "evil," "sickness," and "evil spirits" are intertwined factors, and often interchangeable terms.

The Essence of Sacrifice

What is the essence of sacrifice in Nuer religion? We can say, after Evans-Pritchard, that it is the mechanism of "life for life"—the life of the animal goes to God, the Spirit, then the life of man can stay with him. This is why the Nuer used to say that "the cow shields" (Evans-Pritchard 1956, 220).

To be a substitute for man, the animal was usually treated as a member of the community or family before it was sacrificed. For example, in a ritual of the Paleo-Siberians, bear festival, the animal was first "domesticated" by a human family with whom it lived for a few years (Smith 1987, 203). Of the domesticated animals, they chose the "most *human* in nature," the most valuable, the gentlest, the ones that were most closely attached to man (Girard 1977, 2–3). The Nuer, for whom it was oxen that had sacrificial functions, treated them almost as people, sang songs, and composed poems about them; they not only gave names to the cattle and named themselves after the cattle, but they knew the genealogical tree of each animal, and human clans and animal herds formed a community for generations. During an offering, the sacrificer identified with the particular ox.

Evans-Pritchard wrote that

> the sacrifice is intended to rid the sufferer of the spiritual influence whose activity is apparent in the sickness. There is here a paradox. God is separated from man by an act which brings them together. The solution of the paradox would seem to lie in a distinction between two kinds of union, union on a material plane which is to be dissolved in the moment of sacrifice by bringing about union on a moral plane. This solution is consistent with the Nuer representation of sickness in which the sickness itself, the moral or spiritual state of the sufferer, and the action of Spirit form a complex whole; and also with the essential ambiguity of their conception of God as the source of good and ill. (Evans-Pritchard 1956, 275)

The above observation and the distinction made very precisely correspond to a certain basic issue in the theory of systemic constellations that also sounds like a paradox. Namely, in constellations, we see that there is "a love that brings sickness and a love that heals," and the whole process of therapy often boils down to shifting from one to the other. The first "love" is an unconscious attachment to a person, which often manifests itself at the level of the body in the form of sickness; the latter, on the other hand, is a conscious inner relationship with that person and "taking him into one's heart." Then a "separation through the act that connects" takes place, because we interrupt the unconscious identification through the "face-to-face" relationship. Someone who was until now emotionally alien to me, someone with whom the bond was only manifested through the symptoms of illness, now becomes someone close to me with whom I have a conscious relationship (e.g., a hitherto unknown twin who died in the womb or a long-dead relative). The "union on a material plane" dissolves in favor of "union on a moral plane," that is, on the plane of conscious bond. In such cases, many symptoms and diseases disappear at once.

Furthermore, we have here something very similar to the whole that according to Evans-Pritchard is formed by sickness and the action of the Spirit or God. Sickness is, as it were, in the service of a higher order, for it directs us to the unsettled family matters. So, although we wish to end our sickness, we cannot consider it merely a kind of unnecessary "ulcer"—through it our family conscience speaks to us, and shows us what is important. The bond is independent of time and space, and the related action of the family conscience is beyond our will and control, resembling the action of a "spirit."

In the psyche, as we observe in constellations, primal moral mechanisms dominate, which are closest to the ideas of exchange, atonement, substitution, and transference. A given person wants to relieve someone from his family, carrying their burden together with them. It does not matter to him that the burden is the pain of losing their little brother in childhood, which he cannot do anything about. It does not even matter that the person he wants to relieve is long dead. He unconsciously believes that burdens of this kind are like material burdens—by adding a pair of hands one can relieve the bearer. Or maybe they are something that can be divided in half, so that the other person can carry only part of it?

Someone else wants to destroy his own life, get sick, suffer, and have no life force because his parent, for some reason, does not have it. So he wants to "do" what his parent does so that the parent does not have to do it. "To do," that is, for example, to be stuck in depression. In some constellations, this looks very dramatic, as if the child wants to sacrifice himself to save his parent. Sacrifice, but to what force? The one that attracts the father or mother.

After losing her twin sister, who died in the womb, the one who survived does not know how to act. Should I pay a debt? Am I burdened by sin? Do I have the right to be happy? Am I a victim or a perpetrator? These primal moral dilemmas shape the life, relationships, and disposition of the survivor.

A woman terminated her pregnancy. Now she wishes to die. But why? Does she want to "atone"? Does she want to "connect" with her child? Or does she want everything to be undone? So that with her death, the child, the pain, the "sin," the guilt, and the whole thing cease to exist?

Just as the subconscious dynamics of conscience are not easy to put into words unambiguously, although their "direction" seems clear, the motivations, understanding, and interpretations of rituals cannot be quite so unambiguous. The above dynamics differ, though they certainly have "something in common." The same is true of sacrificial rituals. Their psychological source seems to be best understood by theories that emphasize "life-for-life" substitution. However, other interpretations, seemingly contradictory to those, may also be close to unconscious dynamics. Thomas Gibson disagrees that sacrificial animals are a substitute for humans. Observing the Buid of Mindoro, he found that, according to their beliefs, the most dangerous spirits cannot be satisfied with an animal sacrifice. Instead, during a ritual "its vitality is assimilated by humans in order to drive off the predatory spirits" (Gibson 1986, 179). The author describes the *saysayan babuy* ("swinging pig") ritual meant to cure a child who threw tantrums. The ritual involved suspending a pig from the rafters, swinging it, and then killing it. Two chickens are treated in a similar manner. Further, Gibson states:

> The spirits fear the swaying of the pigs and chickens and their final struggles. Animals normally live on the boundary between the human and non-human worlds. [. . .] In this ritual, they are brought inside the house in order to re-establish the mystical barriers which have been breached by the invading spirits who have taken up residence in human space. [. . .] Only the sacrifice of a pig and two chickens was sufficient to dislodge them. It was not that the animals was being used as a substitute for the children. The Buid specifically denied that any meat would be offered to the evil spirits. In this ritual the vitality of the animals would be wholly appropriated by the children. This vitality was transferred to the children both by their consumption of the broth and by the swinging of the animals over their heads. (Gibson 1986, 159)

The anthropologist was informed that "the swinging of the pig performed the same function as the swaying of the medium present during a séance" (Gibson 1986, 158). So wasn't there a certain identification of the medium and the animal here? Perhaps the medium was "taking on" certain aspects of the child's psychological situation, which in turn were supposed to be transferred to the pig. The pig was then butchered. Of course, no meat was "offered to the evil spirits," it was generally eaten by people. The ritual, as Gibson himself states, was about "vitality."

Murder and Ritual

In ancient Greece, there was a much more brutal practice than the Semitic scapegoating, called *pharmakos*. In times of calamity, a prisoner or slave was chosen and beaten, manhandled, and expelled from the town, and sometimes possibly killed. The community was probably convinced of their guilt and bad influence (the criminal was guilty of something, and the slave probably came from a hostile nation), and their killing brought peace and hope for a change of fortune. Such a person played the role of a "scapegoat" in the broad sense of the word.

Girard argues that there is "no essential difference between human and animal sacrifice," and I believe there is a difference (Girard 1977, 96). We should think of animal sacrifice as something completely different from what *pharmakos* was. The scapegoat in Leviticus (the Leviticus ritual) is a real ritual, a substitutionary action, and a psychological procedure. It is meant to control the need to balance—resulting from guilt or injustice—that is, the urge to harm oneself or others, in the community. People knew they were guilty of something or felt that way. This is different in the case of *pharmakos*, which integrated the community and reinforced its sense of innocence. People did not symbolically put their own guilt on the victim's back, but confirmed their innocence by projecting evil onto the stranger.

In each of these cases—and a whole host of intermediate ones, such as the "killing of a god" (that is, a chosen person) by the Aztecs—different mechanisms of conscience, different circles of it dominate. In rituals, if we can at all use the term ritual here, such as *pharmakos*, we deal with the escalation of the first circle of conscience (individual conscience), and the related need to belong. They work for the cohesion of the group; they are collective processes (the term "individual conscience" is misleading in contexts such as this one) that do not touch the individual psychology of the person. This is different, for example, in most Nuer rituals of ox sacrifice. As Evans-Pritchard consistently emphasizes, Nuer rituals are expressions of personal—and one can also say self-reflective—religiosity. Nothing of the sort occurs in the *pharmakos* practice.

If we regard the Semitic scapegoat and *pharmakos* as the two poles of the sacrificial continuum, then in past cultures there was also a whole host of "intermediate" practices—when people volunteered to be the "scapegoat" themselves, when bloody expressions of one's own penance were offered at the feet of a woman-goddess and then she was killed, and more (Frazer 1996).

A Nuer, in some sense, identified with the ox he was killing, yet he did not consider the ox to be "evil," whereas members of the Greek community were under a "counter-identification" with their victim. Perhaps the Semitic scapegoat was something intermediate between these two poles—one did not identify with it, but it does not seem likely that one had the same attitude toward it that the Greek crowd had toward its victim. One can imagine that the latter was vituperated and beaten, and everyone felt that he was really guilty and despicable. Was something like this done to the goat?

Girard admits that *pharmakos* "does not merely recall the collective persecution [. . .] it *is* it" (Girard 1987, 76). Yes, *pharmakos* is a scapegoating phenomenon in a broad psychosocial, not ritualistic, sense. Of course, the issue is not quite that simple. The *pharmakos* was driven before death or expulsion to various places in order to "sop up impurities" and collect them on his shoulders (Girard 1977, 95). So we have some ritualistic elements here. However, it is collective violence and projection, and not an attempt to ritually control the mechanisms of conscience, that dominate here.

According to the author of *Violence and the Sacred*, the prophylactic effect of animal sacrifice lies in the fact that, containing an appropriate dose of violence, it resembles the primal murder and therefore provides an opportunity for emotional abreaction. Ritual always aims to bring about "the most profound state of peace known to any community: the peace that follows the sacrificial crisis and results from the unanimous accord generated by the surrogate victim" (Girard 1977, 103), that is, after collective murder. According to Girard, the most "real" and shocking event for man is murder. Despite the fact that murder may seem so, I do not agree with this conclusion. It is not the act of killing that is the axis of sacrificial rituals.

Through family constellations, we have been able to see that homicide does indeed have a great impact, especially when it happened within the family. However, we have also learned that the killer himself may not be affected by the consequences of the act as severely as his descendants. In no way does murder bring peace to the community, even if we agree that it may bring peace to the perpetrator. Could religions be based on this limited effect or are they a way of protecting the community from the long-term effects of murder?

In the case of murder among the Nuer, the family of the slain is paid with cattle. This payment "also pacifies the ghost, who may trouble his family and kin" (Evans-Pritchard 1956, 294). While we can easily understand that the compensation prevents revenge on the part of the killed man's family, to say that his "ghost" could "trouble" any member of the killed man's family seems at best a metaphor referring to possible guilt in those persons. And yet, as systemic constellations have irrefutably demonstrated, there are psychological processes much closer to the interpretation of the Nuer than to our previous interpretations. Descendants of both the killer and the killed (often grandchildren) are sometimes strongly attached to both the perpetrator and the victim. This is because homicide activates the urge in the family conscience to link the perpetrator and the victim. Since these persons are usually excluded, the perpetrator from the victim's family and the victim from the perpetrator's family, the unconscious urge of the descendant to identify with the perpetrator and the victim becomes particularly strong, adversely affecting his life. The Nuer seem to be aware, to some extent, that by demanding payment they not only bring about ordinary social justice, but also free the descendants of the victim from the unconscious seeking of compensation ("justice").

Among the Canadian Indians, there was a custom that followed the orders of love even more clearly. When murder took place, the murderer was adopted by the victim's family (Hellinger 2013, 105). So he was consciously included in the family so that he would not have to be unconsciously represented in it.

PARTICIPATION, SCHIZOPHRENIA, POSSESSION

One of the most distinctive features of the myths and thinking of members of aboriginal cultures is that they see the world as full of metamorphoses and changing identities. As Ernst Cassirer stated:

> By a sudden metamorphosis, everything may be turned into everything else. If there is any characteristic and outstanding feature of the mythical world, any law by which it is governed—it is the law of metamorphosis. (Cassirer 1964, 81)

Metamorphoses happen not only in myths; members of traditional cultures perceive also their own identity as extremely prone to change. During dances and rituals, they transform, as they claim, into ancestors, into totemic animals, into plants, or into a stone. Lévy-Bruhl states that for primitive mentality, objects, persons, and phenomena can be "both themselves and something other than themselves. [. . .] they give forth and they receive mystic powers, virtues, qualities, influences, which make themselves felt outside, without ceasing to remain where they are" (Lévy-Bruhl 1966, 61).

Members of industrial societies generally tend to think in very different terms and do not feel the mysterious external influences and transformations of their own identity. Not all, however. As I described in the book *Systemic Constellations: Theory, Practice, and Applications*, people with schizophrenia seem to experience some kind of external influence, as if their identity was not fully crystalized.

Artur Dobosz advanced the hypothesis that the experiencing and functioning of those with schizophrenia is the result of a struggle between two types of thinking, or two realms of mind, which he described as metamorphic-anarchic thinking and thinking in terms of lasting relationships (Dobosz 2013).[7] Based on an extensive analysis of patients' utterances, the author showed that the structure of schizophrenic symptoms is very similar to that of magical-mythical thinking, and that these utterances themselves are something like short myths. So metamorphic-anarchist thinking would also be characteristic of members of traditional cultures.

Similar two types of thinking or logic were already discussed, as we know, by Lévy-Bruhl. Interestingly, he shifted from understanding these types as opposite to a complementary approach and stated that "there is a mystical mentality which is more marked and more easily observable among 'primitive peoples' than in our own societies, but it is present in every human mind" (Lévy-Bruhl 1975, 101). This view corresponds with Dobosz's theory of schizophrenia.

Dobosz not only showed a substantial correspondence between schizophrenic thinking and that of magical societies, but he also found that the experiencing of members of these societies was close to schizophrenic because their sense of individual identity "was not (and is not) developed to the degree that it is developed in representatives of Western culture" (Dobosz 2013, 277). First, a clear distinction between the internal psychic sphere and the external, physical one has not crystallized in them. Thus, it can be said, the author states, that "magical culture in a particular sense of the word was (and is) a schizophrenic culture" (Dobosz 2013, 278). Of course, this comparison is not meant to depreciate traditional cultures. Rather, the point is that both representatives of these cultures and schizophrenic patients "use" a "metamorphic-anarchistic" level of mind more than other people.

This level—here I go further than the author of the theory—is not merely the sphere of bizarre, from the point of view of ordinary logic, reasoning, but is related to processes of perception. The thinking and concepts of members of magical cultures are not manifestations of simple cultural underdevelopment, but expressions of their concentration on the sphere of certain phenomena. The same is true of the thinking of people with schizophrenia—not only do they stray and cannot cope with life, but they also see and feel what remains hidden for healthy people (Janus 2019, 122 et seq.). First, it is heteropsychic influences, connected with the family field. It is under their influence that "primitive" people experience their metamorphoses, possession, feeling the presence of ancestors, and similar phenomena, while schizophrenics construct their own explanations for the influence of Satan, telepaths, or aliens. In fact, both are affected by the family field, the unconscious extra-individual influences.

Every member of magical culture experienced, or feared, external influences on his own psyche. However, there were situations in which this influence was of a specific nature. Anthropologists are familiar with the so-called possession cults, during which their practitioners or priests seek to intentionally connect with the power of the spirits of the dead in order to obtain advice, prophecy, or healing. The Malagasy *chumba* is one of such cults. In the course of this ritual, the spirit of an ancient king, speaking through the medium, reads the causes of the client's failures, ill-health, and other problems. The point of the ritual is to meet the ancestors and participate in their power and wisdom; therefore, the terms "possession" or "haunting," usually used in such contexts, are not applicable here. The Malagasy themselves use the term *mianjaka*, meaning rather "residence" (Marcinkowska 2016, 332–33).

The *chumba* cult has a clearly psychotherapeutic aspect. Instead of "cleansing" the body and "casting out" spirits—the concepts characteristic of many possession cults (for example, the *zâr* cult in Ethiopia and Sudan)—here some attempt is made to understand the life of the individual, and his family connections, friendships, attitude to other people, and lifestyle are most important. The *chumba* session is not intended to "chase out" the cause of misery, but to identify and analyze it.

Also in Christianity, Islam, Judaism, and other religions, the phenomenon of possession is recognized (Janus 2019, 163 et seq.). It takes an extreme form in the Roman Catholic Church—what possesses is the quintessence of evil, "evil personified," Satan. But there are also many examples that suggest that this "entity" is not that "inhuman." Francesco Vaiasuso, who recounted his possession, writes:

> On the evening of March 2, I fell to the ground again. It was the last day of the ordeal that had continued since February 26 and was the cruelest and most

> horrible episode in all the many years I had been possessed.—I'm a soldier in a Nazi concentration camp!—I was screaming, rolling on the ground. [. . .]—I'm an important soldier, I'm in command here!—I was shouting.—I come from a concentration camp! I'm a German soldier! [. . .]—Ratatatat! I'm shooting, I'm shooting! All dead! Do you know how many I've already killed?—Lord, make him go away from here!—asked Daniela as she watched the depressing scene.—I'll never go from here because I have seen a light in this boy and through him I can survive! (Vaiasuso and Rodari 2015, 186–87)

Was it really a demon? Rather, the man "had contact" with a perpetrator of war crimes. Or with his "soul"? In any case—with a memory of him or with the dramatic past related to him. It could have been his ancestor or the experiences of some other person, transformed by the imagination of the "possessed."

WEIGHT OF RELIGION

Fluctuations in Meaning, Shifts in Emphasis

If sacrifices, such as the Nuer's, served their purpose, it was a similar process to that which takes place in constellations. The client can stay alive by leaving what belongs to the parents with the parents and what belongs to the ancestors with the ancestors. He can stop trying to save those of his loved ones who are pursuing death. He can also stop his own unconscious atonement. It is also possible to think in terms of increasing man's life force, as is the case, according to Gibson, with the Buid. Any entanglement with the fate of the ancestors or atonement leads to a lowering of one's strength and life efficiency.

I do not think, however, that we can say that sacrificial rituals regulated the actions of conscience in a perfect or complete way. Rather, they pointed to these mechanisms, sought to recognize them, and tame them. Without a doubt, religions of all cultures and times show similarities, but different cultures have emphasized different elements in the complex phenomenon of religion. Gibson defined the sacrificial rituals of the Buid of Mindoro (Philippines), that he studied, as "the ritual manipulation, killing and commensal consumption of a 'sacred' animal" (Gibson 1986, 151). However, emphasis was not always placed equally on each of these elements (Barnard and Spencer 2002, 498). The Nuer made careful preparations before killing the victim. Moroccan Muslims emphasized the act of killing itself. The Buid minimized the aspect of killing and emphasized sharing the roasted meat with the spirits. The Greeks seemed to focus on what happened to the remains; they were interested, for example, in the smoke from a burnt victim, which was meant to be food for the gods.

Some interpret sacrifice as a kind of communication with supernatural beings. In religious studies, a distinction was made between two types of this communication: low-intensity and high-intensity (Baal 1976, 168). What seems to be fundamental to understanding sacrifice is high-intensity communication, that is, a sacrifice offered in particular life circumstances (rather than an offering made according to the calendar of festivals of the community). In such cases, the intention was to thank, vow, or propitiate a deity. But was it a "deity" in each case? Or what is "deity" at all? The actual target of the sacrifice was always the sacrificer and what was important to him (e.g., his family). But since sacrifice refers to mechanisms that transcend the individual, which are transpersonal and unconscious, one could just as well regard extra-personal forces as the target. And these—as the "god." The Greeks are a good example here—sometimes they understood their gods as abstract forces, and at other times they presented them as human-like beings. Sometimes they begged the gods, and other times they claimed that they "persuade the gods to serve them" (Plato 1992, 39).

The beliefs and rituals of ancient and distant cultures have always been described with concepts available to the researcher. And these were generally not quite adequate to what the indigenous people thought and how they felt. Anthropologists have looked for basic categories, such as "mana," "soul," "mystical participation," "god," with which they could describe early religions, as well as central phenomena around which the worldview of a given culture is built, such as the cult of ancestors or nature spirits, magic. But an interpretation that seemed to be adequate for one culture failed when applied to another culture.

The phenomenon of sacrifice is a perfect example of the fluctuation of meanings on the part of both believers and interpreters. Sacrifice was seen as a gift to the gods from which repayment was expected; as a sign of expiation and propitiation for sins; a votive offering; a communion of men and gods, even a symbolic feasting with them; and finally, food to endear the spirits. In modern times, some see it as a remnant of hunting culture, while others see it as a way of distributing meat in a community or as a ritual way of preparing a feast. Even in ancient Greece, where sacrifice was such an important part of human life, vegetarian authors criticized animal sacrifice, considering it to be little more than an excuse for a meat banquet (Parker 2011, 127). In our time, Paul Veyne has even put forward the thesis that sacrifice cannot be explained, and it is for this reason that it has always been so common—simply because everyone found their own satisfaction in it (Parker 2011, 126).

So neither practitioners nor interpreters share a common understanding of what sacrifice, and—more generally—religion, is. We could conclude from this that it is anything, therefore, nothing, that has real value. I do not think so. Religion has been essential to human survival and the shaping of civilization. However, in the course of its transformation—as one cannot say "evolution"—it began to serve purposes other than the original ones, its robes, and functions changed.

My thesis is that traditional cultures, those living at the most primordial level of development, were the closest to "what works" in religion. I would venture to say that a religion such as that of the Nuer contains more functional and fundamentally humanistic elements than Islam. It is probably closer to the source from which all religions derive. However, it is also important what a researcher is able to notice in a given religion. Nuer religion is what it is also because of what Evans-Pritchard managed to say about it. He wrote:

> Words and gestures transport us to a realm of experience where what the eye sees and the ear hears is not the same as what the mind perceives. Hands are raised to the sky in supplication, but it is not the sky which is supplicated but what it represents to the imagination. Formal respect is paid to an animal not on account of what the animal is in itself but on account of what for some people it stands for in thought as a symbol. (Evans-Pritchard 1956, 321)

If someone sees only heaven and hands raised to it, they fail to see or guess that it is the inner states that are the way to understand religion. Someone like this will understand religion as a primitive way of explaining the external world, not as a way of expressing and managing the internal world. "Though prayer and sacrifice are exterior actions, Nuer religion is ultimately an interior state," Evans-Pritchard writes (Evans-Pritchard 1956, 322).

Much of the rationalist criticism of religion has been born out of the observation of "external states," of monotheistic religions, of the functioning of churches, of increasingly abstract doctrines, and of the mentality of contemporary believers. But the criticism is blind to the very beginnings of religion and knows nothing of its true meaning.

Much of the tendency to trivialize religious issues stems from the strength of thereligious studies discourse we have commonly adopted, which often fails to keep up with phenomena. We take for granted, for example, that members of traditional cultures "deify" their dead, that their funeral rituals aim at "cutting off" dangerous spirits from the living, and that early men "anthropomorphized" their environment. These are all simplifications that sometimes fit better, sometimes worse, and sometimes not at all with what the natives experienced. The Canaques, for example, as Leenhardt sees it, do not anthropomorphize nature; they are too immersed in it to project themselves onto it (Leenhardt 1979, 19 et seq.). They do not deify the dead either. The ancestors-gods, the *bao*, may be the living elders whose "wisdom participates in the wisdom one finds in contact with ancestors and gods" (Leenhardt 1979, 31). At the same time, a stranger may be considered a *bao*, which, in my opinion, points to fluctuations on the part of the natives themselves—they "forget" that the essence of a "god" is being an ancestor and acting as an ancestor. The *bao* are also not a creation of some detached "mythical" thinking. Leenhardt writes that they are born from "an effort of the intellect inspired by the observation that physical life fades while inner life keeps its permanent freshness in the wisdom of the old men or the counsel of the gods" (Leenhardt 1979, 32). Regarding our understanding of the living-dead relationships, the same author wrote:

> We commonly speak of separation rites. By this we indicate the negative aspect of a movement which is however completed in a positive manner. The rites mark a separation from the daily life of the living, but primarily they mark the definitive incorporation of a relative destined to enrich the transcendent world upon which the human world depends. (Leenhardt 1979, 34)

"Spirit," "gods," "God," and "ancestor," just as "soul," "mana," or "mystical participation," are concepts that can be contrasted with each other and many anthropologists have argued about which of these is the most important and will decode religion. However, the concepts can be viewed jointly as attempts to describe the same experience. The common experience that gave rise to and maintained the original religions was the experience of transpersonal influences, telepathy, a mysterious bond with ancestors, and the covert activity of the family conscience capable of affecting our fate—like God or gods—whether we want it to or not.

Psychotherapy of Ancient Times

Roy A. Rappaport wrote that "in the absence of what we, in a common-sense way, call religion, humanity could not have emerged from its pre- or proto-human condition. It is, therefore, plausible to suppose, although beyond demonstration's possibilities, that religion's origins are, if not one with the origins of humanity, closely connected to them" (Rappaport 2002, 1). I fully agree with his thesis on the role of religion in anthropogenesis and the emergence of culture.

Our ancestors, living in traditional cultures, identified the most fundamental and powerful psychological forces that governed their lives, expressing them in the form of beliefs and rituals. This does not mean, however, that all the beliefs and practices of native peoples were adequate responses to psychological reality. They were probably wrong or fantasized in many points; nevertheless, their way of life proved useful and we may owe the survival and expansion of humans on Earth to it altogether. One might say that "mental hygiene" and "psychotherapy" were at the very core of the aboriginal culture, and perhaps should be considered the primary factors that enabled its emergence.

It is not commonly believed that mental disorders are a significant problem for human collectivities. In most people's view, they are niche issues, unlikely to affect the population at large, a dark area of concern for psychiatrists. And the fact that we increasingly hear that "depression will be the second most common cause of disability" and that "one in four people on Earth suffers from a mental or behavioral disorder" does not change this. Either way, psychological problems (and related psychosomatic problems) are not thought to be something that threatens basically every person. And it is even less thought that humans on the threshold of hominization would have encountered these kinds of problems. But perhaps it is that part of our psyche—prone to development but also to disorders, showing such strong connections with the family and ancestors—the transpersonal and telepathic psyche, and not just our reason, that has given rise to man's evolutionary success.

Family constellations must radically change our view of the causes and prevalence of mental disorders. I do not mean to say that they have shown that each of us is "ill" (this has been shown to some extent by psychoanalysis), but they have revealed that much of what we have not associated with dynamic psychological causes or with any causes at all, considering it to be the result of character traits or chance, has a broader causal background. These include all sorts of problems from career blockages to psychosis, and serious somatic illnesses also come into play.

Magical and religious thinking brought a psychological orientation into the lives (seemingly governed mainly by practical tasks) of representatives of traditional cultures. When a Nuer man kills a hippopotamus, he becomes possessed by the river-sprites gathered in the animal and, as a consequence, falls sick.If he, during a healing ceremony, falls into a trance, and the sprites speak through his mouth, the range of his experiences is completely different from that of the average man in Western culture. Even if we consider him to be influenced by religious beliefs, his different psychophysical functioning remains a fact. He has the opportunity for expression that would not be possible in the absence of such beliefs. For representatives of our culture, similar expressions became possible only after psychotherapy was born.

So why have we strayed so far from that vision of reality? It is possible that a different attitude toward psychological processes related to ancestors is responsible for the fundamental differences between us and traditional cultures. Perhaps the focus on coping with these powerful psychological factors resulted in the extreme conservatism of these cultures, and our forgetting of these influences became an important factor driving the development of civilization and its creations. An important role must have been played by monotheistic religion, which, on the one hand, absorbed some of the primordial observations-beliefs and, on the other hand, cut man off from addressing a good part of them, "entrusting his fate to God." This process seems to be demonstrated by the following quotations from the Bible:

> The word of Jehovah came unto me again, saying,
>
> What mean ye, that ye use this proverb concerning the land of Israel, saying, The fathers have eaten sour grapes, and the children's teeth are set on edge?
>
> As I live, saith the Lord Jehovah, ye shall not have occasion any more to use this proverb in Israel.
>
> Behold, all souls are mine; as the soul of the father, so also the soul of the son is mine: the soul that sinneth, it shall die. (Ezek. 18:1–4)
>
> In those days they shall say no more, The fathers have eaten sour grapes, and the children's teeth are set on edge.
>
> But every one shall die for his own iniquity: every man that eateth the sour grapes, his teeth shall be set on edge. (Jer. 31:29–30)
>
> Thou shalt not bow down thyself unto them, nor serve them, for I Jehovah thy God am a jealous God, visiting the iniquity of the fathers upon the children, upon the third and upon the fourth generation of them that hate me,
>
> and showing lovingkindness unto thousands of them that love me and keep my commandments. (Ex. 20:5–6)

The quoted passages separate man from the primordial transgenerational phenomena, but at the same time confirm their existence. They order one to live against these psychological factors or to transgress them. These words seek to form a "new man" for whom transgenerational processes will no longer be the focus of attention as they were in traditional culture.

THE PSYCHE AND RELIGIOUS IDEAS

The Meaning of Suffering

In the modern world, religions are in decline. However, quasi-religious ideas or near-religious behaviors still exist. Are they merely a legacy of religious teaching embedded in the collective consciousness? Or are they something more primordial, inherent in human nature, which itself underlay religious beliefs? I would argue that they are more of the latter.

There is an idea in Christianity that seems erroneous and harmful from the point of view of psychological knowledge. It is the meaning that suffering is said to have in human life. This is expressed by John Paul II when he says that Christ "raised human suffering to the level of the Redemption" and in this way "each man, in his suffering, can also become a sharer in the redemptive suffering of Christ" (John Paul II 1984), and even more emphatically by St. Paul, who states: "I [. . .] fill up on my part that which is lacking of the afflictions of Christ in my flesh" (Col 1:24).

But is this idea solely Christian? The value of suffering and sacrifice is promoted even by completely secular culture. For example, the value of work-related suffering. Reflecting on the phenomenon of treating work (even "meaningless" work) as a value per se, anthropologist David Graeber states:

> But one possibility the sociologists generally overlook is that, if work is a form of self-sacrifice or self-abnegation, then the very awfulness of modern work *is* what makes it possible to see it as an end in itself. [. . .] Workers, in other words, gain feelings of dignity and self-worth *because* they hate their jobs. (Graeber 2018, 242)

The author also cites a nineteenth-century essayist, writing in the era just after the Industrial Revolution, Thomas Carlyle, who argued:

> All work, even cotton spinning, is noble work is alone noble [. . .]. And in like manner too, all dignity is painful. A life of ease is not for any man. . . Our highest religion is named the Worship of Sorrow. For the son of man there is no noble crown, well worn or even ill worn, but there is a crown of thorns! (Carlyle in: Graeber 2018, 244)

Naturally work is an important thing for man; it is also important to be useful to others. But the "Worship of Sorrow"? Here we go a step further. This may involve turning away from life. Hellinger writes that there is "a widespread innocent waiting for one's own death. For example, when we want to die for someone else so that they can be redeemed from their guilt" (Hellinger 2014, 167). Behind this waiting there is a quasi-religious belief that is expressed by the Biblical sentence "Greater love has no one than this: to lay down one's life for one's friends." Did this phrase in the Bible produce this "waiting"? Of course not. But many referred to the Bible and religion to "consecrate" their destructive pursuits. Psychological experience from family constellations shows that the religious valorization of suffering goes together with the primal mechanisms present in the psyche of a child. It is a feeling that one can carry someone else's suffering or make amends for past wrongs with one's suffering. If this kind of interference of the unconscious mechanism and religious recommendation occurs, the situation may become dangerous.

For years, ecclesiastical writers have seen the merit of man precisely in suffering and have even advised against giving it up. One of them wrote that the therapeutic actions of Hellinger, who also worked with cancer patients, were dangerous to their salvation: "Who will intercede for them? There is no will, no depth, no struggle. There is no room here for salvific suffering, for the logic of the cross as the proper solution to the problem of guilt" (Posacki 2007, 160). In constellations, we see that things are very different. It is precisely remaining in suffering that is the state of "no struggle" and many people find it difficult to transgress toward health. To a person who considers these matters only theoretically, it may be surprising that it is the giving up of suffering, rather than continuing it, that is the truly moral act. For in suffering there may be selfishness and laziness; suffering gives a sense of innocence. By suffering—I "do something" without doing anything. And when I offer my suffering for the intentions of the world—whatever I mean by that—I seemingly go toward others, but in reality, I remain where I was. Struggle, responsibility, and growth involve trying to go beyond suffering. Such situations require humility, as we must often let go of the vision of ourselves as someone particularly good and become "ordinary people" who just want to be healthy and need health. It is amazing, but being healthy is sometimes associated with defeat and unbearable mediocrity in one's own life.

Sacrifice in Our Lives

We use phrases like "to devote oneself to something," "to sacrifice something," "to offer up something to someone" and words like "to redeem," "redemption" in many trivial situations, although their genesis seems to be related to a religious cult. Why have the phrases that—albeit implicitly—concern some form of renunciation, loss, or expiation become permanently embedded in the language? The linguistic usage causes that we recall ancient rituals even when we "offer" someone a gift.

We have long thought that the dynamics of "guilt," "atonement," "redemption," and " sacrifice" concern only the religious, overly concerned with their presumed guilt toward God. But it was first shown by psychoanalysis and then, even more fully, by systemic constellations that ruthless ethical impulses concern everyone. Our conscience desires to "repair," and that repair always takes the same form—someone must fail, someone must suffer, lose, or die. We generally inflict this fate on ourselves. In some cases, we try to evade it, and then our children pursue "justice" even more forcefully.

Immeasurable multitudes of people, in the West and the East, have been and are under the influence of sacrificial madness, which comes most to the surface during wars. German soldiers going to the front sang, "We dedicate our death to you as the smallest deed" (Fritz 1997, 161). In a Polish song, the Legions are depicted as a sacrificial pyre, onto which the soldiers throw "their lives." Numerous songs of other nations also glorify sacrificing and dedicating one's life. Is this merely a matter of patriotism? No, these songs reflect the movement of conscience. It is endless because we constantly feel guilty about something and blame someone. We constantly stand up for someone and exclude someone. We also constantly tremble at our own belonging.

However, we have not sacrificed living people on altars or killed sacrificial animals for a long time. Instead, the Christian religion tells us to eat a piece of bread and drink some wine, which it calls "flesh and blood." We do not have slaves and we do not consider people with different skin colors as inferior. Discrimination, exclusion, division are combated everywhere. Seemingly, there is no one to make a victim of any longer, because everyone is under the same protection of the law. Yet, the sacrificial madness continues. Girard wrote:

> We live in a world, as I have pointed out, that constantly reproaches its own violence, and it does this systematically and ritualistically. We are always prepared to translate all our conflicts, even those that don't lend themselves at all to it, into the language of innocent victims. The debate over abortion, for example: whether we are for it or against it, we always have to choose our side in the interest of the "real victims." (Girard 2001, 176)

Mass demonstrations took place in Poland in 2020, to protest against the verdict of the Constitutional Tribunal that declared abortion for fetal anomalies alone to be unconstitutional. Hundreds of thousands of people protested "for women's rights" and for abortion to be permitted. These were perhaps the largest demonstrations in the history of the country that has known many demonstrations. Could protests for any suffering people gather a single per mille of the participants present at the rallies against "women's hell"? The facts show that they could not. It is women, in their procreative function, who are now designated as victims, it is their suffering around which the consciences of so many are centered. The rallies in question involved great levels of aggression, and the most vulgar words were shouted at those in power. Women were the undisputed victims, and the rulers were the oppressors.[8]

The argument that prohibiting abortions was "forcing women to give birth to monsters" was frequently voiced. It was clear that these "monsters" were deprived of the status of human beings. In this, the protesters seemed to be unanimous. It cemented their consciences into one collective conscience. Girard, with ancient cultures in mind, wrote: "The murder by exposure of weak or ill-formed infants was extremely widespread and is certainly associated with the concept of the surrogate victim—that is, with the unanimous basis of all sacrificial rites" (Girard 1977, 96). During the aforementioned protests, unanimity, sense of community, and belief in the rightness and moral superiority of one's own position dominated.

What do constellations show in this regard? Unborn children's deaths are often coupled with the balancing mechanism. It is strange, but a woman may have many abortions because her grandmother lost many children. She unconsciously repeats the grandmother's fate—she loses children. Sometimes the subconscious "pattern" is war victims or certain dramatic events in which many people were killed.

Abortion is a specific act—it is socially acceptable, and citing biology, one can deny its seriousness. At the same time, the unconscious conscience of the woman (and also of the father) reacts to it in an extremely strong way, demanding compensation (which can lead to illness and death). When such balancing does not occur, someone else, such as the living child, feels guilty and ready to atone.

Reincarnation

Hellinger believed in reincarnation, but it must be said that constellations do not provide any evidence for such belief. One of my clients, Sabine, who worked with regression to earlier incarnations, interpreted entanglements and relationships with the older members of the system as her previous incarnations. She said she had been somebody's wife, had had a child with somebody. She felt a connection with the tragic lot of Louis Charles, the son of the guillotined Louis XVI. The client got very emotional about these things and I was far from underestimating them. However, I tried to guide her to see her connections and identifications with the earlier people, and at the same time remember where and when she was now. I could even assume that in her unquestionable sensitivity she connected with the fates of the kings of France, but it was more likely that a child from her system mattered here. Finally, I said, "You are not everywhere. You are here. There are other people too." For in her comments there was some sort of disrespect for other peoples' fates. In fact, her experiences and interpretations were actions of a child—an urge to interfere in the past and take the problems of her ancestors upon herself.

During our work, Sabine would every now and then enter states of consciousness that seemed psychotic to me (when she reportedly received some verbal messages from the past) and then returned to the here and now.

Slowly, however, the systemic orders proved stronger and Sabina became more and more mentally integrated. She balanced on the verge of psychoticism because she was attached to dramatic events in the previous generations, also to the persons who entered the system as a result of murder. She transformed these influences into reincarnation visions and symptoms such as hearing voices (the hypothesis that she was psychotic is supported by the fact that she did not know her father and was strongly influenced by her mother and grandmother).

Constellators Yuri Karpenkov and Nadezhda Matveeva believe that in about 5 percent of constellations, imageries appear that relate to persons from distant eras and places on the globe that are completely alien to the client and his family (Karpenkov and Matveeva 2015, 172). They do not take a definitive stance, but they use the metaphor of previous incarnations.

Personally, I have never encountered a situation in constellations that would suggest reincarnation. It has always involved entanglement in the ancestral past, that is, the memory contained in the field and concerning the ancestors, and not memories of one's "past life." Thus, from the point of view of constellations, it can be hypothesized that the concept of reincarnation arose from observing the experiences of strongly entangled people who repeated their ancestors' fates and shared their feelings or memories. Lynne McTaggart, referring to the concepts of philosopher Ervin Lászlό, writes:

> EEG studies of the brains of children under five show that they permanently function in alpha mode—the state of altered consciousness in an adult—rather than the beta mode of ordinary mature consciousness. Children are open to far more information in The Field than the average adult. In effect, a child walks around in a state of a permanent hallucination. If a small child claims to remember a past life, the child might not be able to distinguish his own experiences from someone else's information, as stored in the Zero Point Field. (McTaggart 2002, 238)

Esotericism, Witchcraft, and Spiritual Search

Mainstream culture does not take this into account, but the fact is that there are hundreds of thousands of people in the world who consider themselves clairvoyant, having special premonitions, access to higher cognition, contact with angels, or at least extraordinary intuition. Systemic constellations can make it possible for them to come down to earth. In constellations, ordinary people become "seers," so the whole "higher dimensions" thing loses some of its spectacularity. I do not claim that systemic constellations explore the whole field covered by the esoteric tradition. However, they provide the most coherent, empirically consistent, and concise explication of much of the field.

One of my female patients, Kamila, became interested in parapsychology at the age of sixteen and reportedly managed to produce some psychokinetic effects. She soon came into contact with people involved in witchcraft, and after a few years, she became one of the few experts on the subject. She came to my office complaining of psychic discomfort, states of apathy, and psychosomatic disorders.

I facilitated a group constellation for her. In the constellation, there was a child to whom the patient and her mother were attached. Kamila was skeptical about the constellation. She said that for a witch it was all dilettantism, that during the constellation a demon was present, with whom she "worked," and so on. Since then I stopped referring to family constellations and we continued her long-term psychotherapy. In its course, Kamila said about herself that she was "demonic," as if she was "not fully human," that she was partly "animal." She meant two things in particular: the strange fantasies she had about eating raw meat and tearing people apart, and her large sexual appetite.

After about three years of psychotherapy she informed me that she was told by several witchcraft practitioners that she had a brother who had died while still in the womb. True to occult terminology, Kamila herself spoke of a "poroniec," "familiars," and "demons."[9] However, she had no respect for that child as a person. Her esoteric beliefs and practices stood in the way of a calm and love-filled encounter with what affected her. Kamila was slowly opening up to this ordinary dimension of the extraordinary phenomena.

Many people talk about and seek spiritual growth. But can it be found, or is it rather that it finds us? The spiritual is that which is purely human. Can we have more or less of that? We often imagine how much we can do in this regard, how much is up to us. We are like the ancient authors who thought it was possible to reach the end of the world or to build a tower reaching the seat of gods. When speaking of spiritual growth, it is important to do it in moderation. In general, when we talk about it for more than a few seconds, hubris appears in us.

Hellinger writes that spiritual growth is a kind of search for fullness, something we still lack, and states:

> There are those who seek God in a specific way, not so ordinarily. And God is sought by those who lack a father. Jesus is an example of this. [. . .] Of course, Jesus must not be reduced to this issue. This we are not allowed to do. His movement or influence is too great. But look at the seekers of God. What do they lack? There are also ascetics who starve, meditate. The Buddha is an example of this. What does the Buddha lack? Who does he find in nirvana? His mother. She died giving birth to him. [. . .] For those who seek God, the search ends when they find their true father and give him a place in their heart. Ascesis

> ends when one finds his mother and she is given a place in his heart. (Hellinger and Nehrebecki 2012, 166)

He also writes:

> I have observed that people who plead spiritual growth and exalt themselves above others are often those who have abandoned a child in need. And when they begin to care for that child, growth becomes superfluous. (Hellinger and Nehrebecki 2012, 166)

GOD

Through constellations, we can see that behind many big words and ideas are hidden causes that boil down to family ties, loyalty, and our conscience. Even such figures as "God" can be represented in constellations. After all, he plays a huge role in the lives of priests and their families, for example. Hellinger states: "When God appears in a system, he is always really someone in the system" (Hellinger 2001, 246). Thus, although "God"—as a collective representation—has great power to influence individual people and whole societies, here he often turns out to represent some specific person.

But is God *merely* an idea and a matter of faith? Or can we find any empirical basis in this issue? For centuries there have been attempts to "prove" the existence of God. There was, for example, the proof from design—the world is arranged in such a way that someone must have put its parts together or designed it. The proof from degrees of perfection—since there are various degrees of "goodness" or "beauty," there must be a maximum degree of these qualities, unattainable by anything earthly. Finally, the "ontological" proof—since there is the very idea of a supremely perfect being, then this being must also exist, for without the attribute of existence, the being would not be supremely perfect at all. Each of these "proofs" can be questioned and in the end, they prove nothing. So many have taken it as indisputable that "God" is merely a dream, a hypostasis of society, or a collective name for all that we do not understand. Then came only ideas that were extremely distrustful, even paranoid, seeing religion as the result of a "priestly conspiracy."

No doubt the aspect of construction and fantasy is considerable in the cultural idea of God. But let us ask again, in slightly different words, our question: Is the supreme reality to which one can/should turn with reverence/respect/hope nothing more than a phantasm? "What if," Rupert Sheldrake asks, "our life is a gift of nature? What if nature herself is a gift? Then we have our deepest obligation to the powers that brought us and everything else into being, and our greatest cause for gratitude" (Sheldrake 2017). Of course, a die-hard materialist will not accept such an argument; he does not think he has anything to be grateful to "blind" nature for. But what is this "blindness" of nature? Without a doubt, it is our brainchild, perhaps an "illumination" once experienced by someone who believed strongly and got disappointed.

Let's ask another question: Can a materialist be grateful to his parents? Probably yes. For raising him, for loving him. And can he be grateful to them for his life? Perhaps. But in that case, does he not deify them? After all, it was not them, in the strict sense, who gave him this life, life came to him "through them." Will he then feel gratitude toward this wider process? If so, how will he differ from the believer?

But perhaps the materialist will find that he can only be grateful to his parents for begetting him. But did they actually beget *him*? They simply decided to have a child. It is difficult to find a basis for deeper gratitude here. Could it be, then, that a materialistic worldview stands in the way of gratitude even toward parents? Is gratitude possible in a world governed by chance? Or does it need to be grounded in a sense of some mystery of a sequence of connections that we cannot understand but nevertheless notice?

Why would the network of connections in the universe not be God to us? Why should we understand it—and we usually do so—as a mechanism? We do not approach ourselves that way, yet we too are a group of interconnected proteins or neurons. And I by no means mean the abstract "God of the philosophers." The "God" I address is a chain of causes and relationships that we can trivialize or feel its mystery. Family constellations have shown that when we deal with the accessible part of this network of invisible relationships, this can have a transformative effect on our lives. Not underestimating it turns out to be important.

Someone could object that I do not speak of God but of family relationships. Yes, but first, people who were not familiar with systemic constellations could associate such phenomena as madness or seeing ghosts with the supernatural sphere, and second, constellations are not, after all, the final word in learning about the network of relationships in which a human being exists, and which reach far beyond the visible.

So we do not need to understand "God" as the Creator of the universe, Pantocrator, Lord, even Father (or Great Mother). All of these, and many more, terms and depictions of "God" are, in my opinion, secondary. So what is my definition of "God"? "God" is: a reality that transcends us; that at the same time has an effect on us; that we can perceive to a certain, and only to a certain, degree; and toward which we can assume a certain emotional attitude; which in turn will affect our lives.

One of the healing elements in systemic constellations is that they build a much more diverse picture of events, full of relationships, compared to what we remember and what we get through family stories. Often we see a kind of secret interaction between perpetrators and victims, abusers and the abused, and the roots of all these events hidden in the past. Often behaviors that are socially condemned lead us to a covert love and loyalty to our ancestors, parents, or siblings. What is unveiled transcends the individual, transcends his consciousness, transcends what he can control.

Hellinger initially worked in such a way that he told the representatives of the perpetrators of crimes to go out the door of the workshop room, which symbolically showed that they "lost their rights" and was supposed to help the descendants stay away from the guilt that remained with the perpetrators. However, he later observed a spontaneous process of reconciliation between the perpetrators and the victims. The perpetrators gravitated toward the victims and the victims toward the perpetrators, and this movement always resulted in peace between them. Hellinger also observed that the same thing happens in the souls of descendants—they want to make room in their hearts for both the perpetrators and the victims. This is what he referred to as spiritual conscience, which undoubtedly transcends ordinary morality. He stated that "Those who come into harmony with the movements of the Spirit cannot help but turn to all equally, with benevolence and love, whatever their fate. This love knows no limits. The spiritual conscience transcends the divisions into better and worse, and into good and evil" (Hellinger 2008, 64). Such situations occur in constellations. We come to know such deep levels of love-driven human behavior that we must withdraw any ordinary judgments.

Hellinger refers to this reality as Spirit or Creative Spirit. In the face of this Spirit,

> many assumptions and ideas that were important for us until now cease to exist. For example, the assumption of free will, the assumption of personal responsibility. And many of the judgments and distinctions that supported our culture disappear.
>
> Here I refer first and foremost to the distinction between good and evil, between right and wrong, between chosen and rejected ones, between above and below, high and low, better and worse, and finally also between life and death.
>
> Yet we continue to make and experience these distinctions. Aren't they also conceived and willed by this spirit as they are? (Hellinger 2008, 12)
>
> No one can do anything without being moved by the absolute Spirit. No evil can come from this Spirit. We imagine that this Spirit must be for us. But he is for

> all equally. . . . When a woman aborted her children, when someone murdered someone, or started a war in which many innocent people were killed, was it only man who acted here? Or was he driven by this greater force? Was he free? Or was he unable to avoid it? Does anyone have the right to feel guilty? Did his act come from him? [. . .] Isn't everyone moved by the same Spiritual force? Isn't this Spirit turned toward all in equal measure? (Hellinger and Nehrebecki 2012, 77–78)[10]

We cannot have a non-judgmental attitude toward reality on a permanent basis. However it may sound, we touch the whole only partially. I find here a similarity to what quantum mechanics teaches us about the world. In the quantum world, it is the whole that determines all possible relationships between its parts, and the quantum state "is inseparable from the context and from the history of the system" (Woszczek 2010, 249). Thus, it can be said that "a part does not exist"—everything is interconnected. However, this wholeness is "always hidden from the perspective of empirical observers" because all cognition, that is, the identification of a certain connection between the "observer" and the "observed," means its destruction, which is due to the nature of measurement (Woszczek 2010, 250). So we deal with the whole, which is hidden, which we can never see directly. Yet it exists.

An advocate of viewing the universe as a unity connected at a deep level was physicist and philosopher David Bohm. He argued that relativity theory and quantum theory agree in that "they both imply the need to look on the world as an *undivided whole*" (Bohm 1981, 11). Starting from both of these theories, he postulated the existence of a hidden basis of reality, which he called *Undivided Wholeness in Flowing Movement* (Bohm 1981, 11). Bohm believed that matter, particles and fields are merely manifestations of this basis. Also, our body and mind are merely projections of this wider basis, which makes them essentially one. In considering these issues, he stated that "it will be ultimately misleading and indeed wrong to suppose, for example, that each human being is an independent actuality who interacts with other human beings and nature. Rather, all these are projections of a single totality" (Bohm 1987, 210).

This is what constellations confront us with. In constellations, in place of plurality and divisions, wholeness emerges, primarily as a result of the collapse of our judging attitude. In short, we see that everyone is driven by love, even when it produces bad results. We also see that everything has its roots, that there are no uncaused "bad" behaviors or emotions. The extensiveness of causal relationships that a constellation provides is far greater than what any traditional psychological analysis can provide. The latter is usually limited by the analyzer's perceptions and values. In constellations, we can see how one situation entails another, how events concerning ancestors shape the feelings, choices, and deeds of descendants.

"God is love; and he that abideth in love abideth in God, and God abideth in him" (1 John 4:16). In constellations, we find the empirical sense of this, seemingly, purely poetic statement. "God" is the network of relationships that love holds together. We are all in him, and he is in us. "God" whose existence we can deny or "see out of the corner of our eye." He is certainly what underlies human discourse about God (whether there is something else too, that I do not know). Is this reducing the God of believers to something that is not really God? I think it is rather a proof of his existence.

In constellation workshops, synchronicities frequently occur and invisible connections between family members come to light. Often, at the moment of resolution and reconciliation, bells begin to toll or a cell phone rings with a cheery tune. Shortly after the constellation, someone in the client's family, who has not called for a long time and was represented during the constellation calls or texts. Workshop participants or trainees observe surprising coincidences of events, dreams, and representations they are involved in. In an ordinary situation, we would not notice all these connections. However, they are noticeable in a "laboratory situation" such as that provided by regular meetings of a training group, where the level of observation and analysis of one's own life, experiences, and behavior is above average.

The sequences of related events in a person's life are his fate, and fate was associated with divine providence (Greek: πρόνοιᾰ). These concepts varied greatly, but what they had in common was that they presented man not as thrown into a chaotic reality, but as existing in a world of supra-individual meaning. Systemic constellations confront us with the phenomena that suggest the existence of a certain order. By this I mean:

- A constellation is of a teleological nature, for example, the essence of the client's problem is manifested spontaneously rather than through the reasoning of the representatives or the therapist.
- Constellations help us observe that the many thoughts, words, and feelings of the participants—including those that occur before or after the constellation—form meaning-related sequences. Without a constellation, these would not be noticed or would be classified as coincidences.
- Constellations seem to "escalate" synchronicities, that is, "physically impossible" connections between the mental world and the material world.
- Constellations confront us with a higher moral level than that of the average individual, which involves a spontaneous reconciliation between perpetrators and victims in every instance.

The course of the constellation is quite different from that of traditional therapy. During the constellation, the therapist intentionally surrenders to certain forces whose source is outside his mind. He also believes, and it never lets him down, that these forces, even without any intervention of his rational mind, will form a coherent pattern, bringing the client relief and resolution. As if they themselves were directed by a superior force. When I cannot grasp what the client's problem actually is, I put a piece of paper in front of him that I define as "What you come to me with/what is most important right now." And then we always get right to the heart of it. What directs this? The "subconscious" of the client? How could I "get into" his subconscious so quickly?

When we become aware of connections and a sense of wholeness comes to us in flashes, silence appears and our judgments lose their force that they have when we look at people as separate and always deciding for themselves. Looking at the wholeness, that our parents, grandparents, perpetrators, victims, winners, and losers were moved by, can bring us peace, and enable us to find our rightful place. We know that in the end "everyone returns to the realm of this Spirit" and "joins the primordial order from whence all life comes and where it ultimately returns" (Hellinger and Nehrebecki 2012, 309). Isn't this the same thing Bohm writes about?

> What we perceive through the senses as empty space is actually the plenum, which is the ground for the existence of everything, including ourselves. The things that appear to our senses are derivative forms and their true meaning can be seen only when we consider the plenum, in which they are generated and sustained, and into which they must ultimately vanish. (Bohm 1987, 192)

NOTES

1. Our father's ex-wife is not our ancestor in the strict sense, but she may turn out to be part of our family system (that is, she may have an influence on us). Also in traditional cultures, "ancestors" sometimes include the spirits of children, sisters, brothers, barren wives, and other persons who were not ancestors in the biological sense (Mbiti 1970, 84).

2. A more neutral view was propounded, for example, by Evans-Pritchard, who wrote that "there is no possibility of his *knowing* whether the spiritual beings of primitive religions or of any others have any existence or not, and since that is the case he [the anthropologist] cannot take the question into consideration. The beliefs are for him sociological facts, not theological facts, and his sole concern is with their relation to each other and to other social facts" (Evans-Pritchard 1965, 17).

3. Here, Turner writes, there is an interpretative equivocality regarding the role and identity of the shade of the deceased ancestor and *Mvweng'i*. In any case, some informants argue that the shade always belongs to a female ancestor and *Mvweng'i* to a male ancestor, and that the shade rouses *Mvweng'i* to jointly harm the victim.

4. Turner says in this context that the woman is persecuted by "by a part or aspect of herself, projected onto the shade" (Turner 2008, 18). However, it is actually aspects of the ancestor that are introjected into the patient's self.

5. Hellinger argued that religion was based on sacrifices, particularly child sacrifices (Hellinger 2014b, 205). Offering a boy, a virgin, a child was supposed to secure the favor of the god and the prosperity of the community. Hellinger gives the example of Jesus, who, if one takes the story literally, was sentenced to death by his father. He also cites the story of Abraham, who was commanded by God to sacrifice his son Isaac. At the same time, he suggests that the phenomenon of offering children is something independent of religious life, that it is based on the unconscious activity of our psyche—the dynamic of "You for me" (Look at the intergenerational traumas for me, take the blame for me), in which the parent can entangle his own child. Nevertheless, Hellinger seems to blame the Christian religion for cultivating the sacrificial trend (Hellinger 2018, 87 et seq.). I do not agree with him. Girard points out that "we must avoid confusing the representation with what is represented" (Girard 2001, 143). If the text of the Bible represents something, it does not necessarily mean that it is "under the sway" of it—the biblical texts address sacrifices, "eating of the flesh" and "drinking of the blood," but in this way they want to lead us beyond these archaic phenomena. Hellinger's attitude toward religion stems from his personal experiences of being a Catholic priest and monk, and his outlook is a critique of the Church rather than an overall view of religion.

6. The source of violence in Girard's theory is a kind of blurring of differences between people, which is caused by mimetic rivalry. Everyone wants to take the "place" of the other, to "be" like him, to "have" what he has. What the other wants becomes desired. At the same time, everyone wants to be "themselves," wants to be the only one. The more I feel that I am different, the more I want to be like someone else and at the same time I want to differ from them. Before I read this author's works, I proposed a concept of a similar mechanism, which I termed "multiplicity" (unpublished). Multiplicity is a fundamental modality of existence of a human being—as the only one and one of many at the same time. We do not usually perceive the tension caused by the situation that man has a "totalizing" and "solipsizing" consciousness and at the same time is a "social being." Besides, multiplicity has three poles: "the only one," "one of many," and "the undifferentiated part," between which our psyche seems to constantly oscillate. I found that it may be the primary source of interpersonal aggression. Nevertheless, I maintain the thesis that, as an external phenomenon, aggression is motivated or directed by conscience.

7. The author referred to the theory of Polish psychiatrist Jan Mazurkiewicz (1871–1947), which in turn is based on the theory of evolution and dissolution of English psychiatrist and neurologist John Hughlings Jackson (1835–1911). According to Mazurkiewicz's theory, the positive symptoms of schizophrenia are not a direct manifestation of the disease process, but of dissolution, as a result of which the patient's mind in a way goes back to "prelogical" thinking.

8. I will not further explore this topic, but I think it was also relevant that the criticized persons in power were men. I saw in the protests a hatred for the father figure.

9. Poroniec—a malicious demon in Slavic mythology originating from a stillborn child.

10. This recalls St. Paul's phrase: "For in him we live, and move, and have our being" (Acts 17:28).

Chapter 8

A Different Picture of Man

KNOWLEDGE OF SCIENCE AND KNOWLEDGE OF PSYCHOTHERAPY

Is It Only Science that Brings Knowledge?

We expect answers to questions about the nature of man from science. It is science that is supposed to tell us what our capabilities are, what is innate in us and what results from nurture, what drives and motivates us, why we fall mentally and physically ill, what we are really afraid of, and even what we should do to be happy. But can it give us answers to all these questions? And is it the only domain we can turn to when exploring these issues?

If we are somewhat familiar with the history and structure of science, and if, like the author of this book, we are well versed in matters about which science has little to say, we must come to the only logical conclusion: science is not the only way of knowing. In the modern world where we are told to believe in science unreservedly, this statement will sound like heresy, but science does not know everything we know. This is especially true with regard to man and the structure and capacity of his psyche. In this area, psychotherapy can take us further than science. Psychotherapy is not just practice; it contains observations and theories about people's experiences and behaviors that can go beyond what science can see. It is also a certain research methodology that makes it possible to systematically collect further observations.

Usually, one tries to compare the conclusions from psychotherapeutic observations with what science has arrived at, as if psychotherapy was just a kind of *bricolage*, and scientific psychology knew the basic and at the same time true processes. This assumption is incorrect. The idea that only science can know the answers to crucial questions about man is a myth that exists only because of the institutional and financial power of science and its social authority. Although the world of inanimate matter will always be described more fully by academic physics than by self-taught experimenters, the issue gets complicated already in the case of biology, not to mention the sciences that are even further from physics, such as psychology. A science journalist, referring to the findings of Trevor Goward, a self-taught biologist who studies lichens, writes:

> Modern science tends to ignore outsiders. But reductionist science is not the only way of knowing things. Naturalists were the forefathers of science. Humans once lived much closer to the land and were keen observers who had a deep understanding of nature's interactions. Today biology tends to be focused on molecules, and failure to look up from instruments in the lab and actually observe how pieces interact in the natural world sometimes undermines discovery. A clinical focus can lead scientists to miss big-picture connections, such as an emerging understanding that networks may be a more enduring life-form than individuals. (Gies 2017, 55–56)

"Science's reductionist focus has made it nearly impossible to fully understand symbiosis" (Gies 2017, 56). I have no doubt that it is similar, but worse, in psychology. Academic psychologists do not notice many of the things that we—clinicians and psychotherapists—see.

However, there is a persistent question about the "scientific grounds" of a given psychotherapeutic method, although this question alone is not clear. Is it about the therapeutic effectiveness? Or demonstrating that the processes postulated by a given therapy really exist? Or does it contain pure dogmatism that states that certain phenomena simply cannot exist because they are "antithetical to science?" Which science would investigate the phenomena that occur during constellations? Psychology? Or maybe physics, biology, history, or genealogy would be better?

Can psychology, for example, examine all possible nuances of feelings of pregnant women? A woman will not admit to the researcher to what she will tell her best friend, and she will probably not tell her everything either.[1] She will not say that when she was lying in bed and listening to the movements of her several-month-old fetus, which were weaker this time, she thought that if this child died, she could have a second, she would have a chance to have a son. She would not say anything about her mixed feelings about her daughters, about all the tangled feelings about the feminine gender, or about the fact that her attitude toward her mother is very problematic. She will not mention that she is disappointed that her love is not simpler and more unambiguous. She will conceal some of these things, she will not remember part of them or associate them with the subject of the study, and she will not be aware of part of them at all. At which point would a psychologist be more cognitively effective than a friend, let alone a psychotherapist?

Academic psychology has not discovered the processes identified by Hellinger because its methodology protects it from such discoveries. They will not appear in statistical studies, laboratory tests, or brain imaging. One should not expect academic psychology to discover complicated intergenerational patterns. To do so, one needs to talk to people in an atmosphere of trust, which is difficult to achieve under study conditions. People will tell more to a therapist than to a scientist for a simple reason—in the case of a therapist, they hope their problems will be solved. Would it be possible to collect the necessary material objectively, without involving the examined person, for example, by studying chronicles, metrics, biographical records, or hospital records? Not many researchers have done this because it is an extremely painstaking job. It would also be difficult to say that one could find out everything that is important in this way. If academic science studied these processes, there would be plenty of generalizations and simplifications that are required by its method-based quantification and statistical data processing.

Because scientific research is widely regarded as the only source of correct knowledge, many people find it difficult to believe that such a simple procedure as a constellation can lead to substantial discoveries. They probably think that if it was really something important, it would have been discovered a long time ago at some university. This was also the case with facilitated communication. Douglas Biklen, professor of special education, states that when he worked with the method, many people did not believe it because they wondered: "How could something so simple not have been discovered much earlier?" (Biklen 1993, 116).

However, it is precisely thanks to the simple and completely nonscientific procedure of "representing" one person by another that we could observe repetitive patterns and discover extremely important factors that shape mood and behavior. Purely subjective diversity or ordinary chaos did not manifest themselves, as we might have expected based on our psychological knowledge. The previously unknown dynamics of hierarchy, bond, and balance emerged, identification processes and subconscious knowledge about the fate of the ancestors came to light.

We should keep our distance from the word "science." Science is not a monolith, but a multitude of disciplines and methodologies. Domains such as evolutionary anthropology, cosmology, or even political science are treated as scientific even though they use completely different tools for research and controlling results, and each of them is far from the golden standard of experimental physics. "It is difficult or impossible to test many of the conjectures of evolutionary psychology" and the discipline has become "more of faith than a science" (Coyne in: Brockman 2007, 19–20). "Cosmology evolves in a direction in which proven philosophical criteria separating scientific hypotheses from non-scientific ones (especially the criterion of falsifiability or observability) are not easily applicable" (Lamża 2015, 28). Theories and investigations in psychology have nothing of the status they have in physics, chemistry, or even biology. A research project, led by psychologist Brian Nosek, reviewed 100 studies in psychology published in major journals, through their replication (Nosek et al. 2015). The obtained psychological effects were half of those reported in the publications, and only thirty-seven replicated studies were statistically significant, although as many as ninety-seven primary studies were statistically significant.

Behind the Paradigm Wall

In many cases, science does not bother to check something, even if the issue seems important to many people. Although it sprang from curiosity about the world and this tendency is still present in it, science also tends to remain unchanged and resists new cognition. This is due, among other things, to paradigms, that is, the framework within which science is practiced. They determine the paths of experimentation and, as general theoretical schemes, enable the development of detailed research (Kuhn 2012, 25). Importantly, a paradigm also defines the set of questions asked and the shape of possible answers, and thus is responsible for what science sees and what it remains blind to. Once it is established, an important part of science becomes its defense, and science itself, as described by Thomas Kuhn, becomes the so-called "normal science," that is, science that does not discover anything fundamentally new, but organizes and detailes what is already known in the outline. Kuhn states:

> No part of the aim of normal science is to call forth new sorts of phenomena; indeed those that will not fit the box are often not seen at all. Nor do scientists normally aim to invent new theories, and they are often intolerant of those invented by others. (Kuhn 2012, 24)

Microbiologist and science theoretician Ludwik Fleck, author of the concept of thought collective, argued similarly: "Once a structurally complete and closed system of opinions consisting of many details and relations has been formed, it offers enduring resistance to anything that contradicts it" (Fleck 1979, 27). This is clearly visible in psychology. In the 1960s, psychologist John Garcia and his colleagues conducted experiments that called into question the smooth assumptions of behaviorists that "everyone can be taught everything," that is, that the mind is a *tabula rasa* (Harris 2007, 11). In examining rats, he found that they learned certain associations with more ease and other associations with more difficulty, they did not learn some of them at all, although it was previously claimed that any unconditioned stimulus could be associated with any other stimulus, creating a conditioned reflex. And, importantly, in this whole matter, the researchers faced great difficulties in publishing their study because journals rejected their article. All considered their conclusions improbable. They did not follow the paradigm of "pure" conditioning. It was difficult for psychologists to admit that their scheme—so "scientific" and beautiful in its simplicity—that everything is learned, was incorrect. They were not open to truly new data.

In science, there are fashions and trends. Researchers' attention is not necessarily focused solely on important or interesting things; it is largely driven by fashion. New, fashionable topics that dominate universities and minds appear every day. An example in recent years is mirror neurons that are used to explain almost everything in an unreflective manner (Hickok 2014). Fashion plays a role even in advanced sciences, and a subject that is not fashionable can be skipped and unexplored. Mathematician and physicist Roger Penrose states that the mechanisms for furthering careers in the world of theoretical physics and other research areas "are strongly biased in favour of the further propagation of already fashionable areas," which contributes to strengthening the status of fashionable theories (Penrose 2016, 88). For the same reason, we read so much about the effectiveness of behavioral-cognitive psychotherapy and the antidepressant effect of chocolate, and so little about family constellations and the antidepressant effect of reconciliation with parents, because cognitive psychology and neurotransmitters are in line with the reductionist paradigm and are fashionable. If something does not fall within the paradigm, it does not evoke such interest, regardless of its contribution to knowledge about man and its usefulness.

Paradigms have their psychological side. The conviction that I know at least roughly how reality works ensures basic mental comfort. Being in the area of a shared worldview gives a sense of group membership. A professor of psychology who addresses parapsychological phenomena in his environment risks not only losing grants but also being excluded. The facts show that the vast majority of us are unable to suffer such difficulties for the "truth." Paradigms are like political parties that people join in order to make others confirm them in their views and to avoid seeing the rest of humanity.

When a scientific paradigm or prevailing ideas collide with a new discovery, it always results in attempts to squash this discovery. Let us look at the history of science and technology. Most concepts faced astonishing resistance that sometimes even involved hostility and hatred. Albert Einstein, with his theory of relativity in mind, said that he had "hardly come to know the wretchedness of mankind better than as a result of this theory and everything connected to it" (Calaprice 2000, 234). Ludwig Boltzmann's atomic physics was ridiculed, which probably contributed to his suicide (Sautoy 2017, 92). The concept of hand disinfection was rejected as absurd and its initiator,

Hungarian obstetrician Ignaz Semmelweis, was degraded and made to stop practicing (Howick 2018, 67). In the field of psychotherapy, neither Carl Simonton aroused much interest in his discovery that patients can have an impact on the course of their illness, nor Salvador Minuchin with the effects he achieved. The latter stated:

> During the psychosomatic study [. . .] I was absolutely convinced that people would be swayed by the empirical evidence. After all, we were reporting 86 percent success rate. I was sure our work would transform the therapeutic approach to anorexia.
>
> I know now that I was under the rationalistic illusion that knowledge produces change. How did people respond to our findings? By defending their own paradigms. (Simon 1992, 83–84)

Adrian Owen confessed:

> The skepticism confused and intrigued me. I knew that we had sent a clear "Are you there?" signal into inner space, and the answer "Yes, I am here" had come back loud and clear. I had no doubt that Carol [the patient under examination] was conscious—a thinking, feeling person trapped within a useless body. How could anyone dispute that? But they did. (Owen 2017, 114)

The most famous Polish clairvoyant—who found about 700 bodies of missing persons, helped to solve several criminal cases and predicted, for example, the crisis of 2008—Krzysztof Jackowski, said:

> After over 30 years of my experience with the gift, properties, or whatever you call what I do, I no longer delude myself, I am completely alone in it, and I admit that I expected something completely different, that at least science would be interested—perhaps not in me, but in what I can do. In the results of my work, hundreds of bodies that I have found. And yet any coincidence is out of the question here. (Jackowski and Janoszka 2018, 9)

These are just a few examples (of varying degrees of "scientificity") from the vast pool of possible ones that demonstrate that humanity has a serious difficulty in recognizing, assimilating, and developing what is important when it is significantly new.

Man who Does Not Err

The evidence of the existence of extrasensory perception provided by systemic constellations is undisputed. The terms "parapsychic" or "paranormal phenomena" actually lose their meaning, as anyone can be a representative in a constellation. In constellations, unusual phenomena are used routinely and instrumentally. As a representative, every person becomes a kind of clairvoyant. Following his movement, he discovers unknown facts from the client's life. As a representative, I can have a feeling that someone is suffering internally, that he is attached to some other person, that something strange is happening to him, and that something makes me suspect a mental illness. I can look down and have the impression that the person represented by me feels guilty. I can also, which is one of the characteristic symptoms, open and clench my hands, which we describe as "the energy of the perpetrator." These and other feelings build a role, making it possible to access deep systemic dynamics that are fundamental to the client's life. Representatives also have more or less clear visualizations and insights. When an unknown person is represented, they have feelings about his gender or guess who he may be in the system. In addition, they experience traumatic events or have feelings like: "There's something sexual about it," "There's a perpetrator and a victim involved here, someone was killed." Often some words come to the representative's mind that the client can connect with certain facts from the family history. A constellation, which is conducted correctly and patiently, reflects 100 percent of the truth about the given person's emotional state, the basic events in his family, and the dominating feelings.

Although access to this kind of work is so easy—it is enough to just start doing it—psychology has tended to have a different opinion of our abilities. According to its paradigm, which we can describe as a model of a "stray man," these types of activities are not possible, they are only illusions, projections, and the result of not thinking critically. Psychology tells me not to trust my own experience, for example, *the sense of being stared at*. And this has happened to me many times when I walked down the street unwittingly peeking into one of the dozens of windows and meeting someone's eyes there. It claims that this is just "biased hypothesis testing," that I simply do not remember dozens of situations when I looked into a window and no one was there. This attitude is not even changed by the fact that this phenomenon was confirmed by experimental research (Radin 2020, 164 et seq.).

In constellations we do the opposite, which leads to substantial cognitive and therapeutic results—I "follow" what I feel and do not question it. Yes, the rational mind sometimes doubts, asking: Isn't what I'm experiencing in the role created by me?" As representatives, we are by no means in an altered state of consciousness and are constantly accompanied by critical thinking. It must, however, eventually accept the fact that the constellation turns out to show what is essential and true.

Mistrust of ourselves is a clear mark of our culture. It is one of the obstacles for science to build a correct picture of ourselves. Biklen said that the biggest barrier preventing the success of facilitated communication is "the tendency to underestimate people's abilities" (Biklen 1993, 193). Our constant tendency to perceive the other person as inferior and less important manifests itself in many situations. This is how academics look at people who use constellations—as more naive, more susceptible to manipulation, less able to draw correct conclusions than they are themselves.

Yes, many studies confirm the view of man as a stray being. But this is only one side of man. In constellations—when working with clients, observing other therapists, and people undergoing training—we discover another side of man, completely unknown to academic psychologists. It turns out that we have a surprising ability to receive, differentiate, and name the subtle emotional states of other people, and we have an innate sense of the systemic orders and the capacity for psychological insight. Constellations show that when people are given the opportunity, not only are they able to feel what is basically happening in them but they usually also accurately describe it. Although these people probably do not go into psychological processes on a daily basis, in this situation they become sensitive observers. The same is true for the clients who, if confronted with the processes that are important to them, without much explanation from the therapist, begin to understand the essence of the ongoing therapy and feel what is good for them, often seeing what the therapist sees. And the solutions referred to are not colloquial and obvious in advance. All of this is different from the vision presented by the mass media, and sometimes psychology, of unbright clients, who can be made believe everything.

Grof speaks of a taboo against knowing that we have clairvoyant abilities, which are in fact something common (Grof 2006, 198–203). The participants of a workshop were instructed to take an object belonging to another person and write down the associations that came to their minds. Grof saw in his imagination a little German town, his medical studies, his thoughts turned to malignant tumors and his work with a cancer patient, and finally he remembered a joke that involved smashing testicles. He did not think that he had parapsychic abilities and doubted whether anything would result from this experiment. The object that Grof was holding was a pendant shaped like the Vitruvian Man, the emblem of a particular workshop center. It turned out that the owner of the object was a German woman, a doctor of medicine, from a little town. At one of the workshops she attended, the participants were told that the pendant would be given to a person who would do "the most outrageous thing" during the workshop. She bit one of the participants on the testicles (the participants were naked) and won the pendant. Several months after the workshop, where Grof was present, she was diagnosed with cancer.

Representing the family and other systems, which takes place during a constellation session, turns out to be a situation that activates our extrasensory perception in an extremely strong and fully repeatable way. I do not know what I could "read" from an object belonging to someone, but when I am part of the represented system or look at my client's family composed of figurines, the range of my perception broadens. When I let the knowing field "hook" to the represented elements, everything becomes clearer. The associations that come to my mind and feelings that appear in my body turn out to be not accidental. I can see the character of the relationship between the mother and the grandmother, although they are represented by simple plastic figurines and the client has not told me anything about it.

Dean Radin, a well-known researcher of psychotronic phenomena, notes that in scientific and academic circles people quickly learn not to raise the subject of psi-type phenomena, even though many of them may be interested in such matters. The attitude of educational institutions is that it is possible "to advance from preschool through postdoctoral positions and never learn about—or in many cases even hear about—serious scientific investigations of psychic or mystical experiences" (Radin 2013, 68). The vision of the psyche propagated by mainstream psychology and medical sciences is extremely impoverished. The prevailing materialistic view needs to change, which is fundamental both theoretically and in relation to the quality of human life (Kelly et al. 2010, xiv).

THE PSYCHE IN PARTICIPATION

The Mind Beyond the Brain

Through a simple procedure, family constellations have shown that our minds function differently than most psychologists and neuroscientists believe. Memories, emotions, and attitudes partly exist "beyond" our brain and even "beyond" our whole person, and are, to a certain degree, accessible to other people's perception. Moreover, some part of our mental life remains even after death.

Those present in a constellation session experience clear psycho-physical reactions, usually in the form of "energy flows" in systemically and emotionally important moments of the session, completely regardless of their mental attitude. And as a result of bringing about the systemic order, a sense of peace and strength appears.

In the majority of participants a session results in permanent life changes, often also in the spheres that seemed to be independent of the client's actions (for example, attitudes of other people toward him, or new chances and opportunities).

Family constellations discredit the foundations of the prevailing paradigm in psychology and neuroscience, according to which all models of the mind considered scientific are created. According to this paradigm, the mind "is contained" in the brain, the minds of individual people are separated from one other, and communication is possible only through the conventional sense channels, so it is not possible to influence one another at a distance.

The psyche and the brain undoubtedly have much in common. But reducing the mind to the mechanics of the brain, as a biochemical or bioelectrical machine, is a great simplification. In such a model, the mind is locked in the skull as if in a sealed jar, which makes it impossible to answer questions such as how representatives access information about unknown people.

Today, we can no longer doubt that the capabilities of our minds transcend the time and space available to our senses (Kelly et al. 2010; Radin 2013; Cardeña 2018). There are also observations of people who function normally even though they have almost no brain, their skulls are filled with cerebrospinal fluid, and their anatomically degenerated brain has at most 10 percent of its normal volume (Lewin 1980; Dossey 2013; Feuillet, Dufour, and Pelletier 2007). People in a state of clinical death (NDE, *Near Death Experience*), when their brains did not function, observed their own bodies and physicians' actions "from above" or "from the side" (Kelly et al. 2010, 387 et seq.). These phenomena cannot be explained within a materialistic view of mind. The existence of certain cognitive abilities in humans is also difficult to explain. For how can one explain the fact that some people develop new intellectual abilities through brain injury? (Padgett and Seaberg 2014).

Many scholars and philosophers have argued against the idea, obvious to others, that the brain produces the mind. Authors such as William James or Ferdinand C. S. Schiller argued for a "transmission model of consciousness," in which the brain is only a kind of filter for the mind (Kelly et al. 2010, 73).

The fact that the brain functions differently than scholars presumed was already demonstrated by the research conducted by neurophysiologist Karl Lashley in the 1920s—memory seemed to be dispersed throughout the entire cerebral cortex rather than located in certain areas.

Such famous neuroscientists as Nobel Prize winner Charles S. Sherrington, neurosurgeon Wilder Penfield, and another Nobel laureate John C. Eccles also argued that the brain may not be a mere "producer" of mind (Kelly et al. 2010, 607 et seq.; Penfield 1975). There may be an autonomous self, and the brain is a transmitter of consciousness rather than its producer. The eminent neuroscientist Roger Sperry held similar views, arguing that the mind "emerges" from the brain but must not be understood based on the physiological functioning of the latter. He argued that mental phenomena emerge from the processes "that have yet to be discovered" but which will turn out to be "different from and more than the neural events of which they are composed" (Davies 2004, 191).

Eccles wrote:

> I think that, for my personal life as a conscious self, the brain is necessary, but it is not sufficient. In liaison with the brain events in World 1, there is the World 2 of my conscious experience, including a personal self at the core of my being. Throughout our lifetime this personal self has continuity despite the failure of liaison with the brain in states of unconsciousness such as dreamless sleep, anesthesia, coma. The brain states are then unsuitable for liaison, but the self can achieve in dreams a partial liaison in the brain states of *REM sleep*. Thus there is evidence that the self in World 2 has an autonomous existence, bridging gaps of unconsciousness when the brain fails to be in a state of liaison. (Eccles 1977, 227)

Roger Penrose and Stuart Hameroff argue that Planck scale (10^{-35} meters) phenomena may play a fundamental role in the brain, and that consciousness is related to the activity of microtubules in axons, which modify space-time locally. This is far from the vision of the brain as an electrochemical machine. Since the mind is related to the quantum level, any situating it in a specific point of space-time—for example, in the brain—cannot be successful.

Rupert Sheldrake talks about the "extended mind." The mind extends beyond the brain, which we can see in the simple act of perception. Vision is usually considered to be the result of light falling on the retina. However, this concept, now so obvious to us, is very imperfect. What does it actually mean that the tree I am looking at "really" is only in my brain? Since I see it there. Anyway, there must be some kind of projection of my perception outward. Sheldrake believes that it is of a very concrete, physical nature. Our sight, or rather our mind, pervades the body. He writes about it this way:

> Through vision, the external world is brought into the mind through the eyes, and the subjective world of experience is projected outwards into the external world through fields of perception and intention.
>
> Our intentions stretch out into the world around us, and also extend into the future. We are linked to our environment and to each other. (Sheldrake 2003, 282)

Sheldrake provides evidence for the existence of fields of perception, referring to experiments which prove that we can sense that someone is looking at us. However, to someone who does not accept this as evidence or does not believe in it, the British biologist's concept must seem bizarre. And yet it accords with those aspects of the mind that we experience during systemic constellations. The mind undoubtedly extends beyond the physical brain. People's memories, emotions, attitudes, and bonds extend beyond the brain. This is why we access them so easily during a constellation.

The Mind in a Network of Connections

Science has a wealth of experimental data suggesting—or actually proving—the existence of unconventional impacts that living organisms can exert on one another or on inanimate matter. For example, Russian researchers have found that there is an informational connection between the cells placed on separate Petri plates. They noted the phenomenon of "shared experiencing" between living cells—a destructive impact on one cell culture caused changes in the cells of another culture isolated from the first one (Dubrov and Pushkin 1989, 120). It also turns out that the isolated DNA reacts to the emotional states of the donor (Braden 2009, 42 et seq.). Cleve Backster's experience on plant perception has been known since the 1960s (McTaggart 2002, 144–45). When Backster destroyed a leaf of one plant, another one reacted, which could be detected with a device testing galvanic response of the leaf.

Jacobo Grinberg-Zylberbaum's experiments proved the existence of spontaneous communication between people at a distance, manifested in the synchronization of their EEG records (Lászlό 2007, 53). Psychologist Charles Tart demonstrated that the sender's pain is unconsciously registered by the "recipient," as reflected in such physiological indicators as blood pressure and pulse (McTaggart 2002, 127–28). William G. Braud and Marilyn Schlitz proved that the mental images of one person can influence the skin-galvanic response of another person remotely (Dossey 1994, 49).

There are also other observations indicating the existence of remote contact between people. For example, the phenomenon of a sudden feeling of the presence of people we know when they die or when their lives are in danger. Most of these events concern the father, mother, or close family (Pearson 2015). Neuropsychiatrist Berthold E. Schwarz observed a similar phenomenon of "linking" with loved ones and described it as "telesomatic" (Dossey 2013). It refers to situations when a person experiences the same physical sensations as another person, separated by a distance. In a typical case, when someone experiences, for example, an injury to the left hand, the partner at the same time feels pain or numbness precisely in the left hand. The so-called syndrome of couvade, when a man co-experiences his wife's labor pains, is similar to this (Pearson 2015, 62). Based on his research on the experiences of people who have undergone clinical death, Pim van Lommel states that "it seems to be possible to have a nonlocal connection with other people's consciousness as well as with the thoughts and feelings of deceased friends and family and to communicate with them by way of thought transfer" (Lommel 2010, 225).

All the above results and phenomena are not unusual for a person familiar with systemic constellations. The representative may feel tingling and even pain in the part of the body that, as it later turns out, is affected in the represented person. We find out about the mental states of people whom we do not know and who are separated by a distance. We also have access to the "memory" of the dead. It would be strange if studies did not show the existence of similar processes.

In trying to understand them, we usually refer to quantum mechanics and concepts such as nonlocality and quantum entanglement. The history of these concepts began in 1935, when Albert Einstein, Boris Podolsky, and Nathan Rosen published an article in which they referred to the absurd—in their opinion—properties of quantum mechanics (Halpern 2015, 133 et seq.). The thought experiment, known as the EPR paradox, was supposed to show that quantum mechanics breaks the principles of relativity theory, so it cannot be correct. However, Alain Aspect's experiments confirmed the existence of links between distant objects (Baggott 2011, 318–27). Russian researchers Alexander Dubrov and Veniamin Pushkin write that if we make the assumption of nonlocality, then all objects of the universe are located in the form of a wave invisible to the observer, at any point of space. If the necessary focusing were achieved, one could detect the hidden wave structures of even very distant objects (Dubrov and Pushkin 1989, 48).

Perhaps this is what obtaining information during representation consists of. It turns out that this "necessary focus" is achieved very simply through intention and following the movement that emerges in the body.

Harald Atmanspacher, Hartmann Römer, and Harald Walach presented a view of quantum mechanics (*Weak Quantum Theory*), in which they consider the phenomena of entanglement and complementarity also in relation to phenomena other than purely physical ones, such as transference and countertransference. They write:

> The basic framework of weak quantum theory offers an interesting perspective for what can happen in transference and countertransference processes even beyond therapeutic applications. For instance, if in a marriage relationship one of the partners "experiences" something which is systemically unconscious, say the wish to separate, then this wish can manifest itself in the other partner's awareness as his or her own wish. The fatal aspect of such a phenomenon is that the corresponding material is mostly taken at face value rather than as a possible indicator of something originally belonging to another person. (Atmanspacher, Römer, and Walach 2001, 23)

This would be the physical basis for the phenomenon that Hellinger repeatedly observed during constellations—one of the spouses leaves because he unconsciously wants to stop the other from leaving the family. The real wish to separate is in the other spouse, but it is realized in the consciousness of the first one.

Influence at a distance does not need to be neutral; it can be healing. When we facilitate family constellations, we constantly hear from our clients about such phenomena. The accounts concern mainly the cases of children who were absent during the constellation and yet stopped having the symptoms on the same day. In other cases, the accounts concern parents who change their attitude after the constellation set up by their adult child, open up and, for example, hug their son or daughter for the first time in years. Therefore, for those who practice and use constellations, the idea of remote healing completely loses its unusual character.

The possibility of healing at a distance has been demonstrated by studies showing the influence of intention and imagery on tissues, cells, or bacteria, and the influence of intercessory prayer for the sick (Dossey 1994, 169–95). Larry Dossey writes that if we analyze "actual experiments in hospitals, clinics, and laboratories, distant prayer does have an effect—in humans and nonhumans, even when the recipient of the prayer is unaware the prayer is being offered" (Dossey 1997, 13). For example, Elisabeth Targ's research indicated that there is a remote effect of intercessory prayer on the condition of patients with AIDS (Dossey 1999, 45–47). McTaggart, on the other hand, involved thousands of people who sent positive intentions to others in her Intention Experiment, and found that these had a healing effect on both the recipients and the senders themselves (McTaggart 2017, 178–79).

Of course, attempts at this type of healing can only be compared to what happens during systemic constellations. Constellations transcend most of the unconventional methods of healing, which are unlikely to solve the causes of problems and do not address the individual's life situation in a deeper way. Instead, they have an element of wishful thinking, and sometimes force things to happen. Perhaps it is for this reason that studies of intercessory prayer for the sick do not produce such unambiguous results as the impact of thoughts and imagery on simple organisms and cells (Spilka and Ladd 2013).

In the context of "distant influences," one should mention the reflections of a Catholic priest (transcommunication researcher), François Brune, who speaks of the theological idea of the communion of saints, that is, the mystical connection of all Christians, living and dead.[2] Here we are even closer to what happens during constellations. Brune writes that the communion of saints assumes that some share others' experiences, not only by providing support but also by experiencing their real suffering and temptations. In doing so, they do not want to replace them but to help them through a mysterious but real "symbiosis," connection at a distance. Some saints are said to have helped the dying by experiencing their last temptations with them (Brune 2011, 344–45).

Father Brune takes quite seriously the statements of some mystics who maintained that they took on the temptations of others or their sufferings, as was the case with St. Faustina Kowalska or Teresa Neumann.

Brune says that the mystic helps the sinner, through specific empathy, to change, develop feelings and spiritual behavior that he was incapable of before (Brune 2011, 348). This is very close to the way we understand how constellations work on absent people, for instance, children. A child's representative triggers something in the child himself that could not spontaneously reveal itself. In this way, he removes blockages and initiates internal development. At the same time, it is important to remember that the strength of this effect does not result, as in most unconventional methods, from a simple action of the therapist's mind on the patient's mind. It emerges as a result of more complex relationships: in addition to a kind of *catharsis per procura*, the therapist, who alternately tunes into the client, into his absent child, and into other people in the family system, enables the mind of the client and his child to be "situated" in a "new place" of the system. And it is precisely the effect of their system that is most healing.

Contemporary physics confirms the existence of "nonlocal" phenomena, and it does not deny the possibility of mental influence on reality. Prominent physicist John Wheeler said that "we are participators in bringing into being not only the near and here but the far away and long ago" (McTaggart 2017, 16). He had in mind the conclusions from the so-called "delayed choice" experiment. This experiment is a modification of the original double-slit experiment.[3] The difference is that Wheeler proposed to check which slit the particle has gone through, and not which slit it is going through now. It turned out—which is beyond normal logic—that particles react to this observation in the same way as they do to the observation made during their going through—when they are observed they go through one of the slits, and when they are not, through both at once. But this time the observation took place—as we normally understand it—after the particle had chosen a way to act!

The double-slit experiments were explained in many ways and none of the explanations was successful. There is no indication that the experiments involve the physical interaction between the detector and the particle. Instead, it seems that the awareness of the observer is important. Since this experience has its own version, in which photons of distant stars would be the examined particles, distance and time do not seem to play a role. Or they definitely play a completely different role than we normally assume.

The Mind in the Field

The field is a physical concept. Does the field known from systemic constellations have anything to do with it? Michael Faraday was the first to speak of "field" in the mid-nineteenth century (Musser 2015, 72). It described the interactions between magnets and electric conductors. Albert Einstein and Leopold Infeld write:

> Starting as a helpful model, the field became more and more real. It helped us to understand old facts and led us to new ones. The attribution of energy to the field is one step farther in the development in which the field concept was stressed more and more, and the concepts of substances, so essential to the mechanical point of view, were more and more suppressed. (Einstein and Infeld 1978, 142)

Fields began to be ubiquitous in physics, and their use led to a vision of reality, in which objects influence one another through invisible forces; moreover, they are somehow constantly connected with one another. When Einstein formulated his concept of the gravity field, space ceased to be an empty stage for events, and the world turned, according to his metaphor, into the "giant mollusk" in which we live. Everything became somewhat connected (despite the elimination of the concept of all-pervading ether).

The knowing field cannot be identified with any particular physical field. However, the basic idea is very similar. The field we feel during constellations is clearly energetic, in some constellations we feel very strongly that "something is coming" from the outside, precisely in the form of "energy" that shapes our feelings and movements during the constellation. The clients are usually surprised by the power of this psychophysical, "energetic" impact. Even if the session is conducted without a group, only with the therapist, who stands on sheets of paper that denote members of the system, the clients start to unexpectedly experience somatic sensations or emotions. These sensations are never accidental, and very often they are some kind of somatic signs of transgenerational phenomena. If it were not for these experiences, I would be skeptical about the concept of "energy," which is present in so many paratherapeutic systems of different quality. However, this concept perfectly describes what we deal with here.

Kurt Lewin and Gestalt psychologists introduced the concept of field to psychology (Hall and Lindzey 1978, 385 et seq.). According to Lewin's field concept, people behave in a given way because they function in the field of forces that push and attract them. Of course, this concept does not take into account the specific interactions that we have learned from systemic constellations, such as invisible loyalties. However, by claiming that a person functions in the field of forces that determine his behavior, he gets close to the understanding we derive from constellations. When the "system of forces" changes in the constellation, because, for example, the mother expresses respect for her mother and the father leaves something that is not his, the client's mood and behavioral tendencies change immediately.

The concept of field is also used by other authors. Harry Stack Sullivan, considered to be the developer of the interpersonal approach in psychiatry, regarded the interpersonal field as the basic unit of psychological analysis (Mitchell and Black 1995, 62 et seq.). Sullivan concentrated on observing human interactions and even came to the conclusion that man's personality or self is not located in the individual, but generated by these interactions. The concept of field is also used by psychoanalysts who use this term to describe the psychic space between the analyst and the patient (Baranger and Baranger 2009). In this field paradigm of psychoanalysis, it is this shared space filled with projections, dreams, and reactions of both the patient and the analyst that is what analysis concentrates on. The field, as the psychodramatic field, is also discussed in psychodrama (Czapów and Czapów 1969, 30).

Brian D. Josephson, a Nobel Prize winner in physics, stated that "genuine physical facts may exist which lie outside the scope of current scientific descriptions. Indeed a new kind of understanding of nature is now emerging, with concepts like implicate order and subject-dependent reality (and now, perhaps formative causation)" (Sheldrake 2009, 21–22). The author of these words referred to the concept of Sheldrake, whose theory of morphic resonance seems to explain much of what we encounter during systemic constellations.

It all began with difficulties in explaining the embryonic development of organisms. How do billions of cells differentiate and interact, and still follow the global plan of body structure? How do they know where and what to do? Biologists began to wonder "whether the traditional mechanistic reductionist approach can ever be successful, based as it is on the particle concept, borrowed from physics. As remarked earlier, physicists no longer regard particles as primary objects anyway. This role is reserved for fields" (Davies 2004, 105).

Three biologists, Aleksander Gurwicz, Hans Spemann (Nobel Prize laureate), and Paul A. Weiss proposed independently of each other the concepts of "development fields" (embryonic, morphogenetic) that would act as controllers of embryonic development. These concepts were developed by Sheldrake. According to him, an organism inherits not only DNA but also the morphic (morphogenetic) field of previous organisms. This enables the formation of its complex structure, which, contrary to what is sometimes presented, is not "contained in the DNA," since deoxyribonucleic acid only codes the structure of proteins.

Morphic fields do not only concern organisms but also make it possible for all systems to form—from atoms and molecules to human societies. At the core of Sheldrake's concept is the assumption that there is a kind of memory that stores information about past structures. This information becomes available to similar structures that are just emerging. When a process, such as the formation of a molecule, begins, its course is determined by the morphic field formed as a result of past processes of formation of similar molecules. The field, through the so-called morphic resonance, shapes the molecule according to the earlier patterns. This explains why certain compounds have this and no other spatial form, even though—given only physical indicators—they could take many other shapes. It also explains the increased stability of some compounds in subsequent syntheses observed by chemists.

Sheldrake's concept also refers to behavioral or social fields that model individual and group behavior. Numerous experiments have been conducted to confirm this concept. Examples include experiments on learning. They use sets of existing and imaginary signs, for example, Japanese writing system and an invented set of lines resembling it. It turns out that people learn existing signs much faster, which is explained by the fact that there is a morphic field related to them that has lasted for decades or hundreds of years and concerned large groups of people (Sheldrake 2009, 227 et seq.).

It goes without saying that morphic fields understood in this way are almost identical to the knowing field. The assertion that an individual or group is influenced by a field related to the experience of similar individuals in the past corresponds perfectly with the fact that our ancestors' experiences shape us and that the family group (and other groups) are related to a certain "spirit" guiding them. Sheldrake (who, by the way, knows systemic constellations and acknowledges them) writes:

> Through morphic resonance, animals and plants are connected with their predecessors. Each individual both draws upon and contributes to the collective memory of the species. Animals and plants inherit the habits of their species and of their breed. The same applies to humans. An extended understanding of heredity changes the way we think of ourselves, the influence of our predecessors, and our effects on generations yet unborn. (Sheldrake 2012, 185)

The Supraindividual Soul?

In systemic constellations, we say that we "enter the field," "work in the field," "feel from the field," and are "captured" by the field. As representatives, we become a receiver of information about strangers; these sensations come to us, as it were, from the outside, they overwhelm us, and—with our permission—they take possession of us to some extent. The persons who observe the constellation sometimes feel drawn into this process—they stand up, enter the constellation, and begin to represent a person who has not been mentioned before. The movements of individual representatives and their sensations can be very strongly correlated—a change in one representative often causes a momentary change in others, even if they have not noticed this change. The representatives form a certain dynamic whole, although they do not coordinate their behavior with one another. How is all this possible? It cannot involve a "from-brain-to-brain" influence. For this reason, we speak of the knowing field as the medium in which the constellation takes place.

In a constellation, initial disorder turns into order. The final pictures are much more coherent and centralized than the initial ones. It seems that if we let people follow the movement that arises in them, they become the expressers of some superior organizing force. The representatives do not peek at one another sneakily to somehow correlate their movements; everything happens spontaneously. Moreover, the final picture does not take all possible forms, but expresses the orders of love, regardless of whether the representatives have heard anything about them.

These are teleological features of the constellation. Similar observations were made by Moreno, who observed that, as experts on the subject wrote, "the interactions between group members typically tend to integrate, to form a whole" (Czapów and Czapów 1969, 292).

The whole, as a determinant of the behavior of the parts, is increasingly recognized in science. For many years, science has evolved, recognizing the bottom-up causality and ignoring the purposeful ("top-down") causes. Today, this is changing and scientists see that many structures cannot be explained without assuming global cooperation of their parts. This cooperation seems to be coordinated, as it were, in a top-down way, as it is difficult to imagine how a given element would coordinate its functioning with other elements. László notes that there is an amazing coherence at all levels of physical existence. From large-scale cosmic structures, through living organisms to subatomic matter, the elements of reality are interconnected in a way that seems to go beyond ordinary connections. He claims that what connects the whole cosmos is the active in-formation field, which he names—using a concept of Indian philosophy—the Akashic field:

> The action of this subtle but real A-field explains the nonlocality of the smallest measurable units of the universe as well as of its largest observable structures. It explains the coherence of living organisms, and their coherence with the milieu in which they live and evolve. It also explains the coherence of the human brain, and of the consciousness associated with it, in regard to the brain and consciousness of other human beings, and even the world at large. And, last but not least, it explains the astounding fact that the physical parameters of the universe are so finely adjusted that living organism can exist and evolve on this planet. (László 2007, 157)

In short, for quanta to act as they do, organisms to live and reproduce, and the cosmos to create large-scale structures, there must be something that makes it possible for the basic elements to be in immediate contact and to "coordinate" their actions. Even in the relatively simple physical experiment with two slits, the particles seem to "know" what will happen to them on their way, although they do not receive any information through the channels we know. So it is as if they are driven by some overriding order. For this reason, Paul Davies writes that "modern physics has a strongly holistic, even teleological flavour" (Davies 2004, 165).

Is there, then, something above the individual mind that would itself have the characteristics of something "mental"? It is often argued, for example, that human societies or crowds acquire certain special qualities, as if their own soul that influences the functioning of individuals. The author who spoke about the "soul of crowds" was the French psychiatrist Gustave Le Bon, who wrote that no matter what human characters are concerned, "the fact that they have been transformed into a crowd puts them in possession of a sort of collective mind which makes them feel, think, and act in a manner quite different from that in which each individual of them would feel, think, and act were he in a state of isolation. There are certain ideas and feelings which do not come into being, or do not transform themselves into acts except in the case of individuals forming a crowd" (Le Bon 2006, 4).

Psychologist Raymond B. Cattell believed that integration tendencies give groups a shape similar to personality, which he termed *syntality*, by analogy with *personality* (Eskola et al. 1988, 49). Bion stated that the hypothesis of a "*group mentality* derives from the fact that the group often functions as a unit, even though its members may not intend this, nor be aware of it" (Grinberg, Sor, and Tabak de Bianchedi 1977, 7).

Before that, the philosopher August Comte said that all mankind is similar to a living being that can experience and create. According to him, humanity is an entity superior to individuals, composed of all living, dead, and not yet born individuals. Individuals interchange in it as cells in the body, without affecting its own existence as a whole. They are its product, and their thoughts, preferences, beliefs, or abilities are derived from the life of this great organism (Kołakowski 2004, 70). The sociologist Émile Durkheim believed that society is a kind of supraindividual mind and that our thinking is the product of that "unique intelligence, where all others meet each other, and after a fashion, come to nourish themselves" (Durkheim 1973, 209).

Already for Aristotle, and even more so for Averroes, the intellect came as if from another world; it was a powerful pure spirit that existed independently of individual people. The Averroists concluded that souls cannot be merely individual and that the rational soul is one for all mankind (Świeżawski 1983, 67, 93). Many centuries later, the author of the most famous equation of quantum physics Erwin Schrödinger "had a deep sense that people share a common soul" (Halpern 2015, 80).

World 3 and the Noosphere

I will now present in more detail two concepts, which refer to supraindividual spheres—or perhaps even "minds"—in which the psyches of individual people participate. We will see that these theories, although developed in completely different contexts, have much in common with Hellinger's concepts and the phenomena we witness during constellations. These are the ideas of Karl R. Popper and Pierre Teilhard de Chardin.

Karl Popper advocated the concept of the "three worlds" and his "world 3" has the characteristics of the supraindividual mind. World 1 is the world of matter and physiology, world 2 is the sphere of the psyche, world 3 is the area of the products of the human mind, knowledge, theory, ideas, and problems.[4] Although the objects of world 3 are produced by the minds of people, they retain their autonomy and objective existence. They feed back into the psyche, that is, world 2. And it is not a minor kind of impact. As Popper writes:

> My central thesis [. . .] is that the self or the ego is anchored in world 3, and that it cannot exist without world 3. (Popper 2000, 129)

> We cannot understand world 2, that is, the world inhabited by our own mental states, without understanding that its main function is to *produce* world 3 objects, and to be acted upon by world 3 objects. (Popper 2000, 7)

> If my thesis is correct then we cannot expect to get anywhere near a solution of the body-mind problem unless we take world 3 into account. For the body-mind problem was the problem of the relationship between worlds 1 and 2. And if it is an important element in this relationship that world 2 functions as an intermediary between worlds 1 and 3, then the body-mind problem must remain incomplete, as it were, until we extend it to cover the interrelationships between all three worlds. (Popper 2000, 7–8)

According to Popper, all three worlds are separate realities. Each of them has its own kind of existence, different from the other two. In short, the psyche, for example, is more like a "soul" than a "product of the brain," because the brain is an object from a completely different world—world 1. However, there are mutual influences and interactions between the worlds. World 3 that exists, as it were, above human heads, is of a different nature than physical objects and individual mental states. It affects the psyche in such a way that, as Popper says, the psyche could not exist without it. Someone might doubt that there is something unusual about it. After all, it is clear that a child needs books, stories, knowledge, riddles, and other symbolic products for his development, and if someone wants to, they can call it world

3. However, Popper underlines that world 3 is not a metaphorical picture of obvious things, but a being of a different nature than the other two. And the mind is "an organ for interacting with the objects of the third world." It is not an ordinary vision. Popper supposed that

> one day we will have to revolutionize psychology by looking at the human mind as an organ for interacting with the objects of the third world; for understanding them, contributing to them, participating in them; and for bringing them to bear on the first world. (Popper 1979, 156)[5]

When we take seriously his two main assumptions: that world 3 is a different kind of existence and that there are important interactions between the world of mind and world 3, we are confronted with the processes that have not yet been studied by academic psychology.[6] However, what Popper says about the interactions of worlds 2 and 3 clearly corresponds to the processes related to the effect of the family field, along with my concept of systemic-psychodynamic transduction—the shaping effect of systemic interactions on the individual psyche.

The Christian philosopher Pierre Teilhard de Chardin wrote about the "noosphere," that is, the mental sphere encompassing all humanity.[7] In addition to the notion of the noosphere, he used the terms "great monad," "soul of the world," "super-humanity," and "soul of the collective" (Pacewicz 2010, 31). Teilhard de Chardin was a soldier during the Great War and it was then that he began to think of humanity as a unity that produces and at the same time inhabits the supraindividual mind. The idea of the noosphere formed in his mind "through prolonged contact with the huge masses of mankind that were then facing one another in the trenches of France" (Teilhard 1978, 31). This is how he wrote about it:

> The atmosphere of "the Front": it was, I am quite sure, from having plunged into that atmosphere—from having been soaked in it for months and months on end—and precisely where it was at its most dense and heavily charged, that I ceased to notice any break (if not any difference) between "physical" and "moral," between "natural" and "artificial." The "Human-million," with its psychic temperature and its internal energy, became for me a magnitude as evolutionary, and therefore as biologically, real as a giant molecule of protein. I was later to be astonished on many occasions to find in my own circle that those who could not agree with me suffered from a complete inability to understand that precisely because the individual human being represents a corpuscular magnitude he must be subject to the same development as every other species of corpuscles in the World: that means that he must coalesce into

physical relationships and groupings that belong to a higher order than his. (Teilhard 1978, 31)

People seemed to Teilhard de Chardin to merge into one superior organism, perhaps into one great spirit—since there was no difference between the physical and the moral—guided by its own will. What took possession of them was greater than themselves. This being lived and was active. Teilhard de Chardin said that he owed the gift of perceiving the "organic" nature of collective objects to the experience of war. He believed that it was a kind of another sense, which for the time being was quite rare in people, but would become more common over time.

Teilhard de Chardin's noosphere is a collective mind emerging in the course of evolution, becoming increasingly complex and personified. A certain part of human knowledge and experience aggregates and organizes itself into a kind of collective memory, which then affects the mind of the child through language, law, science, tradition, and other creations. This, of course, resembles the concept of world 3. The existence of this collective consciousness causes the mind to receive something it would be deprived of if it were left to itself.

The impression of the existence of the noosphere that Teilhard de Chardin got during the war shows that his concept was not the result of rational speculation, but of perceiving and feeling something that really exists (Pacewicz 2010, 32). This resembles Hellinger's vision of the Spirit which moves the world and in which our fates are immersed. The vision that, like that of Teilhard de Chardin, is not the result of mere reflection, but of observation of collective phenomena (representatives during a constellation).

What is the force that binds humanity together? Love, which is "the beginning and the end of all spiritual relationships" and "the more or less conscious cohesion of souls" (Teilhard 1968, 144). Love is not understood in a romantic way, its function is cosmic, which makes it similar to the love that binds systems that we know from family constellations.[8]

Universal Laws

Systemic constellations leave no doubt that beyond the individual consciousness, or even narrowly understood subconscious, there is something that affects our psychic life. We participate in nonindividual processes, independent of our life history, views, or value hierarchy. These processes seem to be universal, identical for all people. They resemble laws—they demand respect, although they are frequently violated, which is not without consequences.

For a mentality shaped by postmodernism, this may be shocking. Postmodernism dominates in the humanities—as well as in psychotherapy and social politics—and puts emphasis on subjectivism and the multiplicity of equivalent points of view. It negates the existence of "natural laws" or "atemporal principles," promoting a vision of variability of norms and values. It emphasizes man's freedom and individuality. While earlier humanities sought to discover the hidden structures that condition the observable phenomena, postmodernism questioned the very existence of such structures. It pointed out that under the surface of the phenomena there are probably no objective mechanisms, but another layer of arbitrary interpretations.

I do not reject all arguments of postmodernism. We need to deconstruct illusions and certainties. We also do this in the course of constellations, when, for instance, we expect the client to "detach" himself from his mother's words that bind him, or from his family's beliefs, and turn toward his own individuality. I am also far from epistemic objectivity that recognizes the existence of knowledge that closely corresponds to the processes of the world—I believe that any knowledge in relation to *real* processes remains a certain construction (Janus 2019, 9–13). Hellinger's discoveries, however, bring to light the incorrectness of total axiological relativism and extreme subjectivism. For it turns out that not everything can be one or the other with the same result; not everything that seems to serve us or our family, in fact, does so; my freedom does not end only where the freedom of another person begins, and in any case not when I want to remain healthy or professionally successful; it is not that for one person it is better to accept his parents and for another to reject them; nor that it is better not to know about the existence of older siblings or that one is adopted.

Underneath the interindividual and transcultural variability there is a common ground. There are laws, psychological or systemic ones, that we are all subject. They are reflected, for example, in how people react to sentences of strength. For instance, the phrase "I am only a child," uttered in a constellation, always has the same effect: a feeling of relief (because of the confirmation of one's right to one's own life, without carrying the burdens of one's ancestors), a sense of strength, and a new beginning (because of respect for the hierarchy and the possibility to derive strength from one's parents and other ancestors). There are no differences in how people respond here. There are no people who feel stronger and better when they say sentences like: "I am bigger and better," "I am not your child," "I am your equal," or "I will do it for you." When the client utters sentences of strength, there are strong positive psychophysical sensations, even if his initial attitude did not correspond to them (e.g., he exalted himself above his parents or rejected them).

So there is something in our thoughts that is independent of the subjectivity of meanings. And this seems obvious—where would the extreme diversity of thinking in individuals with such similar physiology, needs, and common evolutionary history come from? And how would we have formed communities and societies for thousands of years if each of us lived only in our own world? The philosopher and logician Gottlob Frege wrote:

> If every thought requires an owner and belongs to the contents of his consciousness, then the thought has this owner alone; and there is no science common to many on which many could work, but perhaps I have my science, a totality of thoughts whose owner I am, and another person has his. Each of us is concerned with the contents of his own consciousness. [. . .]
>
> So the result seems to be: thoughts are neither things in the external world nor ideas.
>
> A third realm must be recognized. Anything belonging to this realm has it in common with ideas that it cannot be perceived by the senses, but has it in common with things that it does not need an owner so as to belong to the contents of his consciousness. Thus for example the thought we have expressed in the Pythagorean theorem is timelessly true, true independently of whether anyone takes it to be true. (Frege 2003, 336–37)

Frege is against subjectifying everything. It is interesting that we often seem to be blind to this common reality ("third realm"). And yet it is everywhere. Sentences of strength are, in a sense, "thoughts without an owner" or we are all their unaware owners, equally, without subjective differences. The sentence "I accept you as my parents" is equally important for every person. There are no exceptions such as "Because of what you are like, I am cutting myself off from you." Uttering sentences of strength has a different status from that of ordinary statements. Sentences spoken in other situations can be the source of disputes, misunderstandings, superficial consent, or have no transformative effect. In sentences of strength and when they are spoken, the completely universal and nonindividual aspect of language, but also of our existence, manifests itself.

Polish psychiatrist Antoni Kępiński wrote:

> We tend to think that morality is a specifically human creation, that nature is not moral. We try to reduce the laws of animate nature to simple laws of inanimate nature, that is, only physical and chemical. [. . .] However, doesn't this approach narrow our understanding of animate nature, don't we lose sight of what is most important in it? Perhaps one of such important issues of animate nature is the problem of self-controlling systems, a kind of "conscience" of living beings. (Kępiński 2002, 124)[9]

Kępiński believed that nature has a kind of natural law whose imperative is to multiply the good, understood as what serves life, and to reduce entropy (disorder). Such are the systemic dynamics and their superior form—the orders of love. They may have been shaped evolutionarily. The bond is in fact the imperative to be together and to respect the other. Balancing arises from the need to be equal, that is, not to put selfish interest before the good of others and thus of the community. The hierarchy dynamics lead toward the awareness that I am next, so I owe my life to my ancestors. I owe them something, but at the same time I can only pay back my debt by giving to my children. Thus it contributes to the preservation of the species. All these processes are filled with a sense of solidarity that says that "everyone should hold together," which is an expression of the principle of equal belonging for all.

While these laws are not perfect in that they sacrifice individuals, they may have worked for the survival of the community (as, known in evolutionary biology, the law of cumulative adaptation that makes organisms more altruistic). Even such a destructive script as "You for me" can have the same evolutionary meaning. As Hellinger noted, it is usually the mother's inner voice. From an evolutionary perspective, this may be due to the prerogatives that nature has given to parents, mothers in particular. When a mother died, all her offspring died; so she began to be protected at all costs. One child can be sacrificed so that the others would survive.

Evolutionary biologist David Haig speculates that the same genes may act differently depending on whether they are inherited from the father or the mother. Mothers and fathers pursue conflicting interests through epigenetic imprinting of their germ cells. Mothers "silence" the genes that promote the growth of their offspring, while fathers turn off the genes that inhibit their offspring's development and feeding; for example, their genes intensify suckling in infants. Mothers do not want their offspring to consume too much of their own resources, so that enough is left for them and their next children (Haig 1993, 2010). Do these theses correspond to our observations that a child is often safer with his father and that more children are directed toward death because of their mother than their father?

The Presence of the Dead

Family constellations proved that we are "in relationships" not only with the people we are currently communicate with, but also with distant people, with those we do not know about, and even with the dead. When we speak of "relationships" with the dead, do we inexorably enter the territory of religion and faith? It is possible to take a standpoint between religious faith in the incorporeal existence of souls and materialism that reduces the whole issue of the dead to mere memories. This was already addressed in the nineteenth century by the founder of psychophysics, Gustav Theodor Fechner, who wrote:

> Man does not often know from whence his thoughts come to him: he is seized with a longing, a foreboding, or a joy, which he is quite unable to account for;

> he is urged to a force of activity, or a voice warns him away from it, without his being conscious of any special cause. These are the visitations of spirits, which think and act in him from another centre than his own. Their influence is even more manifest in us, when, in abnormal conditions (clairvoyance or mental disorder) the really mutual relation of dependence between them and us is determined in their favor, so that we only passively receive what flows into us from them, without return on our part. (Fechner 1905, 25–26)

Fechner claimed that the spirits of great and well-known figures are of particular significance. Plato's spirit lives in Europeans not only metaphorically—it really exists. What remains of Plato in people's minds is somehow connected, forming a self-aware being that wants to influence these minds. Fechner noted that what moves us internally may come from a "center" other than our own, namely "spirits," active "remnants" of the dead. Of these "apparitions of the dead," Fechner wrote:

> Doctors call them phantasms, hallucinations. So they are for the living, yet, at the same time, they are actual apparitions of the dead, as we call them. For though they be the weaker forms of memory in us, how should they not also be the more pronounced corresponding apparitions. Therefore, why still dispute whether they are the one or the other when they are at once both. (Fechner 1905, 98–99)

The "ghosts" we encounter during constellations are not only memories, even if we counted subconscious knowledge, cryptomnesia, as memories. We do not have the power over them that we could have over memories. This does not mean, however, that we meet a "real being." Spiritists claim that they "summon" a spirit and that this spirit can "remain" among the living after an incorrectly conducted séance, which sometimes results in many difficulties. This does not correspond at all to the observations we make during constellations. In the course of a constellation, we do not test the "spirit world," nor do we "summit" ghosts, and they do not "stay" after the session. It is only possible that a representative "does not entirely leave" the role and—if the role aroused some of his own conflicts in him—some part of the emotional experience of the represented deceased person remains in him for a while.

So one could say that during a constellation, a representative of the deceased person simply plays out his emotional states or personality traits, based on the "record" that is available in the knowing field. However, this picture reduces the experience. When, during a constellation, the client stands in front of the representative of his late mother, he primarily experiences contact with his mother, and not with the person who represents her. This is a common experience, and an average degree of openness is enough to feel it. Whether one believes in the afterlife or not, one has a strong sensation of contact with more than the person just playing the mother or father. Therefore, during constellations, one can fix one's relationship with the deceased parents, and it will be more than a work based on imagination. Looking from this angle, we actually work with the "souls" of the dead. Understanding the above requires going beyond the standard division "real spirit versus product of the psyche."

There is another unusual phenomenon, the understanding of which may also require something similar. It is the phenomenon experienced by climbers, polar explorers, and people who are in fatal danger and referred to as the third man factor. It involves a companion appearing out of nowhere, looking quite real, to provide support and guidance. Wilfrid Noyce, a member of the first successful expedition to Mount Everest, wrote:

> When we are alone or in difficulty it can appear as a personification, though dim, of what we need in order to escape our isolation or helplessness. Because of human association and past experience stored in subconscious memory, it takes the form of another person. I believe that it may indeed be another person, summoned from the deep in which, unknown to conscious mind, we are joined with those others who provided that association and that experience. [. . .] The survival situation struck a spark which in many lay unsuspected or dormant. This spark seems to me to have some essential connection with other people. (Geiger 2009, 251)

The person who appears would be both a product of our subconscious and an autonomous being (it is worth noting that it is often a deceased relative or friend). Perhaps he appears as a result of a need. On the other hand, his knowledge may surpass that of the individual. So who is he?

The existence and role of the dead can be briefly illustrated by the case of Josie who suffered from depression. She lost her son, who committed suicide, and miscarried a child in advanced pregnancy. The constellation enabled her to rid herself of the guilt she had felt because of the son, and the image of the children as siblings who "exist on a certain level" helped her to gradually overcome the trauma and the sense of omnipresent death. Some might think that the suggestion that her children "exist" is a therapeutic trick to comfort the client. However, I learned about the miscarried child myself when, during the constellation, I stood as "what caused her depression" and felt that I represented precisely an excluded child. Josie said that she had completely forgotten about him. Only during this session did she imagine his sex and gave him a name.

The experience of the presence of the deceased is common in people who lost someone dear, especially widows and widowers. Louis E. LaGrand, researcher of the phenomenon of after-death communication (ADC), writes:

> ADCs include sensing the presence of the deceased, feeling a touch, smelling a fragrance, hearing the voice or seeing the deceased, and meeting the loved one in a vision or dream. Messages are also received in symbolic ways, such as finding an object associated with the deceased, unusual appearances or behavior of birds and animals, or other unexplainable happenings which occur at or shortly after the moment of death. (Greer 2004, 73)

LaGrand notes that many such experiences resulted in an immediate change in attitude among those who mourned their dead and helped them better cope with their loss. The simplifying biomedical paradigm would refer to such phenomena as hallucinations or wishful thinking. However, their prevalence, their occurrence in people who are mentally healthy, and their positive and transformative effects contradict this view. For example, even if we acknowledge the transformative and developmental dimension of psychosis, in the case of psychotic hallucinations we will not see such consistency or their directly positive effect. LaGrand concludes that such an experience could be a natural occurrence, part of human nature not yet fully understood.

Near-death experience also involve meeting the departed loved ones, as well as gaining knowledge about the family's past. For example, someone found out that his grandfather was not his great-grandfather's son, which he later checked; another person, in a coma, met his sister who had died in her childhood, and when he asked his parents about it, they confirmed that they had lost their daughter a year before he was born (Rymuszko 2013, 121; Lommel 2010). A woman who went through a near-death experience told them:

> I saw both my dead grandmother and a man who looked at me lovingly but whom I didn't know. Over ten years later my mother confided on her deathbed that I'd been born from an extramarital affair; my biological father was a Jewish man who'd been deported and killed in World War II. My mother showed me a photograph. The unfamiliar man I'd seen more than ten years earlier during my NDE turned out to be my biological father. (Lommel 2010, 32–33)

Those who take part in constellation workshops may recall this moment—the unknown parent or the excluded grandfather is looking with affection and blessing. Most people who went through a near-death experience want to stay in the world "on the other side." In general, a voice or a loved one tells them, "Not yet." This resembles the gravity toward the deceased and death that we witness in constellations along with the feelings of the representatives of the dead that it is something wrong. Some NDEs involve seeing a person or event from a different perspective, which causes a complete change of attitude toward them. Also, almost everyone talks about the all-embracing love they felt "on the other side." In constellations, we operate at a similar level—we see love under the tissue of ordinary or difficult events, and we also uncover the other side of people who were judged long ago.

Development in the Family Field

Isn't there something mysterious about the development of children? For example, the fact that children often appear to be more "adult" than one might assume based on the range of their life experiences. Or the fact that even infants seem to differ not only in what we define as temperament, but even in personality. Where do distinct personalities come from in beings whose lives have just begun? One can reduce it to genes, but genes do not "code" behavior.

And aren't personality differences between siblings raised in the same family puzzling? Where do they come from if genetic difference does not account for them at all? And how can we explain the fact that so many children have completely different "values" and behaviors from those "instilled" in them by their parents? On the other hand, we see the opposite, great similarities and life "coincidences" in members of the same family, even across generations.

As linguist Noam Chomsky noted, a child learning a language can surprisingly early develop the ability to construct a variety of sentences, including those that he has never heard. Therefore, Chomsky assumed that the structures underlying language must be biologically determined and are genetically transmitted to children by their parents (Lyons 1976, 11). But is it really a matter of genes? Based on the knowledge that systemic constellations bring, one must argue that the mediator here is rather the morphic field that the human mind draws from.

Melanie Klein's little patients responded intensely to her interpretations of sexual themes that they could not understand because of their age. When describing psychoanalytically treated children, Klein often says, for instance, "a curiously unchildlike nature" (Klein 1975a, 35), "her behaviour and movements were those of a very sensual girl in her puberty" (Klein 1975a, 53), "boy, who behaved in many respects like an adult obsessional" (Klein 1975a, 66), "the un-childlike, strained expression of his face" (Klein 1975a, 67–68). Although Klein understands it as the effect of drives and defenses, it may be the intrusion of heteropsychic material into the child's psyche. In other words, Klein's patients experienced in their childlike minds the affairs of adults belonging to their family system. The author says that "the child's fear of being devoured, or cut up, or torn to pieces, or its terror of being surrounded and pursued by menacing figures, as a regular component of its mental life" (Klein 1975, 249). The psychoanalyst sees it as fantasies, developed on the basis of the drive life and bodily sensations. Perhaps, however, is it actually fears related to real events? Based on what would small children create an image of "tearing to pieces," if not some real tearing? These children's fears may involve abortions or lost twins (being attacked by "menacing figures") or dramatic events in the family history.

We tend to attribute child development, to hereditary influences, to parental influence. However, the assumption regarding the strength of parental influence, as demonstrated by Harris, is highly questionable. For example, when siblings are separated and raised in different families, their mutual psychological similarity does not decrease or remain constant but may increase (Harris 1998, 36). How can we explain this fact which is completely contrary to the traditional understanding of development? It seems that this can only be answered by a theory that takes into account the participation of siblings in their family field. Siblings separated from the family want to share their fate even more strongly. Without knowing their family on a conscious level, they cling to it on an unconscious level, which shapes character and behavior most strongly. This reduces the degree of their inner freedom and thus makes them more alike.

There are individuals whose development remains particularly puzzling for us, for example, psychopaths. Although in some cases we are able to find events in those people's biographies that could explain their behavior, in other cases, we are not (besides, the factors found can only be an apparent explanation). Psychopaths never feel guilty and are motivated solely by self-interest (Stout 2005). How is it that people who are sometimes raised in normal families can be so different from the average person? Why do we not see their conscience working? Guilt or compassion is sometimes blocked also in people who are not psychopaths, for example, when they experience great traumas or losses, during war, in acts of revenge. Could the psychic structure in psychopaths result from reactions to similar events? If we consider the existence of the family field, the answer is "Yes." The future psychopath, even if he did not experience anything dramatic in his life, may have experienced this in his inner life. This in turn caused a specific reaction in him—it "turned off" his conscience. Perhaps the primal conscience toward the loved ones was blocked first. It is possible that the development of conscience begins with feelings toward parents, siblings, and grandparents. From here it spreads to the closest group of people and then to all people.

Consider the mass of unsettled issues, excluded people, pain, traumas, separation, and incomplete mourning. And try to imagine the great openness of the child's psyche. It is as a result of the combination of these two factors that so many children suffer from various problems: ADHD, lack of concentration, anxieties, nightmares, aggressive behavior, depression, psychosomatic disorders. Very often those who behave worst and, for instance, take drugs, are expelled from schools, get into conflicts with the law—take the most on themselves, are guided by the greatest love. Does the environment see it? Such a child is perceived as selfish, demanding, and ungrateful. Well, led by the unconscious bond and need to balance, he will become like that.

Extraconsciousness and Systemic-Psychodynamic Transduction

By analogy with the concepts of subconsciousness, unconsciousness, or superconsciousness, I introduce the term extraconsciousness, with which I describe certain aspects of the manifestation of the knowing field or the "soul" or "conscience" of the family. One can say that the extraconsciousness is part of the self to an even lesser extent than the unconscious. While we understand the unconscious as a kind of record in the individual's mind, the extraconsciousness goes beyond the individual mind.

Of course, there is the concept of the collective unconscious, which also seems to be beyond the individuum. Therefore, the collective unconscious is a much less unambiguous and verifiable concept. The collective unconscious described by Jung emerges from the interpretation of dreams, patients' statements, as well as myths and religious ideas. Therefore, it is relatively easy to negate its existence—by simply reinterpreting the collected material. It is different with the extraconsciousness. We observe something that cannot be encapsulated in the known concepts. First, representatives who do not know the client at all discover verifiable facts about his life. Second, representatives who are completely unfamiliar with constellations begin to follow the orders of love that emerge spontaneously. Third, the client usually experiences a constellation strongly on an "energetic" and "informational" level (he begins to experience tingling, choking, numbness in the hands, pressure in the head, and other bodily sensations, often clearly related to certain persons or events in the family). Fourth and finally, the constellation generally has a powerfully transformative impact on the client's life. These four cardinal points indicate that we have here a process that, first, transcends the individual (the movement of the representatives and the supraindividual laws—the orders of love) and, second, closely relates to the individual (the client's feelings, the therapeutic change). The vehicle of this process is what I name man's extraconsciousness.

I speak of the "extra-consciousness" to emphasize that this structure is separate from the consciousness, and at the same time to indicate that it interacts with man's ego. It is both part of the mind and something outside the person. It is something intermediate between one's "personality" and the "external environment."

Thus, developmental theories that focus on the mother as the child's early "environment," on parental influence, on the role of peers, on the development of the child's social responses only touch the surface of the matter. The range of active developmental factors turns out to be much richer. The child's mind participates in the field of the family, at some level "contacting" the psychic activity of its other members. This area also includes the deceased, and the rudimentary aspects of their psyche—the memory of the field—are available to the child. All of this is the extraconsciousness.

Conclusions from systemic constellations enable to formulate a new vision of the psychological development process. In the book *Systemic Constellations: Theory, Practice, and Applications* (Janus 2021), I presented the hypothesis of systemic-psychodynamic transduction. It is a process in which "stimuli" received unconsciously from the family field become one of the key factors shaping one's personality, and causing mental disorders. This concept radically changes the understanding of the developmental "environment." The "environment" has turned out to be a much richer area, containing previously unknown factors. At the same time—as evidenced during constellations—many factors that are commonly believed to determine one's mental state are not essential.

In the light of the transduction hypothesis, it becomes clear why so many human behaviors, tendencies, or disorders seem to be completely "causeless," or why their alleged causes are questionable. The factors that are expected to have a fundamental impact on the child in the process of upbringing, that are so often taken into account by traditional therapists and psychologists, turn out to be either marginal or completely irrelevant. Despite the fact that some of them appear to be undeniable devastators of mental life, for example, alcoholism of a parent, divorce, or dramatic quarrels. All of these are unpleasant for the child, they affect the child's emotional state, and in part, his attitude toward certain issues or people in adulthood. However, they are not the ones that underlie the deepest structures of his personality, and they are not the ones that cause someone to fail completely, to be full of resentment, to feel a deep aversion to having children, to be sick, or to display suicidal tendencies.

The real causes of our bad mood, life choices, and attitudes are hidden from the consciousness. We build our explanations based on a very narrow set of data. We often see the actions of parents as the cause of our condition, and we remain blind to the influence of other members of the system, our siblings, parents' former partners, grandparents. We overestimate not only the power of our parents but also the power of external behavior in general, underestimating the impact of mental states.

Such explanations, although erroneous, may seem to be correct. This can be illustrated by the example of a client who felt unloved and unnoticed by her mother, which made her full of resentment. The constellation showed, which the client was unaware of, that her mother felt rejected by her mother as a child, or actually felt that her existence was in danger. Based on the course of the constellation, one could guess that she was threatened with an abortion. The real, or in any case fundamental, source of the overwhelming sadness and sense of abandonment in the client was not the mother's behavior, but the mother's deeply hidden anxiety, which the client shared with her since childhood. Her explanation was also not unfounded, as the client's mother, feeling she was an unwanted child and not having a good internal relationship with her own mother, was unable to show her full affection. However, it did not actually explain the intensity of her negative sentiments.

Much of what the family field is responsible for is nowadays interpreted as gene impact. The "power of genes" is demonstrated, for example, by the observations of monozygotic twins who, despite being separated and brought up in different homes, show astonishing similarities, in the form of shared interests, identical lifestyles, and even the same courses of life. Harris states that the histories of twins raised separately suggest that "genes can control behavior in subtle, intricate ways that cannot be explained in terms of our current understanding of genetic mechanisms and brain neurophysiology" (Harris 1998, 33). Contemporary knowledge cannot explain these phenomena, as it assumes that the only possible effect is transmission through physical genes. It does not take into account the fact that the family field affects the child from the beginning.

The question "Genes or nurture?" is becoming out of date (partly due to the research on epigenetics that has shown that the environment can affect the expression of genes). Children are as they are not only due to their genotype, the influence of their parents, and their environment, but also due to the influence of the bond and loyalty within the family and the affairs of their ancestors. The family system may also include unrelated people, which genetics obviously does not take into consideration. In the course of constellations, we see how strongly the child may be affected, for example, by his father's ex-wife, who he has never met, and whose existence he may not even have known about.

Changes in behavior, preferences, and identity problems observed in people after organ transplantations confirm that the field modifies the psyche. This was the case with Claire Sylvia, who dreamed the name of the unknown donor after the heart transplantation, and her behavior and habits changed (Sylvia and Novak 1997). Michael Hagan, who had a liver transplant, reports similar phenomena (Lego 2015). In cases of transplantation, there is often a sense of gratitude to the donor's family and a sense of guilt for his death., The recipients imagine and think about the donor, they can feel the need to contact his family and actively integrate "the real or imagined personality of the donor into their post-transplant identity" (Mauthner et al. 2014). Usually in such situations, if one does not try to reduce everything to "incorporation fantasies," the term "cellular memory" is used. The concept of cellular memory results from attempts to reconcile these unusual phenomena with the materialistic viewpoint. However, it does not seem possible that an organ can be a carrier of a complex form of memory (with which, in addition, the recipient's brain is connected). The organ is rather a kind of antenna that receives information from the field. The donation of the organ is such a strong connection between the donor and the recipient that the latter is affected by the donor's information field. This, probably together with a subconscious sense of gratitude, leads to new eating preferences or behaviors, "someone else's" memories, and other changes in the psyche. These changes are perhaps more frequent than expected, as most recipients do not want to reflect on and discuss this topic at all (Bunzel and others 1992).

NOTES

1. Recently, other avenues for studying this type of attitudes have emerged—Big Data and search engine analysis (Stephens-Davidowitz 2017). These analyses confirm that many previous studies of psychology and sociology led to erroneous conclusions (for example, about racism or sexual behavior, about which the respondents have not spoken frankly).
2. As Pope Paul VI put it: "We believe in the communion of all the faithful of Christ, those who are pilgrims on earth, the dead who are being purified, and the blessed in heaven, all together forming one Church" (Catechism of the Catholic Church 1994, 250).
3. In the double-slit experiment—sometimes referred to as the most beautiful experiment of physics or the most important experiment of quantum mechanics—particles (photons, electrons) pass through a screen with two very small slits. This experiment shows strange quantum phenomena, such as interference of a particle with itself, dependence of the result on the act of observation. The phenomena shown by this experiment cannot be fully explained.
4. Eccles used the concept of Popper's three worlds in his theories of the self.
5. Popper would perhaps oppose linking his concept to such theories as the Akashic records, the noosphere or the information field. However, when we take the category of family resemblance, the parallels are obvious. Nevertheless, Popper criticized holism or determinism, for example, claiming that many apparent systems are nothing more than a group of chaotic and randomly moving elements. He advocated the "open

society" and argued against historicism. In other words, he negated the existence of overriding laws concerning human societies. One could say that his world 3 has a zero degree of personification—it is far from being a kind of autonomous "intelligence."

6. Neither in this, nor in the rest of his major concepts, is Popper precise. He wants to discuss "states" (physical, mental), not, like Descartes—"substances," and yet he distinguishes three separate worlds (physical, mental, and the world of theory and language), and thus beings completely different from one other. But states are states of something, they have a common basis. The common basis, however, would be monism, and Popper describes himself as a pluralist. Although he identifies three worlds and claims that world 3 is real, other times—when he is forced to do so by the course of the discussion—he says that world 3 should not be taken too literally.

7. The notion of "noosphere" was introduced by Russian chemist and geologist Vladimir Vernadsky, who used it to describe the collective activity of thinking beings, humans, which transforms the geological environment of the planet (Ryszkiewicz 1994, 340 et seq.).

8. Both Popper and Teilhard de Chardin seem inconsistent in presenting their basic concepts. Sometimes the third world appears to be a truly third and different being, and other times it looks almost like just a new term for materially existing books or other products of the mind. The noosphere (although it remains unusual anyway) is sometimes the superconsciousness that connects people on some ethereal level, and other times it is explained as a result of purely technical connections (telephone, radio, and now probably Internet ones). I think that this is mainly due to the fact that both thinkers tried to stay on the rational level of the discourse. Their observation, reflection, and intuition led them toward exotic supraindividual beings, but they tried to remain on the level of commonly known phenomena.

9. Antoni Kępiński (1918–1972)—psychiatrist, founder of the notion of information metabolism (constant exchange of information between the body and the environment), precursor of humanistic psychiatry in Poland and author of phenomenological analyses of mental disorders (schizophrenia, depression, psychopathy, etc.).

Bibliography

Abraham, Nicolas, and Maria Torok. 1994. *The Shell and the Kernel: Renewals of Psychoanalysis*. Chicago: The University of Chicago Press.

Ameln, Falko von, and Jochen Becker-Ebel. 2020. *Fundamentals of Psychodrama*. Singapore: Springer.

Atmanspacher, Harald, Hartmann Römer, and Harald Walach, 2001. *Weak Quantum Theory: Complementarity and Entanglement in Physics and Beyond*. Freiburg. arXiv:quant-ph/0104109v2.

Augsburger, David. 1981. *Caring Enough to Forgive: True Forgiveness*. Ventura, CA: Regal Books.

Awdish, Rana. 2017. *In Shock: My Journey from Death to Recovery and the Redemptive Power of Hope*. New York: Picador, St. Martin's Press.

Baal, Jan van. 1976. "Offering, Sacrifice and Gift." *Numen* 23(3): 161–78.

Baggott, Jim. 2011. *The Quantum Story: A History in 40 Moments*. New York: Oxford University Press.

Baghramian, Arvick. 2015. *The Magic of Shamanism: The Healing Power of the Shamanic Journey*. Barcelona: Guid Publications.

Bandler, Richard, John Grinder, and Virginia Satir. 1976. *Changing With Families: A Book About Further Education for Being Human*. Palo Alto, CA: Science and Behavior Books.

Baranger, Madeleine, and Willy Baranger. 2009. *The Work of Confluence: Listening and Interpreting in the Psychoanalytic Field*. London: Karnac Books.

Barnard, Alan, and Jonathan Spencer (eds.). 2002. *Encyclopedia of Social and Cultural Anthropology*. London and New York: Routledge.

Barrows, Paul. 2008. "Locating the Ghost in the Nursery: The Importance of the Parental Couple." In *What Can the Matter Be?: Therapeutic Interventions with Parents, Infants and Young Children*, edited by Louise Emanuel and Elizabeth Bradley, 171–86. London: Karnac Books.

Bavister, Steve, and Amanda Vickers. 2010. *NLP w praktyce, czyli sztuka kształtowania przyszłości*. Warszawa: Wydawnictwo Edgard.

Bell, John Elderkin. 1975. *Family Therapy*. New York, London: Jason Aronson, Inc.

Bertalanffy, Ludwig von. 2015. *General System Theory: Foundations, Development, Applications*. New York: George Baziller.

Bielańska, Anna. 2009. *Psychodrama. Elementy teorii i praktyki*. Warszawa: ENETEIA.

Biklen, Douglas. 1993. *Communication Unbound: How Facilitated Communication Is Challenging Traditional Views of Autism and Ability/Disability*. New York and London: Teachers College Press.

Bloch, Donald, and Robert Simon. 1982. *The Strength of Family Therapy: Selected Papers of Nathan W. Ackerman*. New York: Brunner/Mazel Publishers.

Blok, Aleksandr. 1974. *Dzienniki 1901–1921*, translated by Maria Leśniewska. Kraków: Wydawnictwo Literackie.

Bloom, Paul. 2013. *Just Babies: The Origins of Good and Evil*. New York: Crown Publishers.

———. 2016. *Against Empathy: The Case for Rational Compassion*. New York: Ecco.

Bohm, David. 1987. *Wholeness and the Implicate Order*. London and New York: ARK Paperbacks.

Bowen, Murray. 2004. *Family Therapy in Clinical Practice*. Lanham, MD: Rowan & Littlefield Publishers.

Boszormenyi-Nagy, Ivan, and Barbara R. Krasner. 1986. *Between Give and Take: A Clinical Guide to Contextual Therapy*. New York: Brunner/Mazel Publishers.

Boszormenyi-Nagy, Ivan, and Geraldine M. Spark. 1984. *Invisible Loyalties: Reciprocity in Intergenerational Family Therapy*. New York: Brunner/Mazel Publishers.

Botkin, Allan, and Craig Hogan. 2014. *Induced After-death Communication: A New Therapy for Healing Grief and Trauma*. Charlottesville, VA: Hampton Roads Publishing.

Braden, Gregg. 2009. *The Divine Matrix: Bridging Time, Space, Miracles, and Belief*. Carlsbad, CA: Hay House.

Brenman, Eric. 2006. *Recovery Of The Lost Good Object*, edited by Gigliola Fornari Spoto. New York and London: Routledge.

Britton, Ronald. 1989. "The Missing Link: Parental Sexuality in the Oedipus Complex." In *The Oedipus Complex Today: Clinical Implications*, edited by J. Steiner, 83–101. London: Karnac Books.

———. 2018. *Sex, Death, and the Superego: Experiences in Psychoanalysis*. New York: Routledge.

Brockman, John (ed.) 2007. *What Is Your Dangerous Idea?: Today's Leading Thinkers on the Unthinkable*. New York, London, Toronto, and Sydney: Harper Perennial.

Brottman, Mikita. 2011. *Phantoms of the Clinic: From Thought-Transference to Projective Identification*. London: Karnac Books. Kindle.

Brune, François. 2011. *Umarli są z nami*. Konstancin-Jeziorna: Wydawnictwo MEDIUM.

Burkert, Walter. 1983. *Homo Necans: The Anthropology of Ancient Greek Sacrificial Ritual and Myth*, translated by Peter Bing. Berkeley, Los Angeles, and London: University of California Press.

Buss, David M. 2005. *The Murderer Next Door: Why the Mind Is Designed to Kill*. New York: Penguin Books.

———. 2016. *Evolutionary Psychology: The New Science of the Mind*. Abingdon and New York: Routledge.

Bychowski, Gustav, and J. Louise Despert (eds.). 1952. *Specialized Techniques in Psychotherapy*. New York: Grove Press.

Calaprice, Alice. 2000. *The Expanded Quotable Einstein*. Princeton and Oxford: Princeton University Press.

Canetti, Elias. 1984. *Crowds and Power*, translated by Carol Stewart. New York: Ferrar, Straus and Giroux.

Cardeña, E. 2018. "The Experimental Evidence for Parapsychological Phenomena: A Review." *American Psychologist* 73(5): 663–77.

Cassirer, Ernst. 1964. *An Essay on Man: An Introduction to a Philosophy of Human Culture*. New Haven, CT: Yale University Press.

Catechism of the Catholic Church. 1994. San Francisco, CA: Ignatius Press.

Chardin, Pierre Teilhard de. 1968. *The Divine Milieu*. New York: Harper& Row.

———. 1978. *Heart of Matter*, translated by René Hague. San Diego: Harcourt Brace & Company.

Chazan, Bogdan, and Witold Simon (eds.). 2009. *Aborcja. Przyczyny, następstwa, terapia*. Wrocław: Wydawnictwo Wektory.

Coles, Prophecy. 2011. *The Uninvited Guest from the Unremembered Past: An Exploration of the Unconscious Transmission of Trauma Across the Generations*. London: Karnac Books.

Cornford, F.M. 2004. *From Religion to Philosophy: A Study in the Origins of Western Speculation*. Mineola, NY: Dover Publications.

Czapów, Gabriela, and Czesław Czapów. 1969. *Psychodrama. Geneza i historia. Teoria i praktyka. Próba oceny*. Warszawa: Państwowe Wydawnictwo Naukowe.

Damasio, Antonio R. 2006. *Descartes' Error: Emotion, Reason, and the Human Brain*. London: Vintage Books.

Davies, Paul. 2004. *The Cosmic Blueprint: New Discoveries in Nature's Creative Ability to Order the Universe*. West Conshohocken, PA: Templeton Foundation Press.

Dawkins, Richard. 2008. *The God Delusion*. Boston and New York: Houghton Mifflin Harcourt.

Dayton, Tian. 1994. *The Drama Within. Psychodrama and Experiential Therapy*. Deerfield Beach, FL: Health Communications.

DeGrandis, Robert, and Linda Schubert. 1989. *Intergenerational Healing: An Intimate Journey Into Forgiveness*. Praising God Catholic Association.

De Masi, Franco. 2018. *Vulnerability to Psychosis: A Psychoanalytic Study of the Nature and Therapy of the Psychotic State*, translated by Philip Slotkin. New York: Routledge.

Dobosz, Artur. 2013. *Myślenie magiczno-mityczne a schizofrenia*. Bydgoszcz: Oficyna Wydawnicza Epigram.

Dolto, Françoise. 2002. *Zrozumieć dziecko. Rozmowy o wychowaniu*, translated by Dorota Ben-Ghorbal and Ewa Pawlikowska. Warszawa: Jacek Santorski & Co.

Dossey, Larry. 1994. *Healing Words: The Power of Prayer and The Practice of Medicine*. New York: HarperSanFrancisco.

———. 1997. *Prayer Is Good Medicine: How to Reap the Healing Benefits of Prayer*. New York: HarperSanFrancisco.

———. 1999. *Reinventing Medicine: Beyond Mind-Body to a New Era of Healing*. New York: HarperCollins Publishers.

———. 2013. *One Mind: How Our Individual Mind Is Part of a Greater Consciousness and Why It Matters*. New York: Hay House.

Dubrov, A. P., and V. N. Pushkin. 1989. *Parapsychologia i współczesne przyrodoznawstwo*. Warszawa: Krajowa Agencja Wydawnicza.

Duhl, Frederick J., David Kantor, and Bunny S. Duhl. 1973. "Learning, Space, and Action in Family Therapy: A Primer of Sculpture." In *Techniques of Family Psychotherapy: A Primer*, edited by Donald A. Bloch, 47–63. New York and London: Grune and Stratton.

Dupreé, Ulrich Emil. 2012. *Ho'oponopono: The Hawaiian Forgiveness Ritual as the Key to Your Life's Fulfillment*, translated by Tony Mitton. Forres: Earthdancer/Findhorn Press.

Durkheim, Émile. 1973. *Emile Durkheim* on *Morality and Society*, edited by Robert N. Bellah. Chicago and London: The University of Chicago Press.

Eccles, John C. 1977. *The Understanding of the Brain*. New York: McGraw-Hill Book Company.

Einstein, Albert, and Leopold Infeld. 1978. *The Evolution of Physics: The Growth of Ideas from Early Concepts to Relativity and Quanta*. Cambridge, London, and Melbourne: Cambridge University Press.

Eisenberger, Naomi I., Matthew D. Lieberman, and Kipling D. Williams. 2003. "Does Rejection Hurt? An fMRI Study of Social Exclusion." *Science* 302: 290–92.

Eisenbud, Jule. 1970. *Psi and Psychoanalysis: Studies in the Psychoanalysis of Psi-conditioned Behavior*. New York and London: Grune & Stratton.

Emmons, Robert A. 2016. *The Little Book of Gratitude: Create a Life of Happiness and Wellbeing by Giving Thanks*. London: Gaia Books.

Epstein, Catherine. 2010. *Model Nazi: Arthur Greiser and the Occupation of Western Poland*. Oxford: Oxford University Press.

Eskola, Antti, Anna Kihlström, David Kivinen, Klaus Weckroth, and Oili-Helena Ylijoki. 1988. *Blind Alleys in Social Psychology: A Search for Ways Out*. Amsterdam, New York, Oxford, and Tokyo: Elsevier Science Publishers.

Evans-Pritchard, E. E. 1956. *Nuer Religion*. Oxford: Oxford University Press.

———. 1965. *Theories of Primitive Religion*. Oxford: Oxford University Press.

Fechner, Gustav Theodor. 1905. *The Little Book of Life After Death*, translated by Mary C. Wadsworth. Boston, MA: Little, Brown, & Company.

Feuillet, Lionel, Henry Dufour, and Jean Pelletier. 2007. "Brain of a White-Collar Worker." *Lancet* 370: 262.

Fields, Leslie Leyland, and Jill Hubbard. 2014. *Forgiving Our Fathers and Mothers: Finding Freedom from Hurt and Hate*. Nashville, TN: W Publishing.

Fink, Bruce. 1997. *A Clinical Introduction to Lacanian Psychoanalysis: Theory and Technique*. Cambridge, MA and London: Harvard University Press.

Fiore, Edith. 2006. *The Unquiet Dead: A Psychologist Treats Spirit Possession*. New York: Ballantine Books.

Fleck, Ludwik. 1979. *Genesis and Development of a Scientific Fact*, translated by Fred Bradley and Thaddeus J. Trenn, edited by Thaddeus J. Trenn and Robert K. Merton. Chicago: The University of Chicago Press.

Foà, Benedetta. 2015. *Imię cierpienia. Żałoba po aborcji dziecka*. Poznań: Wydawnictwo W drodze.

Foor, Daniel. 2017. *Ancestral Medicine: Rituals for Personal and Family Healing*. Rochester: Bear & Company.

Forward, Susan, and Craig Buck. 2002. *Toxic Parents: Overcoming Their Hurtful Legacy and Reclaiming Your Life*. New York, Toronto, London, Sydney, and Auckland: Bantam Books.

Forward, Susan, and Donna Frazier Glynn. 2013. *Mothers Who Can't Love: A Healing Guide for Daughters*. New York: HarperCollins.

Fraiberg, Selma. 1987. *Selected Writings of Selma Fraiberg*, edited by Louis Fraiberg. Columbus, OH: Ohio State University Press.

Framo, James L. 1992. *Family-of-Origin Therapy: An Intergenerational Approach*. New York: Brunner/Mazel Publishers.

Frazer, James. 1996. *The Golden Bough: A Study in Magic and Religion*. London: Penguin Books.

Frege, Gottlob. 2003. "Thought." In *The Frege Reader*, edited by Michael Beaney. Oxford: Blackwell Publishing, 325–45.

Freud, Sigmund. 1946. *Totem and Taboo: Resemblances Between the Psychic Lives of Savages and Neurotics*, translated by A. A. Brill. New York: Vintage Books.

———. 1957. *A General Selection from The Works of Sigmund Freud*, edited by John Rickman. New York: Doubleday Anchor.

———. 1964. *The Sexual Enlightenment of Children*, edited by Philip Rieff. New York: Collier Books.

———. 1975. *Group Psychology and the Analysis of the Ego*, translated by James Strachey. New York: W. W. Norton & Company.

———. 1989. *Leonardo da Vinci and a Memory of His Childhood*, translated by Alan Tyson, edited by James Strachey. New York and London: W. W. Norton & Company.

———. 1989a. *The Future of an Illusion*, translated and edited by James Strachey. New York: W. W. Norton & Company.

———. 1989b. *The Ego and the Id*, translated by Joan Riviere and edited by James Strachey. New York and London: W. W. Norton & Company.

———. 1989c. *Civilization and Its Discontents*, translated and edited by James Strachey. New York: W. W. Norton & Company.

———. 1990. *New Introductory Lectures on Psycho-Analysis*, translated by James Strachey. New York: W. W. Norton & Company.

———. 2001. "Recommendations to Physicians Practising Psycho-Analysis." In *The Standard Edition of the Complete Psychological Works of Sigmund Freud*, translated and edited by James Strachey, vol. 12, 109–20. London: Vintage.

———. 2001a. "The Unconscious." In *The Standard Edition of the Complete Psychological Works of Sigmund Freud*, translated and edited by James Strachey, vol. 14, 159–216. London: Vintage.

———. 2001b. "Economic Problem of Masochism." In *The Standard Edition of the Complete Psychological Works of Sigmund Freud*, translated and edited by James Strachey, vol. 19, 159–70. London: Vintage.

———. 2007. *Psychologia nieświadomości*, translated by Robert Reszke. Warszawa: Wydawnictwo KR.

Fritz, Stephen G. 1997. *Frontsoldaten: The German Soldier in World War II.* Lexington, KY: The University Press of Kentucky.

Geiger, John. 2009. *The Third Man Factor: Surviving the Impossible.* New York: Weinstein Books.

Gendlin, Eugene T. 2003. *Focusing*. London: Rider.

Gennep, Arnold van. 1960. *The Rites of Passage*, translated by Monika B. Vizedom and Gabrielle L. Caffee. Chicago: The University of Chicago Press.

Gies, Erica. 2017. "The Meaning of Lichen: How a Self-taught Naturalist Unearthed Hidden Symbioses in the Wilds of British Columbia—and Helped to Overturn 150 Years of Accepted Scientific Wisdom." *Scientific American* 316(6): 52–59.

Girard, René. 1977. *Violence and the Sacred*, translated by Patrick Gregory. Baltimore, MD, London: Johns Hopkins University Press.

———. 1987. "Generative Scapegoating." In *Violent Origins: On Ritual Killing and Cultural Formation*, edited by Robert G. Hamerton-Kelly, 73–145. Stanford, CA: Stanford University Press.

———. 1987a. *Job, the Victim of His People*, translated by Yvonne Freccero. Stanford, CA: Stanford University Press.

———. 2001. *I See Satan Fall Like Lightning*, translated by James G. Williams. Maryknoll, NY: Orbis Books.

Goldenberg, Herbert, and Irene Goldenberg. 2008. *Family Therapy: An Overview.* Belmont, CA: Thomson Brooks/Cole.

Górniak, Lech, and Barbara Józefik (eds.). 2003. *Ewolucja myślenia systemowego w terapii rodzin. Od metafory cybernetycznej do dialogu i narracji.* Kraków: Wydawnictwo Uniwersytetu Jagiellońskiego.

Graeber, David. 2018. *Bullshit Jobs: A Theory.* New York: Simon & Schuster.

Green, André, and Gregorio Kohon. 2005. *Love and its Vicissitudes.* London, New York: Routledge.

Greer, Jane. 2004. *The Afterlife Connection: A Therapist Reveals How to Communicate with Departed Loved Ones.* New York: St. Martin's Press.

Grinberg, Leon, Dario Sor, and Elizabeth Tabak de Bianchedi. 1977. *Introduction to the Work of Bion: Groups, Knowledge, Psychosis, Thought, Transformations, Psychoanalytic Practice*, translated by Alberto Hahn. New York: Jason Aronson.

Grof, Stanislav. 1988. *The Adventure of Self-Discovery: Dimensions of Consciousness and New Perspectives in Psychotherapy and Inner Exploration.* New York: State University of New York Press.

———. 2006. *When the Impossible Happens: Adventures in Non-Ordinary Realities*. Boulder CO: Sounds True.

Grotowski, Jerzy. 2002. *Towards a Poor Theatre*, edited by Eugenio Barba. New York: Routledge.

Guzowski, Krzysztof (ed.). 2015. *Obciążenia pokoleniowe – uzdrowienie*. Warszawa: Wydawnictwo Monumen.

Haig, David. 1993. "Genetic Conflicts in Human Pregnancy." *The Quarterly Review of Biology* 68(4): 495–532.

———. 2010. "Transfers and Transitions: Parent–Offspring Conflict, Genomic Imprinting, and the Evolution of Human Life History." *PNAS* 107(suppl. 1): 1731–35.

Hall, Calvin S., and Gardner Lindzey. 1978. *Theories of Personality*. New York, Chichester, Brisbane, Toronto, and Singapore: John Wiley & Sons.

Halpern, Paul. 2015. *Einstein's Dice and Schrödinger's Cat How Two Great Minds Battled Quantum Randomness to Create a Unified Theory of Physics*. New York: Basic Books.

Harris, Adrienne, Margery Kalb, and Susan Klebanoff (eds.). 2016. *Ghosts in the Consulting Room: Echoes of Trauma in Psychoanalysis*. London and New York: Routledge.

———. 2017. *Demons in the Consulting Room: Echoes of Genocide, Slavery, and Extreme Trauma in Psychoanalytic Practice*. London and New York: Routledge.

Harris, Judith Rich. 1995. "Where Is the Child's Environment? A Group Socialization Theory of Development." *Psychological Review* 102(3): 458–89.

———. 1998. *The Nurture Assumption: Why Children Turn Out the Way They Do*. New York: The Free Press.

———. 2007. *No Two Alike: Human Nature and Human Individuality*. New York and London: W. W. Norton & Company.

Harrison, Elizabeth G. 2008. "I Can Only Move My Feet towards mizuko kuyō: Memorial Services for Dead Children in Japan." In *Magic, Witchcraft, and Religion: An Anthropological Study of the Supernatural*, edited by Pamela A. Moro, James E. Myers, and Arthur C. Lehmann. New York: McGraw-Hill.

Healy, Mary. 2015. *Healing: Bringing the Gift of God's Mercy to the World*. Huntington, IN: Our Sunday Visitor.

Heimann, Paula. 1989. *About Children and Children-No-Longer: Collected Papers 1942–80*, edited by Margaret Tonnesmann. London and New York: Routledge.

Heinze, Ruth-Inge. 1999. "Multiplicity in Cross-Cultural Perspective." In *The Plural Self: Multiplicity in Everyday Life*, edited by John Rowan and Mick Cooper, 151–67. London, Thousand Oaks, CA, and New Delhi: SAGE Publications.

Hellinger, Bert. 2001. *Love's Own Truths: Bonding and Balancing in Close Relationships*, translated by Maureen Oberli-Turner and Hunter Beaumont. Phoenix: Zeig, Tucker & Theisen.

———. 2003. *To the Heart of the Matter: Brief Therapies*, translated by Colleen Beaumont. Heidelberg: Carl-Auer-Systeme Verlag.

———. 2006. *Sumienie miał czyste. Wykłady i opowieści*. Warszawa: Wydawnictwo Jacek Santorski & Co.

———. 2008. *Die Liebe des Geistes: Was zu ihr führt und wie sie gelingt*. Bischofswiesen: Hellinger Publications.

———. 2011. *Laws of Healing: Getting Well, Staying Well*, translated by Angelika Schenk and edited by Suzi Tucker. Bischofswiesen: Hellinger Publications.

———. 2013. *The Churches and their God*, translated by Angelika Schenk. Bischofswiesen: Hellinger Publications.

———. 2014. *Neue Geschichten: Eins*. Bischofswiesen: Hellinger Publications.

———. 2014a. *Neue Geschichten: Zwei*. Bischofswiesen: Hellinger Publications.

———. 2014b. *Neue Geschichten: Drei*. Bischofswiesen: Hellinger Publications.

———. 2014c. *Nowa świadomość. Duchowy wymiar ustawień rodzin*, translated by Katarzyna Preiss-Jastrzębska. Warszawa: Wydawnictwo Czarna Owca.

Hellinger, Bert, and Andrzej Nehrebecki. 2012. *Miłość zaklęta w chorobie*. Kraków: Wydawnictwo Pocieszka.

Hellinger, Bert, and Gabriele ten Hövel. 2007. *Anerkennen was ist: Gespräche über Verstrickung und Lösung*. München: Wilhelm Goldmann Verlag.

Hellinger, Bert, Gunthard Weber, and Hunter Beaumont. 1989. *Love's Hidden Symmetry: What Makes Love Work in Relationships*. Phoenix, AZ: Zeig, Tucker & Theisen.

Hellinger, Bert, and Hanne-Lore Heilmann. 2018. *Mein Leben. Mein Werk*. München: Ariston Verlag.

Hickok, Gregory. 2014. *The Myth of Mirror Neurons: The Real Neuroscience of Communication and Cognition*. New York: W. W. Norton & Company.

Holy Bible: American Standard Version – New & Old Testament. 2018. Kindle.

Horney, Karen. 1991. *Final Lectures*, edited by Douglas H. Ingram. New York, London: W. W. Norton & Company.

Houston, Gaie. 2003. *Brief Gestalt Therapy*. London, Thousand Oaks, CA, and New Delhi: SAGE Publications.

Howick, Jeremy. 2018. *Doktor Ty. O wewnętrznej sile organizmu i zdolności do samouzdrawiania*, translated by Aleksandra Żak. Kraków: Wydawnictwo Otwarte.

Hulme, Thomas Ernest. 2003. *Selected Writings*, edited by Patrick McGuinness. New York: Routledge.

Jackowski, Krzysztof, and Krzysztof Janoszka. 2018. *Jasnowidz na policyjnym etacie*. Kraków: Wydawnictwo SQN.

Janus, Damian. 2019. *Psychopathology and Religion: Structural Convergences between Mental Disorders and Religion*, translated by Barbara Gąstoł. Lanham, Boulder, CO, New York, and London: Lexington Books.

———. 2021. *Systemic Constellations: Theory, Practice, and Applications*, translated by Barbara Gąstoł. Lanham, Boulder, CO, New York, and London: Lexington Books.

John Paul II. 1984. "Apostolic Letter Salvifici Doloris." Accessed June 29, 2021. https://www.vatican.va/content/john-paul-ii/en/apost_letters/1984/documents/hf_jp-ii_apl_11021984_salvifici-doloris.html.

Jung, Carl Gustav. 1960. *Answer to Job*, translated by R. F. C. Hull. New York: Meridian Books.

———. 1978. *The Collected Works of C. G. Jung: Volume 10: Civilization in Transition*, translated by R. F. C. Hull. Princeton, NJ: Princeton University Press.

Kampenhout, Daan van. 2006. *Rytuały szamańskie a ustawienia rodzinne*, translated by Małgorzata Baworowska. Katowice: Wydawnictwo KOS.

Karpenkov, Yuri, and Nadezhda Matveeva. 2015. *Ustawienia systemowe*, translated by Alla A. Chrzanowska. Białystok: Ars Scripti-2.

Karwat, Paweł. 2015. *Ho'oponopono. Wprowadzanie wewnętrznej harmonii*. Gliwice: Wydawnictwo Helion.

Kelly, Edward F., Emily Williams Kelly, Adam Crabtree, Alan Gauld, Michael Grosso, and Bruce Greyson. *Irreducible Mind: Toward a Psychology for the 21st Century*. Lanham, Boulder, CO, New York, Toronto, and Plymouth: Rowman & Littlefield.

Kępiński, Antoni. 2002. *Lęk*. Kraków: Wydawnictwo Literackie.

Klein, Melanie. 1975. *Love, Guilt and Reparation: And Other Works 1921–1945*. New York: The Free Press.

———. 1975a. *The Psycho-Analysis of Children*, translated by Alix Strachey. New York: Dell Publishing.

———. 1977. *Envy and Gratitude and Other Works, 1946–1963*. New York: Dell Publishing.

Kohon, Gregorio (ed.). 1999. *The Dead Mother: The Work of André Green*. London: Routledge.

Kołakowski, Leszek. 2004. *Filozofia pozytywistyczna*. Warszawa: Wydawnictwo Naukowe PWN.

Konkolÿ-Thege, Barna, Carla Petroll, Carlos Rivas, and Salome Scholtens. 2021. "The Effectiveness of Family Constellation Therapy in Improving Mental Health: A Systematic Review." *Family Process* 60(2): 409–23.

Kubitsky, Jacek. 2010. *Vademecum terapeuty rodzinnego*. Warszawa: Wydawnictwo Lekarskie PZWL.

Kuhn, Thomas. 2012. *The Structure of Scientific Revolutions*. Chicago: The University of Chicago Press.

Lacadée, Philippe. 2019. *Nieporozumienie wokół dziecka. Co mówią nam dzisiejsze dzieci i nastolatki?* Translated by Małgorzata Gorzula. Kraków.

Lacan, Jacques. 1979. "The Neurotic's Individual Myth." *Psychoanalytic Quarterly* 48: 405–25.

———. 2002. *Écrits*, translated by Bruce Fink, Héloïse Fink, and Russell Grigg. New York and London: W. W. Norton & Company.

———. 2015. *Mit indywidualny neurotyka albo Poezja i prawda w nerwicy*, translated by Tomasz Gajda, Janusz Kotara, and Jacek Waga. Warszawa: Wydawnictwo Naukowe PWN.

———. 2018. "Note on the Child," translated by Russell Grigg. *The Lacanian Review*, no. 4 (2018), 13-14.

Lake, Medicine Grizzlybear (Robert G.). 2006. *Native Healer: Initiation Into an Ancient Art*. Wheaton, IL: Quest Books.

Lamża, Łukasz. 2015. *Granice kosmosu – granice kosmologii*. Kraków: Copernicus Center Press.

László, Ervin. 1972. *The Systems View of the World: The Natural Philosophy of the New Developments in the Sciences*. New York: George Braziller.

———. 2007. *Science and the Akashic Field. An Integral Theory of Everything*. Rochester, NY: Inner Traditions.

Le Bon, Gustave. 2006. *The Crowd: A Study of the Popular Mind.* New York: Cosimo.

Lederer, William J., and Don D. Jackson. 1990. *The Mirages of Marriage.* New York and London: W. W. Norton & Company.

Leenhardt, Maurice. 1979. *Do Kamo: Person and Myth in the Melanesian World*, translated by Basia Miller Gulati. Chicago: University of Chicago Press.

Lemoine, Bernadette. 2016. *Przebaczenie źródłem uzdrowienia*, translated by Maria Żurowska. Kraków: Wydawnictwo Esprit.

Lévi-Strauss, Claude. 1961. *Tristes Tropiques*, translated by John Russell. New York: Criterion Books.

Levine, Peter A. 2015. *Trauma and Memory: Brain and Body in a Search for the Living Past: A Practical Guide for Understanding and Working with Traumatic Memory.* Berkeley, CA: North Atlantic Books. Kindle.

Lévy-Bruhl, Lucien. 1966. *How Natives Think*, translated by Lilian A. Clare. New York: Washington Square Press.

———. 1975. *The Notebooks on Primitive Mentality*, translated by Peter Rivière. Oxford: Blackwell.

Lewin, R. 1980. "Is Your Brain Really Necessary?" *Science* 210(4475): 1232–34.

Loewald, Hans W. 1960. "On the Therapeutic Action of Psycho-Analysis." *The International Journal of Psychoanalysis* 41: 16–33.

Lommel, Pim van. 2010. *Consciousness Beyond Life: The Science of the Near-Death Experience*, translated by Laura Vroomen. New York: HarperOne.

Lowen, Alexander. 1993. *Depression and the Body: The Biological Basis of Faith and Reality.* New York: Arkana.

———. 2003. *Fear of Life.* Alachua, FL: Bioenergetics Press.

Ludewig, Kurt. 1995. *Terapia systemowa. Podstawy teoretyczne i praktyka.* Gdańsk: Gdańskie Wydawnictwo Psychologiczne.

Lyons, John. 1976. *Chomsky.* Glasgow: Fontana / Collins.

Malinowski, Bronisław. 1954. *Magic, Science and Religion.* Garden City, NY: Doubleday Anchor Books.

———. 1962. *Sex, Culture, and Myth.* New York: Harcourt, Brace & World.

Marcinkowska, Karolina. 2016. *Od-tworzyć przeszłość. Kult czumba na Madagaskarze.* Gdańsk: Wydawnictwo Naukowe Katedra.

Mauss, Marcel. 1967. *The Gift: Forms and Functions of Exchange in Archaic Societies*, translated by Ian Cunnison. New York: W. W. Norton & Company.

———. 2001. *A General Theory of Magic*, translated by Robert Brain. London and New York: Routledge.

———. 2002. *The Gift: The Form and Reason for Exchange in Archaic Societies*, translated by W. D. Halls. London and New York: Routledge.

Mauthner, Oliver E., Enza De Luca, Jennifer M. Poole, Susan E. Abbey, Margrit Shildrick, Mena Gewarges, and Heather J. Ross. 2014. "Heart Transplants: Identity Disruption, Bodily Integrity and Interconnectedness." *Health* 19(6): 578–94. doi: 10.1177/1363459314560067.

Mbiti, John S. 1970. *African Religions and Philosophy.* Oxford: Heinemann Educational Publishers.

McAll, Kenneth. 1986. *Healing the Family Tree.* London: Sheldon Press.

McDougall, William. 1927. *The Group Mind: A Sketch of the Principles of Collective Psychology With Some Attempt to Apply Them to the Interpretation of National Life and Character*. Cambridge: Cambridge University Press.
McGoldrick, Monica, Randy Gerson, and Sylvia Shellenberger. 1999. *Genograms: Assessment and Intervention*. New York and London: W. W. Norton & Company.
McTaggart, Lynne. 2002. *The Field: The Quest for the Secret Force of the Universe*. New York: HaprerCollins Publishers.
———. 2017. *The Bond: How to Fix Your Falling-Down World*. New York: Atria Paperback.
Mijolla de, Alain. 2003. *Les visiteurs du moi: Fantasmes d'identification*. Paris: Les Belles Lettres.
Milgram, Stanley. 2009. *Obedience to Authority: An Experimental View*. New York: Harper Perennial Modern Thought.
Miller, Alice. 1981. *The Drama of the Gifted Child: How Narcissistic Parents Form and Deform the Emotional Lives of Their Talented Children*, translated by Ruth Ward. New York: Basic Books.
———. 1990. *For Your Own Good: Hidden Cruelty in Child-Rearing and the Roots of Violence*, translated by Hildegarde Hannum and Hunter Hannum. New York: The Noonday Press, Farrar, Straus and Giroux.
———. 1997. *Breaking Down the Wall of Silence: The Liberating Experience of Facing Painful Truth*, translated by Simon Worrall. New York: Penguin Books.
———. 1998. *Thou Shalt Not Be Aware: Society's Betrayal of the Child*, translated by Hildegarde Hannum and Hunter Hannum. New York: Farrar, Straus and Giroux.
Miller, Martin. 2018. *The True "Drama of the Gifted Child": The Phantom Alice Miller—The Real Person*, translated by Barbara Rogers and Rebecca Peterson. Columbia, SC: Martin Miller.
Minuchin, Salvador. 1975. *Families and Family Therapy*. Cambridge: Harvard University Press.
Minuchin, Salvador, and H. Charles Fishman. 1981. *Family Therapy Techniques*. Cambridge and London: Harvard University Press.
Moody, Raymond, and Paul Perry. 1993. *Reunions: Visionary Encounters with Departed Loved Ones*. New York: Villard Books.
Moreno, Jacob Levy. 2019. *Psychodrama, Volume I*. Princeton, NJ: Psychodrama Press.
Moreno, Jacob Levy, and Zerka T. Moreno. 2011. *Psychodrama: Second Volume: Foundations of Psychotherapy*. Manchester: The North-West Psychodrama Association.
Musser, George. 2015. *Spooky Action at a Distance. The Phenomenon That Reimagines Space and Time-and What It Means for Black Holes, the Big Bang, and Theories of Everything*. New York: Scientific American/Farrar, Straus and Giroux.
Namysłowska, Irena. 1997. *Terapia rodzin*. Warszawa: Springer PWN.
Neuhauser, Johannes (ed.). 2001. *Supporting Love: How Love Works in Couple Relationships: Bert Hellinger's Work with Couples*, translated by Colleen Beaumont. Phoenix, AZ: Zeig, Tucker & Theisen.
Nietzsche, Friedrich. 1998. *On the Genealogy of Morality*, translated by Maudemarie Clark and Alan J. Swensen. Indianapolis, IN: Hackett Publishing Company.

Nosek, Brian A., Johanna Cohoon, Mallory Kidwell, Marcel van Assen, Chris Hartgerink, Robbie van Aert, Fred Hasselman, and Sacha Epskamp. 2015. "Estimating the Reproducibility of Psychological Science. Open Science Collaboration." *Science* 349: aac4716. doi: 10.1126/science.aac4716.

Nowaczyk, Małgorzata. 2007. *Rodzinne drzewo zdrowia. Genetyka dla każdego.* Warszawa: Państwowy Instytut Wydawniczy.

Osiński, Zbigniew. 1980. *Grotowski i jego Laboratorium.* Warszawa: Państwowy Instytut Wydawniczy.

Owen, Adrian. 2017. *Into the Gray Zone: A Neuroscientist Explores the Border Between Life and Death.* New York, London, Toronto, Sydney, and New Delhi: Scribner.

Pacewicz, Grzegorz. 2010. *Koncepcja noosfery w myśli Pierre'a Teilharda de Chardin.* Olsztyn: Instytut Filozofii Uniwersytetu Warmińsko-Mazurskiego w Olsztynie.

Padgett, Jason, and Maureen Ann Seaberg. 2014. *Struck by Genius: How a Brain Injury Made Me a Mathematical Marvel.* New York: Houghton Mifflin Harcourt.

Parker, Robert. 2011. *On Greek Religion.* Ithaca and London: Cornell University Press.

Pawlik, Jerzy (ed.). 2012. *Psychodrama i techniki niewerbalne.* Warszawa: ENETEIA.

Pearson, Patricia. 2015. *Opening the Heaven's Door: What the Dying Are Trying to Say about Where They're Going.* New York: Atria Paperback.

Penfield Wilder. 1975. *Mystery of the Mind: A Critical Study of Consciousness and the Human Brain.* Princeton, NJ: Princeton University Press.

Penrose, Roger. 2016. *Fashion, Faith, and Fantasy in the New Physics of the Universe.* Princeton, NJ: Princeton University Press.

Plato. 1992. *Republic*, translated by G.M.A. Grube. Indianapolis, IN, Cambridge: Hackett Publishing Company.

———. 1995. *Phaedrus*, translated by Alexander Nehamas and Paul Woodruff. Indianapolis, IN, Cambridge: Hackett Publishing Company.

Popper, Karl R. 1979. *Objective Knowledge: An Evolutionary Approach.* New York: Oxford University Press.

———. 2000. *Knowledge and the Body-Mind Problem: In Defence of Interaction*, edited by M.A. Notturno. London and New York: Routledge.

Posacki, Aleksander. 2007. *Psychologia i New Age. Psychologiczne terapie czy okultystyczne inicjacje?* Gdańsk: Wydawnictwo Arka Noego.

Quinodoz, Jean-Michel. 2008. *Listening to Hanna Segal: Her Contribution to Psychoanalysis*, translated by David Alcorn, edited by Dana Birksted-Breen. London and New York: Routledge.

Radcliffe-Brown, A. R. 2013. *The Andaman Islanders.* Cambridge: Cambridge University Press.

Radin, Dean. 2006. *Entangled Minds: Extrasensory Experiences in Quantum Reality.* New York: Paraview Pocket Books.

———. 2013. *Supernormal: Science, Yoga, and the Evidence for Extraordinary Psychic Abilities.* New York: Deepak Chopra Books.

———. 2020. *Prawdziwa magia. Starożytna mądrość, współczesna nauka i tajemnicza moc Wszechświata*, translated by Iwona Szuwalska. Wrocław: Wydawnictwo Manendra.

Rank, Otto. 2014. *The Trauma of Birth*. London, New York: Routledge.

Rappaport, Roy A. 2002. *Ritual and Religion in the Making of Humanity*. Cambridge: Cambridge University Press.

Ratzinger, Joseph. 2000. *The Spirit of the Liturgy*, translated by John Saward. San Francisco: Ignatius Press.

Reik, Theodor. 1948. *Listening with the Third Ear*. New York: Grove Press.

Roberto, Laura Giat. 1992. *Transgenerational Family Therapies*. New York and London: The Guilford Press.

Rogers, Jenny. 2012. *Coaching Skills: A Handbook*. Maidenhead: Open University Press.

Røine, Eva. 1997. *Psychodrama: Group Psychotherapy as Experimental Theatre: Playing the Leading Role in Your Own Life*, translated by Ann Zwik. London, Bristol, and Pennsylvania: Jessica Kingsley Publishers.

Rosenfeld, Herbert. 1990. *Impasse and Interpretation: Therapeutic and Anti-Therapeutic Factors in the Psychoanalytic Treatment of Psychotic, Borderline, and Neurotic Patients*. London and New York: Routledge.

Rymuszko, Marek (ed.) 2013. *Polskie życie po życiu. Relacje ludzi uratowanych ze stanu śmierci klinicznej*. Warszawa: Wydawnictwo "Nieznany Świat".

Ryszkiewicz, Marcin. 1994. *Matka Ziemia w przyjaznym kosmosie. Gaja i zasada antropiczna w dziejach myśli przyrodniczej*. Warszawa: Wydawnictwo Naukowe PWN.

Safouan, Moustafa. 2004. *Four Lessons of Psychoanalysis*, edited by Anna Shane. New York: Other Press.

Satir, Virginia. 1972. *Peoplemaking*. Palo Alto, CA: Science and Behavior Books.

———. 1983. *Conjoint Family Therapy*. Palo Alto, CA: Science and Behavior Books.

———. 1988. *The New Peoplemaking*. Mountain View, CA: Science and Behavior Books.

Satir, Virginia, James Stachowiak, and Harvey A. Taschman. 1990. *Helping Families to Change*. Northvale, NJ, and London: Jason Aronson.

Sautoy, Marcus du. 2017. *What We Cannot Know: From Consciousness to the Cosmos, the Cutting Edge of Science Explained*. London: 4th Estate.

Schopenhauer, Arthur. 1995. *On the Basis of Morality*, translated by E.F.J. Payne. Indianapolis, IN, Cambridge: Hackett Publishing Company.

Schützenberger, Anne Ancelin. 1998. *The Ancestor Syndrome: Transgenerational Psychotherapy and the Hidden Links in the Family Tree*, translated by Anne Trager. London and New York: Routledge.

———. 2017. *Psychogenealogia w praktyce*. Warszawa: Wydawnictwo Virgo.

Segal, Hanna. 1990. *The Work of Hanna Segal: A Kleinian Approach to Clinical Practice*. North Vale, NJ, and London: Jason Aronson Inc.

———. 2018. *Introduction to the Work of Melanie Klein*. New York: Routledge.

Selvini Palazzoli, Mara, Luigi Boscolo, Gianfranco Cecchin, and Giuliana Prata. 1978. *Paradox and Counterparadox: A New Model in the Therapy of the Family in Schizophrenic Transaction*. New York and London: Jason Aronson.

Sheldrake, Rupert. 2003. *The Sense of Being Stared At: And Other Aspects of the Extended Mind*. London: Arrow Books.

———. 2009. *A New Science of Life: The Hypothesis of Morphic Resonance*. London: Icon Books.

———. 2012. *Science Set Free: 10 Paths to New Discovery*. New York: Deepak Chopra Books.

———. 2017. *Science and Spiritual Practices: Reconnecting Through Direct Experience*. London: Coronet. Kindle.

Simon, Richard. 1992. *One on One: Conversations with the Shapers of Family Therapy*. Washington, DC: Family Therapy Networker; New York: Guilford Press.

Somé, Malidoma Patrice. 1995. *Of Water and the Spirit: Ritual, Magic, and Initiation in the Life of an African Shaman*. New York: Penguin Compass.

Smith, Jonathan Z. 1987. "The Domestication of Sacrifice." In *Violent Origins: On Ritual Killing and Cultural Formation*, edited by Robert G. Hamerton-Kelly, 191–235. Stanford, CA: Stanford University Press.

Spilka, Bernard and Kevin L. Ladd. 2013. *The Psychology of Prayer: A Scientific Approach*. New York and London: The Guilford Press.

Spork, Peter. 2011. *Drugi kod. Epigenetyka, czyli jak możemy sterować własnymi genotypami*. Warszawa: Wydawnictwo W.A.B.

Stadler, Christian. 2018. *Psychodrama w teorii i praktyce*, translated by Iwona Kowal. Warszawa: ENETEIA.

Stanislavski, Konstantin. 2010. *An Actor's Work on a Role*, translated and edited by Jean Benedetti. London and New York: Routledge.

Stark, Heinz. 2005. *Systemic Constellation Work is an Art: About Deep Dimensions of Family Therapy*. Rapid City: Many Kites Press.

Stephens-Davidowitz, Seth. 2019. *Everybody Lies: Big Data, New Data, and What the Internet Can Tell Us About Who We Really Are*. New York: HarperCollins Publishers.

Stout, Martha. 2005. *The Sociopath Next Door*. New York: Broadway Books.

Strenger, Carlo. 1989. "The Classic and the Romantic Vision in Psychoanalysis." *International Journal of Psychoanalysis* 70: 593–610.

Styron, William. 1992. *Darkness Visible: A Memoir of Madness*. New York: Vintage Books.

Świeżawski, Stefan. 1983. *Dzieje filozofii europejskiej XV wieku, vol. 6, Człowiek*. Warszawa: Akademia Teologii Katolickiej.

Sylvia, Claire, and William Novak. 1997. *A Change of Heart: A Memoir*. New York: Warner Books.

Symington, Neville. 1993. *Narcissism: A New Theory*. London: Karnac.

Szulc, Anna. 2009. "Pola Psychościemy." *Przekrój* 44: 10–15.

Szyjewski, Artur. 2005. *Religie czarnej Afryki*. Kraków: Wydawnictwo WAM.

Target, Mary, and Peter Fonagy. 2002. "Fathers in Modern Psychoanalysis and in Society: The Role of the Father and Child Development." In *The Importance of*

Fathers: A Psychoanalytic Re-evaluation, edited by Judith Trowell and Alicia Etchegoyen, 45–66. Hove: Brunner-Routledge.

Taub-Bynum, Edward Bruce. 1994. *The Family Unconscious: An Invisible Bond.* London: Theosophical Publishing House.

The New American Bible: Revised Edition. 2012. Harper Catholic Bibles.

Tipping, Colin. 2009. *Radical Forgiveness: A Revolutionary Five-Stage Process to Heal Relationships, Let Go of Anger & Blame, Find Peace in Any Situation.* Boulder, CO: Sounds True.

Turner, Victor. 2008. *The Ritual Process: Structure and Anti-Structure.* New Brunswick and London: Aldine Transaction.

Vaiasuso, Francesco, and Paolo Rodari. 2015. *Moje opętanie. Relacja człowieka opętanego od dzieciństwa*, translated by Anna Flisiak Zdziarska. Kraków: Esprit.

Vitale, Joe. 2013. *At Zero: The Quest for Miracles Through Ho'oponopono.* Hoboken, NJ: Wiley.

Volkan, Vamik D., and Gabriele Ast. 2018. *Siblings in the Unconscious and Psychopathology: Womb Fantasies, Claustrophobias, Fear of Pregnancy, Murderous Rage, Animal Symbolism, Christmas and ... or Identifications with Sisters and Brothers.* London: Karnac Books.

Walewska, Katarzyna (ed.). 2007. *Psychoanaliza współcześnie. Nurt francuski.* Warszawa: MediPage, IPP "Dialogi".

Wasilewski, Bohdan, and Liliana Engel. 2011. *Grupowy trening balintowski. Teoria i zastosowania.* Warszawa: ENETEIA.

Wegscheider-Cruse, Sharon. 1981. *Another Chance: Hope and Health for the Alcoholic Family.* Palo Alto, CA: Science and Behavior Books.

Wegscheider-Cruse, Sharon, Kathy Higby, Ted Klontz, and Ann Rainey. 1994. *Family Reconstruction: The Living Theater Model.* Palo Alto, CA: Science & Behavior Books.

Welch, Martha G. 1989. *Holding Time: How to Eliminate Conflict, Temper, Tantrums, and Sibling Rivalry and Raise Happy, Loving, Successful Children.* New York: Simon & Schuster.

Welldon, Estela V. 2018. *Mother, Madonna, Whore: The Idealization and Denigration of Motherhood.* New York: Routledge.

Whitaker, Carl. 1976. "A Family is a Four-Dimensional Relationship." In *Family Therapy: Theory and Practice*, edited by Philip J. Guerin: 182–92. New York: Gardner Press.

Winnicott, Donald Woods. 1986. *Home is Where We Start From: Essays by a Psychoanalyst*, edited by Clare Winnicott, Ray Shepherd, and Madeleine Davis. New York: W. W. Norton & Company.

Wojciszke, Bogdan. 2017. *Psychologia społeczna.* Warszawa: Wydawnictwo Naukowe Scholar.

Woszczek, Marek. 2010. *Ukryta całość przyrody a mikrofizyka.* Poznań: Wydawnictwo Naukowe Instytutu Filozofii UAM.

Zaremba Bielawski, Maciej. 2011. *Higieniści. Z dziejów eugeniki.* Wołowiec: Wydawnictwo Czarne.

Zazzo, René (ed.). 1978. *Przywiązanie*, translated by Tadeusz Gałkowski. Warszawa: Państwowe Wydawnictwo Naukowe.

Index

About the Author

Damian Janus graduated from the faculties of psychology, philosophy, and religious studies at the Jagiellonian University (Krakow, Poland) and has specializations in clinical psychology and psycho-oncology. He participated in training courses in Gestalt psychotherapy, bodywork, psychodynamic psychotherapy, and Lacanian psychoanalysis. He completed trainings in family constellations and new family constellations. He worked in a psychiatric ward, mental health clinic, addiction treatment clinic, and has a private psychotherapeutic practice. He has been working as a psychotherapist for almost twenty years. He is interested in physics and the history of science and technology.

www.ingramcontent.com/pod-product-compliance
Ingram Content Group UK Ltd.
Pitfield, Milton Keynes, MK11 3LW, UK
UKHW041833031026
15587UKWH00002B/737

9 781793 627421